he use be *S*omebody

A JOURNEY INTO ALZHEIMER'S DISEASE
THROUGH THE EYES OF A CAREGIVER

Beverly Bigtree Murphy

Gibbs Associates • Boulder, Colorado USA

DISCLAIMER

Unless permission was expressly given for the use of real names of persons mentioned in this publication, names, locations, genders, and initials were disguised to protect the anonymity of those people mentioned in the course of actual events chronicled in the life of Thomas Murphy and Beverly Bigtree Murphy as related in this publication.

Support group conversations chronicled in this publication have been fictionalized with regard to person and place and are not to be viewed as actual Alzheimer's support group meetings that occurred. However, the dialogues are based on actual commentary made by caregivers in other settings and are a compilation of those comments. The dialogues are meant to represent what occurs in support groups amongst Alzheimer family members and that integrity has been maintained. The subject matter portrayed is common to caregivers in general and therefore not specific to any one group or individual.

Printed in
Boulder, Colorado USA

© Copyright 1995, by Gibbs Associates
P.O. Box 706, Boulder, CO 80306-0706 USA
(303)444-6032   ISBN 0-943909-14-7

TABLE OF CONTENTS

ACKNOWLEDGMENTS

I wish to specially thank Betty Gibbs, my publisher, and Lancia Smith, my editor. These two women formed a bond with me that was directed towards excellence in both the producing of this book and the enrichment of our lives as sentient beings. We have formed an alliance that goes beyond mere friendship.

I wish to thank Tom's friends who contributed their memories of him and their encouragement to me. Jordan, Schiller, O'Leary, Dobson, and Poe head the list and since Tom always referred to them by their last names I feel it is fitting to continue the tradition out of his affection for them as friends and colleagues.

I wish to single out Tom's brothers, James, Paul, and John who supported my effort completely and who were loved by Tom and who obviously love him.

I wish to remember my sisters Norma and Sandy who supported me when the going got rough and my sons Norman and Laszlo who not only hung in there with me, but who make sure the walk is shoveled, the plumbing is fixed, the car is taken care of and who stop by mornings to make sure I have someone to share coffee with.

And most of all, I wish to thank my parents, Norman Bigtree and Mary Wolniak Bigtree who first taught me about the meaning of the dance.

℘ ☙❦❧ ℰ

DEDICATION

This book is dedicated to Jim O'Leary and his wife Rosemary. Jim was enthusiastic about the prospect of this book being written and was one of the first to give his time and memories to this effort. He spent hours with me on the phone and took an equal amount of time to write the letters that helped me form a more complete vision of Tom Murphy, the man I married. Jim was one of Tom's closest friends and colleagues and a man he trusted without question.

Jim suffered a near drowning after an accident plunged his car into water on December 8, 1991. He is now severely brain damaged and needs 24 hour care. His wife Rosemary describes him as being locked in his own body, an ironic turn of events for these two friends, since I would also describe Tom in those terms. Rosemary and their children, Ann and Paul, decided to bring Jim home after he was released from rehabilitation. With the help of home health aides and personal effort they have managed to adjust to his care needs and keep him a part of the everyday life of their family. He is now able to recognize his family and his surroundings and Rosemary tells me he still responds to a request for a kiss, which is more confirmation that the loving continues even when the ability to speak leaves. He is only 60 years old.

Rosemary has joined the ranks of those of us who have learned how tenuous life is and how completely it can change in the flash of an instant. She, like millions of others in this country, has faced the unexpected head on and learned more than any of us ever wished to know about the long term care of someone we love. I have come to count her as my friend.

℘ ❧ ℘

iv

FOREWORD

It was 8:30 in the evening in mid-July. I was in my cottage on a Maine island and stepped out the back door, which faces west, to go to my boat and pick up one of my sons, who was working the late shift at a yacht club on the mainland. What I saw as I opened the cottage door was so extraordinary that I stood transfixed.

The ball of the sun had disappeared over the horizon and had just begun its final show for the day. This night it was a gold display. Into a cloudless sky it sent back brilliant rays of pure gold. And the reflection of the sky created a golden sea below.

Seeing that sky and sea was as perfect a moment as any in my life. I couldn't wait to get into my boat and ride on that golden sea. So I ran down the 82 steps to the beach, hurriedly rowed to the boat, started the engine and prepared to go the five miles to the mainland very slowly so I might absorb and fully experience that most spectacular moment.

With the throttle forward the boat slowly crept along, but I noticed the gold was ahead of me. So I went a little faster to catch it. Still the gold stayed ahead of me. I increased the speed until I was at full throttle, skimming across the bay at 35 miles an hour, but I could never catch the gold.

I met my son and, still feeling unsettled as I returned to the island, I spilled out the experience to my wife. "That's interesting," she said. "I stood on the bank and watched you go across the bay, and I thought, 'Isn't Art lucky to be on that golden sea.' You were in the middle of the gold and you didn't even know it."

Looking down from the hill, she had had a higher perspective. Her observation helped me to clearly see what I had not seen before, that every moment we are alive is really a golden moment, that every era is a golden era, that we are always surrounded by gold but we don't know it.

I knew Tom Murphy when he was a somebody, a bright, wide-eyed, thoughtful, generous and sometimes devilish man who is so delightful that if you met him on the street when you were in a hurry you wouldn't mind being late to have just a few minutes with him.

In the purest sense he still is that same somebody, but what Alzheimer's Disease has done to him is to camouflage the real Tom Murphy so he appears to have been replaced with a shadow, a strange and troubled look-alike. His wife, Beverly, has chosen to see the real person behind the facade. Seeing and loving the original man makes it possible for her to manage herself among the frustrations and stresses of dealing with the replacement man.

When Beverly was considering marrying Tom I was one of those who persisted with the hard questions about what she was getting into, and whether she might be taking on more than she expected or wanted to deal with. I had serious doubts about the wisdom of her decision. But these concerns have been buried. She clearly made the right decision. Tom needs her and has her fully. She also needs Tom, not because he is able to be a normal and loving and supportive husband, but because his condition calls out in her a level of loving and a need for growth that can happen only in this relationship. Beverly had unknown resources for caring which needed to be tapped. Through Tom's illness the creative source of the Universe was calling to the core of her being for her to fulfill whoever she is and is meant to be.

Beverly needed to write this story, not only because it helped her to dig deep into herself, but also for the rest of us. We learn, are stretched and summoned to growth as we read this story of a woman who in choosing to relate to a daunting challenge has unlocked the doors to the greatness of the human spirit. She is discovering that we have more resources, more spiritual and emotional wealth, more capacity for empathy and compassion than most of us have ever touched.

Beverly is realizing that she is surrounded by the gold, that she has every resource needed to do what she must do. That this time is the golden era of her life.

Dr. Arthur Caliandro
Minister, Marble Collegiate Church
New York City

Dr. Arthur Caliandro can be seen on the VISN cable network throughout the country on Sunday mornings bringing his message - Make Your Life Count - to millions.

"Rage, rage against the dying of the light"
Dylan Thomas

About Tom Murphy

Tom Murphy was always color blind, gender blind, and age blind. He was someone who believed so strongly that if he did his best then you would do your best, that in many instances, his blind faith was strong enough for those of us who worked with him to raise ourselves up to challenges we never anticipated. We were granted an unspoken assumption of excellence in our thinking and doing simply because he believed in us and trusted in us. If I were to characterize him in terms of his greatest strength it was that he gave people the opportunity to be the best they could be.

I was one to whom he gave such an opportunity. When I met Tom I was teaching first grade for the armed forces in Europe with no notion of changing occupations. But circumstances sometimes change and he told me to contact him if I ever needed help finding a job. When that day came he offered me the task of organizing his operation, a job that meant keeping multifaceted international projects, personnel, materials, and everything else that impacted on the flow of business in Tom's life, in the air, at once. I had no specific experience but I now believe he saw abilities in me that I didn't know I had. In many ways he gave me the beginnings of faith in myself, a faith that permeated every facet of my life. Over the years that followed I found myself doing much more than running his office. I found myself giving presentations to hundreds of people on major projects and proposals. I set up trade shows, one of which was with Russian ministries in Moscow where we represented several U.S. manufacturers. I was Tom's liaison and directly involved with NASA during the development of the Space Shuttle program and his front man in the project which resulted in the sale of a hover transport to be used for exploration on the Dead Sea. I became the first woman to market the heavy equipment used in the mining, oil and transporting industries in the world arena.

He gave me challenges to stretch farther than I sometimes had the nerve to go. The words, "Just do it!", still ring in my ears. He once told me that if I waited until I had every detail I thought I needed, I would never take the first step. Today, I often find myself carrying the bravado I learned from him when entering into complicated negotiations. He was someone to watch and he was someone to learn from.

Tom was blatantly honest about who he was. There was never a hidden agenda with him, he was exactly as he portrayed himself. He was also someone who had a deepened sense of equality in the value of every person he met. He had the same anticipation of regard for the superintendent in his building as he had for the Prince of Brunei, and his generosity and his humanity towards those who crossed his path are legendary. Tom was someone for whom the word 'friend' had a special meaning and to be counted as his friend did not only encompass a feeling of goodwill and camaraderie, it was to be endowed with his respect, and loyalty, and confidence. He was my friend and that never wavered no matter how our life paths moved and changed. To say I really value the impact his friendship had on me somehow falls short of my regard and love for this man.

Judith Jordan

 C3 ಹಿo✿ ಙ

THOMAS MURPHY

EXECUTIVE SUMMARY

Proven capabilities in general management. Strong financial background with complete profit and loss responsibilities as a Chief Executive Officer, including highly sophisticated lease and financial transactions. Skilled negotiator and planner with extensive contracts within major international companies and an understanding of the political requirements for successful business relationships in Europe, the Middle East and South America.

PROFESSIONAL ACCOMPLISHMENTS

INTERNATIONAL

MIDDLE EAST: Successfully directed Tiger's studies for a potential joint venture with large American and Arab banks for the leasing of construction equipment and heavy machinery in the Middle East. His studies determined the viability, profitability and the long term market potential of this project and, upon completing five year investment and profitability projections, the three partners agreed to proceed.

UNITED ARAB EMIRATES, ABU DHABI, 1965-1982: Responsible for engineering projects, purchasing from multi-national sources, and the distribution of sales within the Emirates. Worked directly with Arab Emirates in development of their drilling, transporting, and refineries. Developed purchase and leasing packages, involved in maintenance of equipment.

Developed a system of training, using color coding and the breaking down of very complex tasks into small step by step units that allowed non English speaking, multi nationals from India, Pakistani, Egypt and the Saudi/Arabian peninsula to learn to operate and maintain the complex heavy equipment used in the building of the pipeline from the oil fields in Oman for Royal Dutch Shell in the early '60s. When the word went out that Royal Dutch was hiring, men began drifting out of the desert on foot or on camel, carrying a sword, a rifle, a dagger and a stick. Some of them brought their animals. None of them spoke English and few were able to communicate with others than those in their own language group. Within six weeks they were trained to operate hydraulic cranes, weighing over 60,000 pounds, 22 feet long and 12 feet wide, with six

ix

gears forward and six reverse. This at a time when roads within the Emirates were nearly non existent.

Sponsored and actively participated in United States Arab Chamber's 1978 business tour of major American Cities by Arab Businessmen and served as moderator for their Chicago Panel.

KOREA: Designed a lease/purchase method for Korean contractors working in Saudi Arabia.

Negotiated lease contract for equipment necessary to modernize a major shipyard in Korea. This company is still acquiring equipment under the original "Equipment Application and Engineered Lease Program".

Conceptualized the plan to utilize the high tides to move water in and out of the newly proposed dry dock, thus saving on the use of highly expensive hydraulic equipment.

SOUTHEAST ASIA: Consultant to óur government during Vietnam. Involved in the concept and utilization of the plan to stop the theft of equipment and supplies during the war. Conceived and implemented an underwater parking ground where ship containers were held until needed. Placement of containers was set on a graph, scuba divers connected containers to crane equipment which then lifted them on the dock for disbursement. The cranes were also 'parked' in the bay. Theft was almost totally alleviated.

Member of the Fact-Finding Mission to Southeast Asia in 1975, sponsored by the U.S. Council for Southeast Asian Trade and Investment. The purpose of the mission was to encourage and foster good relations and trade between the business community of the United States and the peoples, governments and business sectors of Asia.

As a result of this tour, he became involved with the "Committee for Organizing the Pa Hmong Project" in the Mekong Basin. Was then President of Bell Worldwide, Inc. He remained behind to gather data, have a firsthand look at the dam site and reservoir area. It was his view that private financing was the only way that Pa Mong would ever be built in any timely fashion. The dam was essential to the re-development of the Mekong Basin area and essential to the further development of the very rich oil fields. His plan to involve private financing with all members, Government including, having equal votes, with a majority vote essential so that no group could take action independent of the other, or hold up work, was unprecedented at that time. He was given carte blanche by Thailand and Laos to move ahead with his concept as quickly as possible, and he was credited with a major innovative breakthrough for the post-war development of the Mekong Basin. Due to political changes in Southeast Asia the project was dropped.

IRELAND: By seeing the increasing need for larger tower cranes and their application in high rise construction and other government projects such as missile sites and NASA, and by pushing for construction of that equipment to meet the potential demand he facilitated expansion of the Liebherr factory in Killarny Ireland. The increased revenue to the German based manufacturer of cranes and tower cranes and the improvement in the economic standing of that area of Ireland was substantial.

CURACAO: Secured a unique lease contract for all construction and materials handling equipment used in Royal Dutch Shell's Curacao refinery. This contract is still acknowledged as one of the most innovative concepts to have been implemented in this industry and is as effective today in supplying all equipment with full maintenance to this 5000,000 BPD refinery, as it was when first conceived over 20 years ago. As of 1962 the refinery was approximately half its present size, and required 41 cranes for maintenance purposes. Today it functions with only 18 cranes.

CANADA: Consultant for a major Canadian mining company to conceive, design, manufacture, deliver and put into service a complete unit for cleaning their industrial dump, enabling them to expand their facilities. This unit was marketed on a leased basis and the sales of recovered scrap and other waste material far exceeded the overall cost to the lessee.

RUSSIA: Made several trips to Russia wherein he initiated and completed a major engineering and equipment seminar in June 1978 to Russian ministries of Oil, Gas, Construction, Railroad, Marine, and Highway.

Negotiated a lease project with the Russian Government and acted as consultant on their natural gas line. Held responsibility for the recruitment of necessary personnel to operate and maintain equipment for the pipeline, which ran from Siberia to Italy.

MEXICO: Designed a unique (due to offshore funding and tax problems) lease purchase method for supplying the pipe laying equipment used by contractors on Mexico's 48" natural gas pipeline. The tons of equipment no longer needed in Alaska were re-tooled, adjusted to climate and terrain changes and adapted for use in Mexico. The lease package saved the Mexican Government millions in costs, and millions of dollars in the clean up of Alaska after their line was completed.

UNITED STATES

ALASKA: Consultant for Alyeska Pipeline Service Company, owners of the Alaskan Pipeline.

Responsibilities Included: Supplying Alyeska with the first 12 month operational system to cross the Yukon River. This assignment included the concept, design, manufacture, placing into service, and the management contract for the operation of this system which carried all materials needed for construction of the 300 plus miles of pipeline north of the Yukon. The Yukon River presented a major obstacle to the continued movement of pipe throughout the years because of harsh winters and erratic summer conditions. The Yukon Bridge which was only in planning stages would take at least a year to two years to complete. The projected cost of interrupting services was astronomical.

The resulting concept was The Hover Craft, or A.C.T. (Air Cushion Technology) Ferry System. It was the first of it's kind in the world. The two ACT's he had built were capable of delivering a payload of 160 tons every thirty minutes. In other words, it carried four fully loaded trucks north, and six empty ones on the return trip. **"I HOVERED THE YUKON"** bumper stickers started appearing all over the world as truckers announced they had become a part of the elite group to work this project.

The ACT's design was flexible enough to operate in arctic winters and mild summers while adjusting to the conditions brought about by the unpredictable Yukon River. It operated over water or ice, was ecologically sound in an area that was ecologically vulnerable and saved millions of dollars over the two year period it was in operation. The system was operated with a winch and cable system which propelled the ACT's to their destinations. A total of 42,800 feet of cable was strung across the Yukon River and traveled in excess of 24 miles every 24 hours.

Consultant for the drilling program for above ground support of pipeline and the $200 million lease program for construction equipment and housing for all personnel.

Adapted a fork lift truck that enabled the operator to move an entire load of pipe on and off the trucks in one operation, thus saving on the traffic in an ecologically vulnerable area. The first person to drive the entire length of the All Weather Highway from the Yukon River to Prudhoe Bay inspecting the line and the success of the underpasses constructed to enable migrating herds of caribou to continue unimpeded.

Initiated American Management Team Planning Process for Alyeska and took management though the process to improve pervious inadequate planning and budget methods.

SOUTH CAROLINA: Consulted and supplied, on an engineered lease basis, the materials handling equipment for first German steel mill built in the United States in Georgetown, South Carolina. Involved in the creation of a package that resulted in economic recovery in that area. Developed the concept for the lease, the mill and the long term operation of the mill.

MASSACHUSETTS: Developed a unique handling of his shore containers in the port of Boston which is still in operation.

- Conceived and marketed first complete equipment packages for erection of major offshore industrial complexes by American contractors in the following countries: **TURKEY, BELGIUM, WALES, PHILIPPINES, BORNEO, VENEZUELA AND OTHERS.**

- Involved in the building of the Pan Am Building in New York City, among other notable projects there. He worked on major building sites, dam constructions and mining projects across the nation.

- One of the first to recognize the potential for hydraulic cranes. Almost single-handedly, through his marketing and sales instincts helped his industry recognize the potential and future for that equipment.

- Inventor and holder of patents for specialized equipment used by oil refineries for the maintenance of heat exchangers, most notably the Tube Bundle Pulling machine.

- Recognized the potential for large capacity tower cranes used in the construction of atomic energy plants and secured the first orders for this type of crane in this country. Held an exclusive contract to market the Liebherr equipment in the USA and Canada. Was also responsible for direction and management for three of Pettibone's largest operating units. (Pettibone Corporation is an international manufacturer of construction, materials handling, mining, foundry and railroad equipment.)

- Invented a system for the handling of double T-type pre-stressed concrete beams for the construction of LaGuardia Airport's new runway. These beams were five feet wide, three feet long, weighing over ten tons and had to be cast upside down. The problem was to remove the finished beam from the mold, turn it right side up and move it to the runway site. The adaptation of existing equipment was superior to other methods then available and resulted in savings in man hours as well as expense.

- Equipment consultant and supplier of the equipment needed for construction and activation of Atlas and Minuteman Missile sites.

- Consultant to NASA and the Space Shuttle Program.

- Consultant to a substantial number of energy organizations including:

      QUEBEC IRON & TITANIUM, TIN AND ASSOC. MINERALS
      ROYAL DUTCH SHELL
      COLVAC INTERNATIONAL
      PACIFIC TIN
      ALYESKA PIPELINE SERVICE CO.

MEMBERSHIPS:

AMERICAN MANAGEMENT ASSOCIATION
PRESIDENT'S ASSOCIATION AMA
U.S./ARAB CHAMBER OF COMMERCE
THE MINING CLUB, N.Y.C.
BOARD OF DIRECTORS, C.I.M.A. (Construction Industry Manufacturers Assoc.)
AMERICAN WINE SOCIETY
SHAKO (One of founders: International organization for business men involved in oil and mining)

PUBLICATIONS:

A CHANGING MARKET PLACE
HOORAY FOR THE FALLING DOLLAR

STARDUST

And now the purple dust of twilight time
Steals across the meadows of my heart.
High up in the sky the little stars climb,
Always reminding me that we're apart.
You wandered down the lane and far away,
Leaving me a song that will not die.
Love is now the stardust of yesterday,
The music of the years gone by.

Sometimes I wonder why I spend the lonely night,
... dreaming of a song.
The melody, haunts my reverie
... and I am once again with you.
When our love was new,
And each kiss an inspiration,
But that was long ago,
And now my consolation,
... is in the stardust of a song.

Beside a garden wall, when stars are bright,
... you are in my arms.
The nightingale, tells his fairy tale,
... a paradise where roses grew.
Though I dream in vain,
In my heart it will remain,
My stardust melody,
... a memory of love's refrain.

words by: Mitchell Parish   *music by: Hoagy Carmichael*

PROLOGUE

If I were to name what influenced my outlook on life the most I'd have to say it was the movies. My parents began taking me to them before I was born and anyone who says cognitive memory begins only after birth is wrong because I was born knowing all the old songs. While I was still an infant my mother marveled at how my eyes would fill with tears as those old ballads of the Depression and the War Years played on the radio. It only took a few strains of "I'll Get By", or "Sentimental Journey", or "Once In Awhile", and I'd be overwhelmed with feelings much too complicated for anyone my age to understand and my eyes would fill with tears.

It was such a mystery for her that she'd often have me cry for visitors. I sometimes wonder if the relatives and family friends who witnessed this behavior thought us just a tad odd but then, conforming to the norm was never a lesson my parents stressed very much. As for those tears, they never really stopped flowing. I found as I grew older, they were always just below surface and it took very little for them to start. People laugh when I tell them I've been known to cry in Popeye Cartoons. I have. They will surface at almost any expression of deep feeling from anyone, anywhere, at anytime and it's not because I'm unhappy or weak. On the contrary I see myself as just the opposite.

The uncontrollable flow of water is probably why I developed such a high sense of the ridiculous and learned to appreciate irony so early in my life. As long as I could turn things around and laugh, the tears stayed out of view and out of my way. I learned very quickly that people tend to judge tears in ways they never judge laughter. As for those old ballads, I have yet to listen to any one of them without feeling some sense of melancholy and distant loss. It has always been totally unexplainable and remains so to this day. Perhaps it was the emotion my parents attached to those songs.

My earliest memories as a child are of sitting on my Dad's lap in the Franklin Theater in Syracuse, New York. To say I was weaned on "Casablanca" and "The Road To Zanzibar" would not be an exaggeration. The movies were my family's biggest form of entertainment and we saw them all. The strains of Brahms Lullaby still echo in my memory as the last showing ended and my father carried me to the car. Once television came to our home things changed. Its not that we went to the movies less, its that we were now able to watch those that predated my birth in our living room. I'll never forget Ann Miller tapping her little heart out on a series of tom toms in "Reveille With Beverly". My legs were black and blue for weeks after I tried to duplicate it on a bunch of crates I'd set up in our basement. The only time my sisters and I were allowed to miss church was when an old musical was scheduled on the TV at the same time.

If those movies grew to serve as a microcosm of life for me, then so be it! Learning is where you find it. I not only learned what rising to the occasion was all about from them, I also learned to expect heroics from myself and those around me. I knew that true love was waiting for me when the time was right, and sacrifice for someone I loved was just another word for commitment. Most of all, I learned that love could be magical. I also realized at a fairly young age that I had an abnormally high suspension of disbelief. It never bothered me that a full orchestra was in the wings or that Fred and Ginger always knew those intricate routines flawlessly. Something greater was happening. Their dance wasn't just a dance anymore, it was a symbolic expression of life. And isn't that what life is all about? Isn't it about moving to a rhythm, following a lead, measuring the distance you're expected to leap, and if it's with a partner you trust and love then isn't it just as simple as this, isn't it a dance?

Tom and I met at precisely the right moment in our cumulative experience. We were ready for each other. We were also blessed with an instantaneous acceptance of each other's strengths and weaknesses. We saw each other in all of our colors and the colors were just fine. I doubt that lives are orchestrated by some outside cosmic force but I do believe there are times when a turn in life is destined to be acted out. We met, we recognized each other, and we didn't agonize over what it all meant, we simply got on with the dance ... and oh how he could dance. Falling into step with each other was as simple as breathing. There was a commonality we felt from each other and an understanding of needs that went beyond mere words.

If there was any major difference between us, it was that Tom self-actualized his dreams whereas I allowed myself many reasons for reneging on mine. The reason, as I saw it, was that I had never learned to fully trust life whereas Tom was born knowing that life was to be lived and nothing to fear. He was someone who truly lived in the moment and I was aware enough to recognize that and covet it. Even with the changes that were already occurring in him, he was still the most dynamic, centered person I had ever met.

The condition that had already sealed our fate would be given the rather ambiguous title of Dementia: Unknown Etiology. Even at this late date the doctors are reluctant to list it as anything other than probable Alzheimer's Disease. The truth is we may never know the real reason for Tom's problems. The only thing doctors agreed upon was that there was no frame of reference for our future together, not in time left for a quality life or in predictability of the illness. Tom might live a few years or he might live out his entire life span. I could expect Alzheimer's-like symptoms however, and they were correct in that assessment. The symptoms have been relentless. From this vantage point, I doubt if putting a name on the horror will make much difference to either of us anymore because we now know "It", whatever "It" is, is killing him.

The effects of his illness impacted us and those around us in ways we could never have anticipated. While he was still able to make decisions Tom talked about his desire to tell our story. It was important to him that even this aspect of his life should have meaning. His desire afforded me the opportunity to reach into myself and find the words that became this book. Tom's confidence in my ability to complete this task was his greatest gift to me. He simply told me to do it.

If I have any regrets concerning this life of ours together, it's not having been a part of Tom's earlier history. Tom at full speed must have been something else to watch. I missed that part of his life and part of my reason for writing this book was to find and verify my image of the man I married. It's been a vicarious expedition but one which served to enhance and enrich my sense of him.

We became part of a dance that neither of us could quit from the moment we met. Time and the ravages of his illness were unable to change the commitment we made to each other and on that count we were both fortunate. However, I do have a burning desire to attach the memories of who Tom was with the reality of who he is now. Tom was so much more than the emaciated man who spends his days confined to a recliner in our living room because he is unable to stand or walk anymore and who is now unable to express even his most basic needs. He was someone who loved, and worked, and created, as have the 8,000,000 others who now face this illness. I want people to know this man's story. I want people to know what happens when a person is faced with a disease that robs them slowly and insidiously of all they were, and of the journey we have taken and are still facing, together.

IT ONLY HAPPENS WHEN I DANCE WITH YOU

It only happens
   when I dance with you,
That trip to heaven
   till the dance is through,
With no one else do the heavens
   seem quite so near.
Why does it happen dear,
   only with you?

Two cheeks together
   can be so divine
But only when those cheeks
   are yours and mine.
I've danced with dozens of others
   the whole night through,
But the thrill that comes with spring
When anything could happen,

That only happens with you.

words and music by: Irving Berlin

CHAPTER ONE

* Every now and again I've happened across someone who lives in the moment. They're a rare breed. In fact, I can count the times I've encountered such people on the fingers of one hand. They come from all walks of life bringing with them their unique brand of experience and focus. They are people who not only see the truth in life's tapestry, they also live it. They are successful at whatever they to do because they have no fear of the future and their ability to draw from experience is quick and clean because they have no regrets about their past. Their choices therefore are simple for them. If they share any commonality it is this: When they appear their presence is felt. They are either loved or hated, but they are never ignored. They walk with such assurance that their footsteps create an undeniable rhythm and I have heard a distant drum beat in the center of my being when I've encountered such people. It's as if each footstep is connected to the center of the earth. They may not be saints, but they are I think, old souls. *

It was Tom's second visit to my union's dental clinic in mid-town Manhattan. He had been there for a routine visit six months earlier, just after our marriage. He was now 5½ years into his symptoms and already moving out of the early stage of dementia. He was still keeping appointments on his own then. By the time his second visit had rolled around things had already begun to change. It was difficult for me to know whether his vision and memory had deteriorated further or whether I'd just become more aware of his existing deficits, but I no longer felt secure letting him go into what I perceived as unfamiliar territory to him, alone.

During those first six months of our marriage I'd had the intimate experience of observing how he found his way around the city. It was an arduous and often painful thing to watch. He could still find places he knew on his own but for new locations it was quite a different story. He'd hold the address in his hand and ask directions every block or so, usually arriving late. Even if we were together he'd insist on asking directions. I'd assure him over and over that I knew where we were going but he still had to satisfy his own needs to define his territory. That territory consisted of no more than two blocks at a time. What bothered me most about this behavior was the expression on his face as he asked people for help, a combination of resolve, because come hell or high water he was going to get where he had to go on his own, and on occasion there was an expression of deep sadness. This had been a man for whom territory had meant the farthest reaches of the world.

The dawning of the enormity of Tom's problems was a frightening thing for me to behold. If I'd had any misgivings and fears before our marriage, I couldn't begin to describe the feelings and fears that confronted me after watching what had transpired in only six months into that marriage.

My life had already become one of protecting Tom. I was protecting him from fear, embarrassment, disappointment and the truth, although from this perspective I was protecting myself from those things as well. Tom's ability to navigate his world was shrinking and it had become my task to hold that fact all back. That meant arranging his life in a way that allowed him to move through it as effortlessly as possible for as long as possible. If it meant being in his presence to save him the effort and time it took him to get to an unfamiliar address or jump in to complete a thought he'd left hanging in mid air, or making sure his tie was straight before he left the apartment then that is what I did. It was also foolish of me to think Tom didn't know what was going on. He was aware of my constant hovering and sometimes rebelled but he was also comfortable with the results my attention afforded him. He needed to explain himself less to others with my running shotgun. The goal was to keep life as 'normal' as possible and preserve what was left of his image.

To that degree we were living a lie, but the lie was also essential to our survival. We were trying to stuff as much love and laughter and history into our scenario as humanly possible. We were newlyweds and time wasn't on our side. Instead I stuffed my tears and fears and kept them to myself. I saved them for while I was driving to work, or in the shower, or after he'd fallen asleep. Seeing those tears would have spoiled the illusion.

... so there we stood. Tom was insisting he could go to the dentist by himself while I insisted on going with him. Marriage to me had meant major changes for him in more ways than one. Not only was the concept of going to a dental clinic new to his way of life, so was having someone actually say no to him. He could deal with the clinic a lot easier than he could deal with not having his own way. It's not that he had a problem with the concept of going to a clinic, he wasn't that sort of snob, the problem was in waiting. He hated to wait for anything. He had spent his entire life making things happen. Waiting just wasn't in his frame of reference. Knowing how that clinic operated I had every reason to believe he would not be a happy camper if left to his own devices. At the very least, I'd be faced with setting another appointment and we had waited five weeks for that one. My fears in this instance were groundless. It turned out to be the first time I actually watched Tom in full bloom.

This clinic was in our lives because they accepted my insurance plan and it was the least expensive way I knew to get good dental care in New York. It was clean and neat and populated by retired dentists working part time and young dentists just starting out. The treatment was always excellent. It was also impersonal. I never got the same dentist twice and it always took at least twenty minutes to locate my file because I could never remember the last dentist's name. The card which carried his name was usually long lost in the recesses of my purse.

I'd arrive on time, stand at the counter and wait for a receptionist to get off the phone. Without looking up she'd ask which plan I carried, push a clip board under my nose with the appropriate form, take it when I was finished and tell me to have a seat. Thirty minutes later, a dentist I'd never seen before would call my name and lead me back to his office. The receptionists had been there for years, something of an employment record in New York, and they had that operation down to where they could phone it in. There was no unnecessary expenditure of energy on their part and if the wait was longer than liked or the treatment less than nurturing, well this was New York, it was just part of the every day torture of living there.

As I mentioned earlier, this was Tom's second visit. I walked ahead of him to the counter, running interference as usual. As he came through the door the receptionist at the far end of the counter stood up and broke into a smile ...

"Why Mr. Murphy, how good to see you again, how are you doing?"

The other three ladies behind the counter looked up and chimed in their greeting, four bright faces in expectation of a good time. Tom responded;

"If I were any better, I couldn't stand myself".

He offered this with his usual bravado and just a hint of an Irish brogue. When the giggling subsided, the flurry of activity that followed ended with his chart on it's way to the hygienist in what had to have been record time. I remember thinking ...

... and what is this? ... Charm! ... They're oozing charm! My memory bank started flashing episodes of all those years I'd waltzed into that office, episodes with my children who weren't easily forgotten in their own right. I had yet to achieve eye contact with any of them.

Tom was not only remembered but his file had been assigned to the owner of the clinic who came out personally to greet him. I could hear them laughing as they walked back to the office. The whole sequence of events happened without Tom demanding a thing. He simply walked into their presence wearing his usual affable charm.

It took them twenty minutes to locate my chart because I couldn't remember my dentist's name, but marriage to Tom was not without it's perks and both the chart and I were transferred to 'his' dentist by the time it was found. When my turn came to see the hygienist (first stop on that particular treadmill) she did little but talk of Tom. She told me how nice he was, how helpful he was, how handsome he was, how he listened. Apparently the seeds had been sown on his first visit six months earlier. In what had to have been a few short minutes per person he became someone they simply would not forget.

Over the years I've known and loved him, I've watched him move through life and I've seen incidents like the above happen over and over. Until he was unable to speak, Tom managed to enter people's lives. God knows he certainly entered mine.

My sisters and I were allowed to miss church on Sundays to watch those old musicals for good reason. We were professional performers and in my Mom's opinion those movies had as much to offer us as church did. She'd sit with us and bubble about the dance routines that were about to move across our very small television screen. She loved those movies. It was no surprise to us because she and my dad could have been professional dancers themselves. I vividly remember the way they took over a dance floor. My father would hold her in his arms, their eyes locked on each other as they spun around the floor moving everyone out of their way, and then they'd just fly. They were simply amazing.

Thanks to my mother I learned to watch those movies with a practiced eye and much of what I absorbed made its way into our sister act. We were fast outgrowing what the local dance teachers could give us and by the time I was twelve I did all the choreography and the vocal arrangements for our group. I was somewhat precocious for my age. I could reproduce a tap step by listening to it and I could remember a dance routine by just watching it. My younger sister Norma and I often spent an entire Saturday in a movie theater watching the same film over and over in order to copy a routine. We'd piece it together in the ladies room dashing back into the theater during the next showing in order to pick up what we missed. Those were the days when fifty cents allowed you to sit through a movie as many times as you could stand it.

We were regulars on local radio and television in Syracuse, New York, during the 40's and 50's. We were billed as "The Bigtree Sisters", and we played every town between Buffalo and White Plains, and as far north as Kingston, Ontario. It was an interesting life for us. We performed in just about every circumstance you can imagine from concert halls, to barns, to the back of a truck. I remember one job at a county fair where it had been raining for days. Mud squirted up through the makeshift floor that was to serve as our stage. We were doing our version of a clog dance and were covered with mud by the time we finished but we never missed a step. The audience loved it. For the record, the answer is yes! It is possible to "open" a parking lot, and no! It was not fun to follow Miss Ellie and her Wonder Horse with an acrobatic dance.

We were extremely organized and motivated as children, we had to be. Ours was a life of deadlines and performance and we learned very early that we could produce ... we could always meet that deadline. I grew up knowing I could handle a crisis better than most and that laughter was a necessary ingredient to survival. Nothing got my creative juices pumping faster than a deadline, a trait that has kept me in good stead all my life.

Our parents believed that when one door closed another door opened but, in all honesty, it was a lot of years before I actually subscribed to that belief. I was well into adulthood before I noticed an internal clock that told me when it was time for door closing, or door slamming as the occasion warranted, or that the door closing depended upon my making the decision to do so. Once I recognized the need for change however, change just seemed to happen. I learned to trust that clock, acknowledging in the process that life had a way of working out for me. It was December 1984 and another door was about to open in my life.

There are some who might think what followed was not so wonderful. Some might even call it rotten luck. What happened was the chance to test my limits and learn what living in the moment is really all about. In some ways the ride has been almost magical.

1984 had been a year that resulted in several changes in my life. By the time Christmas arrived I had made decisions I'd put off for too long and was even feeling a vague sense of anticipation about the coming year. My youngest sister Sandy and her husband Phil, who were on their way to London for two years of graduate study, had scheduled a few days in New York in order to spend time with me and catch the Christmas scene before leaving the country. The visit promised to be a fun few days. Not having been to church in years and knowing they would like to attend services before doing the sights, I asked a friend to make a suggestion. He suggested Marble Collegiate Church on Fifth Avenue both for the architecture and because it was also the pulpit from which Norman Vincent Peale had carried his message on 'Positive Thinking'. It was the Sunday between Christmas and New Years. I expected the church to be packed. It was.

The drive from Staten Island where I lived, took much longer than we expected and we reached 'Marble' about ten minutes before the start of the service. There was an open parking space right in front of the church, (minor miracle number one).

   * *Finding parking in New York is very much like finding true love. You live in anticipation of the event, but with very little confidence in attaining it.* *

We walked up the steps of the church and down the center aisle somehow missing an usher. There was a completely empty pew a few rows from the front. When I opened the gate to sit down an usher came running over. I thought perhaps the pew was being saved since it was the only empty space in the entire church, but no, the gate had been stuck all morning and he wondered what I had done to free it. It had clicked and simply swung open when I pulled (minor miracle number two).

The experience of the service was like coming home for me. The familiarity of the hymns, and the fact that I didn't fall asleep during the sermon was compelling but what caught me most was the complete abandon with which the congregation sang. They sang full out, all the stops pulled, harmony filling the highest corners and the tiniest of crannies. Dr. Peale had retired that year and Arthur Caliandro had replaced him. He had an easy manner and was easy to listen to. I felt comfortable with what he had to say. Best of all, a myriad of activities were listed in a folder in the pew, activities designed to bring people together in the many volunteer programs Marble ran and specialty groups designed to develop fellowship and support. There was also a coffee hour every Sunday after service. I returned by myself the following week (minor miracle number three).

I had ended an eight year relationship that year. As often happens when his friends become your friends, he gets to keep custody of the friends and you get to start from scratch. I wasn't so interested in meeting Mr. Right at that point in my life as much as I was looking to find something to get me moving again. Actually, the statistics in New York were that I probably had a better chance of finding Mr. Jack the Ripper than of finding Mr. Right, and frankly the process of dating in New York City was not something I cared to think about at the time. In any event, I was bored with feeling sorry for myself, I was tired of just working and going home.

What I needed was a place where I could meet people. Marble offered that opportunity. There were a number of volunteer programs that interested me but my main objective was to make friends. Thanks to the life style I had enjoyed with my former gentleman friend, I had learned the basic skills essential to survival in a room full of strangers and it was during one of my passes through the coffee room, that second Sunday, that I heard someone utter the magic word ... brunch.

> *   *Brunch ... an activity with a contained group of people who are often a captive audience due to the confines of a table. If you seat yourself strategically you have contact with the greatest number of people at all times.* *

"Brunch ... Is this a particular group of people or can anyone go?"

"No, Tom Murphy generally gets a group together after coffee and whoever is available goes." (long pause) "Would you like to join us?"

"Gosh, I'd just love to." As if I had any intention of going away.

About eight of us moved to the Abbey Tavern, a restaurant in the neighborhood, and two hours later I headed home to Staten Island. The following Sunday I cornered the first person I recognized during coffee hour and asked about the brunch ...

"Hi, it's really nice to see you again ... wasn't the sermon wonderful ... is anyone going to ... brunch, this week?"

The gentleman didn't know. He didn't think so because Murphy hadn't come that day. Not to be undaunted I asked a number of others from the group about joining me and finally found three people who wanted to go anyway ... Murphy or no Murphy.

From that point on, brunch on Sunday became my personal pursuit. I was settling into a very comfortable existence. I was making friends and people had begun to recognize me and come to me to set up the Sunday group in Tom's absence. I was considering joining the church and I had begun to look into various volunteer groups. Sunday had become the high point of my life every week and from that first day I never missed a service. It wasn't just the coffee hour and the extended activities that drew me there however, the sermons were living lessons I could draw from throughout the week. I started to feel a great deal of the anger I'd been living with for years begin to drain off. I felt happier.

I still didn't know who this Tom Murphy was but I did have some curiosity especially since his name came up in conversation so often. I remember wondering who the rather handsome, impeccably dressed, white-haired gentleman was who worked the 'main room' the half hour before the service. He was there every Sunday talking to many of the older people sitting in their pews near the front of the sanctuary. He always seemed to have a good line because everyone laughed as he moved on to the next person. There was always a touch for whomever he was talking to and an occasional kiss on the cheek for the ladies which was sometimes followed by a little giggle. Whoever he was, he seemed very much at ease and very much a part of the church scene. He was of course, Tom. It's odd now that I recall this because until I actually met others who were also prominent in the church social hierarchy, he was the only one I'd noticed.

It was now February 1985, and Tom had just buried his only sister Mary. His absences were due to his visits to see her and to help settle her estate. I learned this after walking in on a conversation he was having with someone during coffee one Sunday. She had died of cancer and his feelings about her death were so articulated that the person he was speaking to felt pressured to say something. When he muttered something that included the words "the will of God", Tom blazed back with a verbal tirade so intense he literally startled the man. My father had died of cancer and I had understood what Tom had meant. He wasn't asking why and he most certainly wasn't expecting any answers. The gentleman's mistake was in feeling obligated to make any comment at all. As he melted back into the crowd leaving Tom alone, I moved forward and introduced myself, finally meeting *Himself.*

From that point on, Tom would be someone I watched. He was an extremely intense person and there was no denying his presence when he entered a room. He was a wonderful story teller and he was obviously comfortable in that role. He was also born to wear clothes and between the English tailoring, the shock of white hair on his head, the French Regimental Beret he sported when he was outdoors and his attitude, he was in the very least flamboyant. He once asked me if he looked too dapper. I laughed. If there was anyone who could carry off dapper in this world it was Tom, and then there were those bagpipes. There were days when numbers of us heard them as Tom marched down the street ahead of us. If you believe in reincarnation I'd offer that we experienced some distant memory of Tom in another place, another time. If not, well perhaps we simply experienced a collective fantasy.

We weren't often seated at the same table at brunch but I could always hear him. He seemed to love controversy and he was always making proclamations and statements that I began to refer to under my breath, as 'History according to Tom Murphy'. He especially loved to rail at smokers, being a reformed one himself, and every time we entered a restaurant his grandiose request to be seated away from any smokers made everyone's eyes roll. I say grandiose, because this was New York, there were no smoking restrictions in those days and for most of us, making such a request was a pointless exercise in futility. Tom didn't see it that way. There were times when he stalked out of a restaurant in search of a more accommodating one with most of us in tow. There was head shaking but I think most of us were somewhat captivated by his bravado. I know I was. The posturing seemed more an act than anything else to me anyway, something he did to stir things up and fill up time. He impressed me as being a loner and at the same time needing people around him. We were a lot alike in that regard.

There were occasions when I left for home wondering what he was all about. People seemed to know little about him except that he was an international business man who had once been very successful but at what they couldn't say. He always seemed in good humor and was always helpful to others but he rarely spoke about himself. However, the little pearls he dropped in conversation let you know he was no fool, he was extremely intelligent, and he had a keen insight and a deep sense of himself. Most of all, he was fun to be with, a real New York character in the finest sense of the expression.

Tom was very active in a number of volunteer groups in the church and I observed that he seemed to function with little regard for 'the drill'. I think this did not endear him to some. He had a way of taking charge when a situation arose without clearing things through the hierarchy, only stopping later to remark to me that he might have stepped on a few toes in the process. More then once I watched him soothe the waters before resentments were allowed to fester. He was extremely adept in getting people to tolerate him. In Tom's eye, he saw a need and answered it. In other's eyes, he was probably viewed as something of a loose cannon. They had no way of knowing this was just another example of how he functioned in general. He had a way of claiming position without ever coveting it. I don't think Tom ever coveted much of anything in life. It was a facet of his personality that could be very threatening to people of lesser confidence, and on occasion I suppose it was.

While he could have spent his Sundays networking, and in the company of the rich and famous in the congregation, Tom turned his attention elsewhere. He spent the coffee hour in search of the new person standing alone and the regular attender who never seemed to talk to anyone. He'd introduce people, bring them together and invite them to brunch. I found myself doing much the same thing when he wasn't around. We both understood how difficult it was for some people to break the ice.

Several more weeks went by, Easter came and went, and then one Sunday it all changed. Tom got the group together as usual and about eight of us piled into a restaurant a few blocks from the church. As often happened during those lunches, someone asked what had brought us all to "Marble". One by one we related our stories and then it came to Tom. He was asked:

"With a name like Murphy, you must be Irish, Tom. You must have been brought up as a Catholic. What made you join Marble?" Tom responded:

"When my Catholic priest, wouldn't give me a Catholic divorce".

I countered with: "Ha! You and Henry VIII."

I remember it so clearly because Tom looked up and at me and our eyes locked. Other things were said around the table. I know everyone was laughing but our eyes were locked together. It was as if we really 'saw' each other for the first time. It was as if we were looking into each other's soul. It was the most intense experience I've ever had. It was just like the movies. Everything seemed to fade, and sound became distant, and everything slowed down and every cell in my being was locked on every cell in his being. It was instant recognition, the thunder bolt, love at first sight. It was happening to me.

Gradually the sound came up, and color returned, and conversation continued as though there had been no interruption but

Tom had moved one person closer to me. The repartee seemed wittier than usual that afternoon, especially that emanating from Tom and myself. I can't remember being so clever and everything he said had such an air of dash. In the midst of all the laughter I'd catch him watching me and I'd have had to be dead to not notice he moved closer to me every time someone left. By the time he was sitting next to me the electricity was so intense that when his sleeve accidentally brushed my arm, I felt as though I was held in space, every chance touch and glance giving off the most delicious waves of delight.

The party was winding down and I didn't want it to end. I knew I was high but not on wine. When we finally left the restaurant I asked Tom if he'd like to stop off for a cup of coffee before going home. He very dryly stated that he didn't care for coffee, but would I care to stop by his place for a last glass of wine. I didn't decline the offer.

I know it's going to be hard to believe but I didn't go to his place to make love to him. Really! I was old enough and secure enough to handle such things in the first place and second, I really didn't feel that's why I was asked. I felt that he as much as I, had to find out who this other person was and if the moment wasn't grabbed we'd pass each other and never catch that moment again.

Tom directed me to his apartment and I entered one of the most beautifully restored cast iron buildings in New York City. He told me the history of the building as we rode the elevator to his place and after a brief tour of the apartment he poured us both a glass of wine and we settled in the living room.

To say his place was beautiful is an understatement. Everything was placed with the utmost in taste, a taste that reflected a person who required a certain standard of living and who was totally at ease among his things. He talked about his antiques in terms of where he found them and how he acquired them and not what he paid for them. It impressed me that he gave equal importance to the lamps he had found on the street and rewired. He made a point of saying his furniture was meant to be lived in, not just looked at. To emphasize the point he sat in the arm chair on the right of the sofa, put his feet on the coffee table and waited for me to decide where I was going to sit. I chose the end of the sofa nearest his chair. We indulged in the usual banter for a while and then Tom spoke ...

"Something was happening in that restaurant wasn't it."

It was phrased as a statement. I nodded.

"There are some things you should know".

He then proceeded to tell me about his divorce in 1981, describing his part in the drama in terms of a straight forward, *'just the facts'* manner with little embellishment or need to absolve himself of blame. But then divorce was hardly an unusual happening in life and why would I be interested in any of the details anyway? I was just happy he wasn't still married and playing around. His children were adults, children he spoke of with warmth and affection. After making his marriage status clear, he refilled his glass and moved to the chair facing me.

> * *In group dynamics, this position is one of confrontation. The person who chooses the seat across from the therapist is generally ready to challenge.* *

There was reason for this move because he then told me about Jordan, or Judith as she was called by everyone else. He and Judith had been through a long involvement, as friends, colleagues and lovers. They planned to marry after his divorce and had bought the apartment we were presently in, in fact, I was surprised to learn Judith was still living in the apartment. However, things had begun to change in his life. The oil business was dying, at least for him it was and he made some vague reference about things in general being different for him. He returned from a business trip one day and Judith told him she couldn't marry him. They went to dinner that evening, talked things out and decided they made better friends than lovers. They agreed to continue living together since it was unfeasible for both of them to sell the apartment at the time. They'd lead their own lives and respect the privacy of each other. She was presently in China running a marathon. He hoped she'd meet someone who deserved her. They'd always be the best of friends but that was all their relationship was and would be. He added that he had dated a number of women since they made that decision but the women always broke it off before it got very serious. He added they never really explained why.

He rose from his chair, refilled our glasses and moved to the chair placed at the left end of the sofa. He settled back and waited.

I hadn't spoken at all through this but to say I appreciated his honesty was an understatement. In a world of half truths and half commitments, his willingness to lay the cards on the table was something to value. It had to do with being fair. If there was one thing I hated it was having to play games and the dating game was right at the top of my list. It was obvious that all of this could have been learned anyway through other sources at Marble. There really was nothing to be gained by keeping a live-in female friend to himself except to play out the rest of the afternoon. The thing is, others might have played out the afternoon. Could I have met someone who also didn't play games?

[Be still my heart.]

His move signaled that it was my turn to talk. He obviously knew how to deal with silence because he just watched me and waited. I remember thinking to myself, keep it simple. I knew well that everyone had a story and Tom's was probably more involved than either of us had time or energy for at that time. Mine could take on the aspects of an epic poem complete with a full string orchestra and stereophonic sound.

I finally began to relate the high points of my life, the last eight years with my friend and my reasons for the break up which revolved around a differing definition of the word commitment. I had also been in a marriage that ended in divorce 10 years earlier. My two children were pushing adulthood, the eldest already independent, my youngest with one more year of high school to finish. Being a single parent wasn't easy in New York but I had managed. I had done the best I could, paid my bills and was out of debt for the first time since my divorce. Things were beginning to look up in general.

In the midst of all of the above I had continued with my career as a rehabilitation counselor, received my masters degree in Guidance and Counseling, and had managed to keep my sense of humor. I was looking forward to accomplishing some other things in my life. My 'former gentleman caller' was a prominent architect in New York and he was instrumental in helping me get my first major commission as an artist with New York Life Insurance. I now had two 6'x9' tapestries hanging in a corporate media building in Washington, DC I had generated a few smaller commissions since that job and rather enjoyed using my creative abilities in a new way.

I remember telling Tom that I could handle anything as long as it was the truth. He looked at me for a few seconds and then moved to the far end of the sofa while remarking ...

"I guess we've both been through a few wars".

"What do you do for fun, Tom?"

"I work."

At that point we both got up to go to the bathroom. After all that wine it was the only thing to do. Men are always faster than women and when I returned he was seated next to my place on the sofa. As I sat down he moved in closer. He put his arm around me and he kissed me.

Three hours later we emerged from the bedroom to find our clothes had been scattered in a trail from the sofa to the bed, where we hadn't slept. We both laughed since neither of us recalled the move off the sofa and neither of us could ignore the evidence of wild abandonment which had obviously occurred. He made the observation that both of us were taking a real chance considering the amount of wine we'd consumed and there was a very real possibility that the whole thing might have been a real disaster. I recall noting I wasn't aware making love was an Olympic sport, although the thought crossed my mind that if he attacked his work with the same level of competency and imagination that had been manifested in the past three hours, he was at the very least, formidable in his business dealings.

I was wearing his robe. He was content walking around as he was. He had the most beautiful body I'd ever seen on a man, at any age. We moved into the kitchen where he prepared dinner and while he was cooking he asked what time I had to leave. I told him I didn't. He stopped what he was doing and laughed ...

"You know, there is something to be said for being older."

We spent the rest of the evening talking and listening to records. We fell asleep in each other's arms. When we awoke the next morning we were still wrapped in each other's arms. It had been a soft, comfortable night with a familiarity between us that I couldn't explain. There was intensity but no desperation or fear attached to it. It was just blissfully comfortable.

He was having some minor surgery on his eyes that day. He had been having problems with his vision for some time and he was at a loss to figure out what was going on. He had been to a number of doctors and hoped the procedure he was about to undergo would help the condition. That evening he phoned to let me know it was a success, much to his relief.

I know I was taken aback by the happenings of the previous day. It was easy to mistrust the intensity of the whole experience and wonder if it had only been one sided. Flight crossed my mind more than once as I waited for his call. It also concerned me, even at my age, that I would be thought of as 'easy'. He didn't disappoint me.

"I want you to know Beverly, that I'm not accustomed to going to bed with everyone who passes by. Yesterday was one of the most loving and giving experiences of my life. I hope you don't mind my saying it was also one of the most enjoyable. I can't wait to see you again."

Lord, where has this man been all my life? Please let me know I can trust my feelings about him. Six months! I'm giving him six months to figure it out. If it's not the same for him by then, then let me know it's time to move on. If nothing else, let us have the wisdom to let this thing just happen.

We decided to keep our involvement out of Marble. He offered that we'd be too visible if our friendship didn't work out and it might then be difficult for either of us to continue there comfortably. Considering that he was living with one woman and had been recently involved with another, I, as new girl on the block did not need to be considered part of Tom's harem. Both of us had a vested interest in maintaining a low profile.

Over the summer we spent every available minute with each other. When Judith was out of town we stayed at his place, when she was home we stayed at mine. Most importantly, we talked and we learned about each other. However, much of his history remained in bits and pieces. He told me the past was over. He had taken on projects others would not or could not handle and once a project was completed his direction was always towards the next challenge. It was how he had always lived his life.

I do not, and will not believe his career was ever motivated by money or power. He had too obvious a contempt for those motivated by such needs and his dealings with such people has been described as ruthless. For Tom it was always the personal sense of accomplishment and an obsessive need to be the best he could be.

In 1988, a therapist asked Tom what he regretted most about his illness. Tom, without a second of thought stated ...

"I hate the thought that I won't be able to realize my full potential before I die. I feel as though my talent is going to waste. I hate the thought of that waste".

I once asked him how he'd characterize his success in life. He told me he was never afraid of failure. He learned early in life that once he envisioned a goal it was as good as done. He reached adulthood knowing there was nothing he couldn't accomplish once he set his sights and his accomplishments speak for themselves. His expectations were always positive. How often have I heard that life responds to your expectations? However, wanting to live your life that way and actually living it that way are often two different things. Tom said it was as simple as walking through a door. He couldn't imagine being any other way.

There was something else about this man that drew me in. He had that very rare capacity to see right to the core of a problem. Time after time I'd watch him listening to someone's problem. He'd let them talk for awhile to get the gist of where they were headed, interrupt them with a couple of questions and then relate what the real problem was and what the only viable alternatives of action could be. He was concise, clear, and basic in his approach to everything. It didn't matter what the subject was, he dealt with it with equal facility and it wasn't with a know-it-all attitude, although I fear many saw it that way. As for me, well I saw a clarity in his thought process that spoke of wisdom. He was someone I wanted to be around. I had to wonder what I might have accomplished in my lifetime if he'd come into it sooner. He became more than a lover to me. He became my mentor, and he became my best friend.

Six months after that first encounter he phoned and asked me to meet him on the Staten Island side of the ferry. He arrived carrying a bottle of his good wine under his arm. He opened the wine when we got to my place, poured us both a glass, and leaned back on my sofa.

"Well, Beverly, are we going to make a commitment to each other or do we just continue to screw around?"

He wiggled his finger in the air when he came to the word 'screw'. I asked him what he meant by a commitment, adding that I already knew the meaning of screwing around. He said ...

"I want to be married to you. I think we need time to consider it but that's my intention. I've had this intention since our second date but I needed to work some other things out first and I wasn't sure how you felt. I love you and I'd like you to be my wife."

Thank You, Lord!!!

In January 1986 he formally asked me to marry him. We set a date in October because that's when my sister was returning from England. We came out of the closet at 'Marble'. He and Judith put the apartment on the market and we started making plans to spend the rest of our lives together. "I love you," are the first and last words we have said to each other every day, since that day.

LONG AGO AND FAR AWAY

Long ago and far away
I dreamed a dream one day
  And now ...
      That dream is here beside me.

Long the skies were overcast
But now the clouds have passed
  You're here ...
      At last ...

Chills run up and down my spine
Aladdin's lamp is mine
  The dream I dreamed ...
      Was not denied me ...

Just one look and then I knew
That all I longed for
  Long ago ...
      Was you ...

words by: Ira Gershwin   music by: Jerome Kern

CHAPTER TWO

January 1988

Dear Tom,

This is the first letter I have ever written to you. I have a few things that I want to say. Let's go back 40 years. You grew up so very fast, and I, just a little younger, but far behind you in the late 30s and early 40s. I am going to refresh your mind about the time you saved our brother John's life and I am sure you don't remember. I am the only one that knows that John is alive today because of your bravery.

We were in Pennsburg, you eleven, me nine, and John five. It was winter and the three of us went for a walk on the pond. The ice cracked and we all went in the water. You and I were only a few feet from shore and got to the bank. John was six or seven feet out, you jumped back in, grabbed his hand and got him to shore. That pond was eight to twelve feet deep. One minute of hesitation and John would have been gone.

We went back to the hotel, and just said we fell in some water. We were never together growing up. Times were hard, you went to Uncle Bobs and then to war. I can't remember you and me going any place together. Pop's drinking didn't help, but I still love him as my father and when I talk to God I pray for Pop and Mom.

I always loved you as my brother and you are always in my prayers. I hope we see each other soon.

Your brother
Paul

During my twenty five years as a Rehabilitation Counselor with the State of New York, I had occasion to observe the following:

* *Environment can teach us the basic amenities of social behavior within the context of a culture and not much else. It also dictates the level of education we receive because of the limits money and social position impose and therefore influences the careers open to us. It might even measure the amount of polish or sophistication we ultimately end up with, although that's probably debatable, but in the final analysis it really*

makes little difference in how we function as individuals. The behaviors we bring with us at birth are the same behaviors we have to work with throughout our lives and given the fact that we do indeed have choices in how we live that life experience, how we approach life remains basically the same. *

I have a photograph of Tom at the age of three that now hangs on our living room wall. He's sitting on a bench with his legs crossed. He's wearing short pants and his long golden curls are falling over his shoulder. His head is turned towards the light and he has an expression on his face that rivals Puck's in sweetness and deviltry. You can see the spark in those eyes and the activity that was raging behind them. In fact, I recognize those eyes. They haven't changed a whole lot since that picture was taken.

He must have been a handful as a child, if the stories I've heard are true. There's little doubt in my mind that he's been a handful his entire life. And, there is no doubt in my mind that the man I married is still very much the same person he was in that child's body, in that photograph.

Tom was one of five children in a family whose roots went back to Killarny, Ireland. His father, James Francis, was a Murphy, his mother Mary, a McLaughlin, and his frame of reference was well steeped in the Irish tradition of Philadelphia where he was born. His eldest brother Jim told me that Tom moved directly from crawling to leaping and running, both at full speed. Tom said the first word he spoke after the obligatory Mom and Pop was 'why'. I remember Jim's laugher as Tom shared that bit of news with me. He described himself as being inquisitive to a fault and remembered his aunts and uncles rolling their eyes the minute he came into sight while remarking, "Here comes Tom with all the questions.".

He was born on Columbus Day, 1928 and maybe it's of note that for the first few years of his life he thought the Columbus Day Parade was held in his honor. (A sense of self has been sown by stranger circumstances.) However, by the time the full effect of the Depression had set in he was old enough to know how life had a way of changing and how desperate it could become. Like so many children who came out of that era he has few memories of being a child and he often remarked that he was born old. As times got harder in Philadelphia, Tom and his brothers were literally farmed out to relatives who were in a position to help or provide work.

His Uncle Gene took Tom and his brothers to stay at his hotel in Pennsburg, Pennsylvania for a while. It was at his Uncle Gene's that the boys fell into that icy pond. It was a time that marked a turning point for Tom.

Studies have shown that in the history of successful men there was always someone who manifested the role of mentor somewhere in their background. For Tom, Uncle Gene was that man. He was the first person to acknowledge Tom's smartness in terms of intelligence. Until then, Tom interpreted his activity level as being mostly a bother to the adults in his life. He knew he had a busy mind, he just never associated it with being smart, clever maybe, but not smart.

The day Tom and his brothers arrived, his uncle took him into his library where he had all the classics as well as reference books and encyclopedias. He picked a book from his collection and handed it to Tom. As Tom related it, the conversation went something like this ...

"You're a smart lad, Tom, and you've got the potential to get far in this life but it's really up to you how far you get. You've got a lot of energy and a lot of time on your hands. I suggest you start putting it to good use. You can come in here anytime you want and as often as you like. You might not completely understand what I'm saying Tom, but the very best advice I can give you is to start reading."

Tom read everything he could get his hands on during that visit developing an appetite for learning he never lost. He also discovered there was very little that didn't interest him and by the time he left Pennsburg, he had a somewhat expanded view of life and himself.

His stay with another uncle was a different story. The man was wealthy by depression standards, owning a farm as well as an auto service station and general store. Tom spent summers working the farm and helping in the auto shop. Tom spoke of those summers in terms of bondage. He worked from sun up until sundown and the salary he received for his entire summer's work was $5.00. As Tom put it, "I was fed". He said he was always mindful of that man's cheapness and his willingness to take advantage of someone young and in need. In some ways that lesson was as valuable to him as his time with his Uncle Gene. Both experiences stayed with him throughout his life and both experiences colored how he viewed and responded to those around him.

As for his parent's influence on his life ... well, it was difficult for Tom to say the words 'my mother' without including the word 'saint' somewhere in the comment. She embodied what was good and solid in his life and that image of her never faltered. He never spoke of her with anything less than unconditional love in his eyes and his voice. His brothers Jim and John both echo his devotion to her and his concern and help during her final years.

When I asked Tom about his father his response was somewhat different.

"Pop was the greatest salesman who ever lived. He was self assured and glib with the capacity to turn stone into cash. No one was as charismatic as Pop. He was very handsome, with a shock of black hair, a swagger in his walk, and an Irish Brogue he could turn on and off at will. He was a great raconteur and the 'party' started when Pop arrived. He could charm you into anything and make it seem like your idea. He was some piece of work to watch."

As Tom described his father, I was struck by the animation and the spark of that description.

"Sounds a lot like you Tom."

"Yes, except I didn't waste it all drinking."

Tom and his older sister Mary were the only ones who seemed able to handle their father when he was drinking, especially after their oldest brother left home. Tom recalled that from the time he and Mary were children, they were sent to track Dad down to try to get money from him before it was all gone. Tom said they both knew the urgency attached to being successful at that task and both of them had become fairly adept at it. However, Tom said he felt humiliated having to convince his dad in front of his cohorts to turn over money for food and bills and was often teased and tormented during those encounters. One time his dad told him he could have a few dollars for his mother but only if he sang for it. Tom recalled feeling like an idiot standing on the bar with everyone carrying on, but sing he did. He grabbed the money when he finished and literally ran home.

But that was only part of it. He and his sister still had the chore of getting him into bed when he finally got home. What their mother didn't say and what Tom already knew is that she was afraid of his father when he was drunk, they all were for that matter. Mary was the safest because she was the favorite and his mother was left alone as long as she didn't interfere. Instead, he picked on the younger boys, especially Tom. He had had more than his share of beatings and was accused, more than he cared to remember, of having a smart mouth. Tom admitted that he did have a smart mouth. He found the whole situation beyond tolerance, realizing at the same time how trapped they all were.

He said he decided at an early age that he was not going to give in to him, not ever. He also felt as if he was the self-appointed protector of the family. His oldest brother Jim, who had done what he could to help support the family had already left for war and his younger brothers were too small to be anything but victims. By the time Tom was fourteen he was big enough and angry enough to take his father on. One day, in the midst of yet another rage, he struck his father and warned him he'd kill him if he ever touched anyone in the family again. Tom said it was the first time his father backed off and both of them knew Tom meant it.

Their relationship was never mended. Tom would often speak of his dad but it was always with regret. He once told me that what bothered him most about his father was the waste of the man's talent. "He could have owned the world", he said.

Tom had just turned fifteen the day he enlisted in the army. He saw enlistment as a way of getting out of a bad home situation and his mother agreed to lie about his age in order to accommodate his wishes. She also wanted him away from what she feared was going to be a major confrontation between he and his father if he stayed.

It's no wonder that Tom described himself as having been born old. A lot had been crammed into those fifteen years. His brother Jim told me he was always on the move, always thinking, always planning. From the time he could put three words together he was concerned with making money, money which he turned over to his mother for the family. By the time he was four he had made his own shoe shine box and whenever he wasn't in school or doing chores he was busy shining shoes. At the age of nine he hit upon another idea.

He realized there was too much involved in collecting and turning in pop and beer bottles by himself, a chore most kids tried some time in their lives. The few pennies that resulted weren't worth the work. He decided to consolidate the neighborhood into one operation. His! He offered the neighborhood kids a third of the going rate if they'd bring him all their bottles. He'd do the washing, sorting and delivering and make two third's profit. He somehow managed to get hold of a beat up red wagon and with a gang of kids collecting bottles for him, he went into the contracting business.

Several months into his 'business' his wagon was run over by a trolley. Tom, expecting the usual stop had already started across the track when the accident happened. Some bystander jokingly told him to go sue the transit authority. Tom who recognized advice when he heard it, picked up pieces of the wagon, walked downtown to the Philadelphia Transit Authority, demanded to see someone in 'authority' and told the receptionist he was going to sue them. After several hours wait he was finally called upstairs to one of the executive offices. The gentleman behind the desk had a smirk on his face when Tom entered his office.

"I hear you're the young man who's planning to sue the Transit Authority".

"Yes, Sir. Your trolley went through a scheduled stop. I've witnesses who'll testify and I have your schedule showing it was a stop. My wagon was destroyed."

The man looked Tom over and after further comments back and forth asked ...

"What do your think the wagon was worth?"

"It was an old wagon and it was probably only worth a few dollars."

"Would $5.00 cover the cost of replacing the wagon?"

"Yes ..." But as Tom spoke the word yes, a light went on in his head and he remembered thinking ... "this is too easy".

Without skipping a beat he added: "... but, there is also the loss of my business".

He then proceeded to describe his business. He calculated how much it would take to pay off the boys who worked for him, the cost of the broken bottles, as well as the days of work he'd lose while he replaced the wagon and reorganized his workers. They shook hands after the deal was struck and Tom walked out of the office with a fair amount of cash in his pocket. I can see the expression on that man's face as Tom left the office. I can imagine the thoughts that went through his mind while he wondered what Tom was going to be like in a few years. Not so many years later, Tom would actualize more than that man could possibly have dreamed.

He was discharged after the war, at the age of 17 with a 'purple heart', having been wounded in action and returned to the front four weeks after his injury. He entered the war near the end and so was part of the occupation forces in Germany. He discovered he had facility with languages and returned to Philadelphia speaking enough German to have functioned as an interpreter for his unit before his discharge. He would eventually add French and some Arabic to his repertoire.

A few years later he joined a heavy equipment firm whose owner was German, as were many of the firm's customers. Tom's co-workers would wonder how he brought in so many accounts. What they didn't know was that he had an edge. When customers slipped into German with each other in order to speak candidly, Tom understood what they were saying. He neglected to tell anyone of his particular skill at the time. Needless to say, the customers and the owner were amazed at his 'intuitive' understanding of their needs. It was while he was with that firm that he spotted a "little hydraulic crane" in the inventory.

[We ran three to four miles every evening while we lived in New York. We were jogging up Park Avenue during one of those runs and had just passed the address where that firm had once had offices. It was then that he started reminiscing about his years with that firm. As he uttered those three words his eyes lit up, his face broke into a smile and his hands came together in the air as if that little hydraulic crane could actually fit in the palms of his hands. I had never seen anyone speak so tenderly of heavy equipment before.]

He had been competing for territory with other salesmen in his field for contracts. He liked what he was doing, his boss liked him and he was making real money for the first time in his life. Cranes in those days were chain driven, subject to frequent breakdown and expensive to maintain. He had been looking at that crane in the inventory for some time. It never seemed to move. He went to his boss and told him he thought there was a real market for that piece of equipment but his boss wasn't interested. Most of his colleagues laughed at him. Why screw around with something new and untried when the market was already proven? He then went to the owner of the company and told him he wanted a contract to market that crane exclusively. He wouldn't sell any other piece of equipment in the inventory leaving the chain driven territory open to all his other competitors, but no one else could have access to sales on that crane. The owner thought he was crazy but Tom got his contract.

At the end of the year he not only outsold everyone else in the firm, earning a record in commissions for that year, but he had demonstrated that the future was in hydraulics. Within a short period of time chain driven cranes became obsolete. Some years later when he was honored at a convention in California for being one of the forerunners in hydraulics, now holding patents on several inventions of his own, he was greeted with a standing ovation as he approached the dais.

However, at the end of the war all this was yet to happen. He was seventeen and a man. He, like so many of the returning servicemen turned his attention to school. The G.I. Bill provided tests to circumvent the high school diploma he hadn't received, tests he passed with little effort. He did four years of college in half the time which was standard for most of the returning servicemen. He majored in mechanical engineering at Columbia and Temple University and continued his studies through the years at a number of other institutions all over the world. He often enrolled in courses if he knew he was going to be based in an area for any period of time. In the end he accumulated at least a master's level of study in marketing and engineering, often teaching courses, but in reality he told me he never actually received his bachelor's degree. He was too busy working.

I once asked Tom why he never started his own equipment business. He replied he really wasn't interested in manufacturing. Owning that type of business made demands that didn't interest him. He'd have had to spend his time watching people like himself, and he was the one having all the fun. He loved his work almost more than anything else in his life.

He added that his need to do things his own way was why he left National Cash Register, his first job after college. Tom made great strides in that corporation having risen from Sales Trainee to Senior Sales Representative in less than two years. In spite of the accounts and business he brought in he was always on the carpet for not conforming. It was by mutual agreement that he finally left.

By the time 1952 rolled around he had defined his vocational choice, realizing he had a real talent for marketing. He had no doubts about his abilities and he knew his fear level was abnormally low because leaving N.C.R. gave him a sense of elation instead of dread over what his next job would be. He added that he always viewed leaving a job as a new opportunity and a chance to do something better. He was ready to embark on a career path that would be defined only by the scope of his imagination and his personal drive.

His friend Heinz Schiller probably put it best in trying to describe how Tom operated. Heinz first met Tom at the Hannover Fair in Germany in 1965. Liebherr, the company he represented, had built a factory in Killarney, Ireland for the construction of tower cranes. Tom had negotiated with that firm to exclusively market those cranes in America and Canada and was so successful that the firm had to hire more workers, benefiting not only the manufacturers but much of Killarney's County Kerry.

He also realized the high rise construction market, now booming in this country, required ever larger cranes, and saw the potential for their use in the building of nuclear power stations therefore pushing forward the design effort even further. His efforts in the American market had a significant influence on the entire industry. Heinz was then Technical Director of the Irish factory and started traveling with Tom, then head of Bell Equipment, to some of his more important customers. Eventually he relocated to America and brought his representation of Liebherr into Tom's organization.

I always asked Tom's friends to share their memories of him when we got together. Heinz was no exception. It was over lunch one day that Heinz and Tom were reminiscing. We were laughing at some of the antics the two of them had shared when a very young waitress approached and asked if we were ready to order. We got as far as the salads when Tom asked what the house dressing was. She became flustered. It was her first day on the job, we were her first customers and she wasn't sure what it was but she would find out. She made a bee line for the kitchen and disappeared.

After she left, Heinz made the following statement ...

"If that had been Tom Murphy he'd have said, 'Oh it has imported olive oil, some herbs, a dash of vinegar, a little mustard and a dollop of heavy cream ... trust me on this, you will love it!' He'd have then returned to the kitchen, handed the order to the cook and said ... This is what I sold, now make it."

In July of 1981, Tom was driving to his office in Houston. He pulled up behind a line of cars to wait for a light to change when he spotted a car in his rear view mirror. He realized it wasn't going to stop in time to avoid hitting him. Tom pressed his foot on the brake in order to avoid a chain reaction of collisions with the cars in front of him. In doing so he absorbed most of the impact himself. He was thrown around his front seat his head hitting the windshield, the side window and the rear view mirror then snapping backwards into the seat. He claims he wasn't knocked unconscious but he had little recall of the events immediately following the accident. He insisted on going to work instead of the hospital after giving the police his report but his behavior was erratic enough to cause concern from his co-workers and they insisted he go to the emergency room. A colleague drove him since it was felt that Tom wasn't in any condition to drive himself.

Feeling that everyone was over-reacting he minimized his symptoms only mentioning the pain in his back and shoulder. He was never checked for a concussion and never given an EEG because there were no obvious cuts or scraps on his head. When queried about dizziness he told the doctor he had bumped his head but denied any confusion or dizziness. He never mentioned the headache thinking it was just a temporary condition that would soon go away. He was also concerned about wasting time in the emergency unit when he was in the midst of planning a business trip to the Middle East and there were a number of other projects that had to be dealt with before he left. He was cautioned about the symptoms of a concussion and told to put a cold pack on his bump and released.

The headache did not go away as he expected and was quite severe for several days following the accident. It was severe enough to interrupt his sleep pattern, something that was unknown to him. Tom decided the best treatment for the headache was no treatment, the same approach he used for colds and the flu. He decided to ignore it. Eventually it did go away and Tom forgot about it. However, the continuing pain in his shoulder and back did not go away and that concerned him because it interfered with his mobility.

Anything that slowed him down was of concern and the day of his flight to the Middle East he agreed to a cortisone shot. The flight turned into a nightmare because he had an adverse reaction to the cortisone and landed in worse shape than ever. He was not someone who spent much time with doctors and the reaction to the cortisone shot only added to his basic distrust of treatment in general. He was in terrible pain and refusing to go to the doctor. A friend finally convinced him to at least try his acupuncturist. Tom said they carried him into the office. An hour later he walked out. He would experience residual pain but the treatments allowed him to conduct his business while on that trip and that is what mattered to him. He continued with an acupuncturist when he returned to the States and except for his yearly checkups which were routine and required by his insurance, he felt no need to see a doctor again and didn't.

However, the residual back pain did interfere with his climbing and inspecting the heavy drilling and rig equipment he marketed while on that trip, not that it stopped him from trying. It was also during that trip that he first experienced visual distortions. Along with the pain in his back he experienced what he called vertigo while on a rig. He suddenly felt he didn't know where his hands and feet were. He said it was as if his brain and his body had been disconnected. He knew he was climbing, he could see his hands were where they were supposed to be but he couldn't feel them. If he looked away he couldn't tell where they were. The experience was very unsettling. He became very frightened but managed to make his way down the rig. Tom said he was never able to go up again and this really bothered him because he'd never had a fear of heights. He couldn't figure out why this suddenly happened. He also felt his credibility was at stake. It didn't matter if others could do that task for him, what mattered was that he couldn't do it any longer. He assumed full responsibility for what he sold and leased and that, he felt, required his personal involvement.

It's interesting that Tom regarded that incident as the primary reason for his contract with the United Arab Emirates being discontinued. It was, of course, something tangible he could pin point. However, other things were also happening that went unnoticed by him.

If changes in Tom's performance were noted by staff and friends after the accident, one has to keep in mind those changes were minimal, erratic, and easily justified. Everyone knew the pressure under which he operated. He was entitled to an occasional bad day once in a while. People had come to expect the unexpected from him. He'd land on his feet again, he always did. Who could suspect that something more insidious was going on? Tom, was the 'Idea Man' in his organization. His knowledge of finance and the intricate workings of international nuances was unequaled. His responsibilities included the design of proposals for equipment and lease packages on international projects in mining, oil and construction that were in the hundred million dollar range.

He could read and absorb reams of material and relate it intact and relevantly. He was able to speak extemporaneously for hours and his friend Bill Poe told me he was noted for heading very complex seminars and proposals with few if ever any notes. He had the sort of mind that forgot little, could organize facts and concepts easily and make relevant conclusions with ease. Sometimes, a spark of an idea he had not only changed the scope of his industry, but how others in his industry measured their careers.

Friends told me his reputation pictured him as formidable and he was. He was a dynamo who expected his staff to function according to his needs and the loyalty he inspired and the care with which he chose people of vision to work with him resulted in accomplishments that stand today as a measure of what can be done. Those same people also added that he was fair and someone it was impossible to dislike as long as you held up your end of the job. For those who didn't hold up their end, or who placed blame for their inadequacies on others, or who were fearful of being displaced from their little empires, or who were lazy and uninspired, he could be their worst nightmare. In spite of his impressive record of achievement he was someone who by the sheer nature of his drive made enemies.

The difficulties Tom began having after the accident left him vulnerable for the first time in his life. Those who were covetous of his position were now able to gain leverage and undermine his effectiveness. One year after the accident the contract with his American based firm was also dropped. Years later when inquiries were made on behalf of the law suit that was finally coming to court regarding the car accident, the reason stated for his firing was incompetence. It's important to note that at the time his contract was dropped Tom was also in the midst of charging patent infringements against that firm. He felt the firm owed him thousands of dollars for use of his inventions, money which he never received while employed there and which was never paid because the firm went into bankruptcy before his case could be litigated. It's my belief that the firm took advantage of his situation and used whatever they could to get him out of their hair.

After our marriage I had occasion to read the deposition he gave in 1984 during proceedings against the company. He didn't conduct it effectively. The language was there, his intent was there, but he fell prey to the intricacies of the questions and did himself in. To say this was unlike him is an understatement. His patent lawyer told me he had been very upset by Tom's performance, and concerned for him. In the end his claim died, a small putt considering his career wasn't far behind.

Judith said changes became noticeable by 1982. He was forgetting to follow through on tasks, leaving instructions incomplete, arriving late for appointments or missing them altogether. Little things became cumulative and no matter how much his staff tried, they weren't able to cover all the holes. After his contract was dropped, he was without a support system altogether because he no longer had a staff. What followed was a steady decline in earning capacity and growing fears about himself. Physically he felt the same. There just were those visual problems. *It*, whatever *it* was, was unnamed and terrible.

Between 1983 and 1985 he changed jobs four times, the first a major change of field from Marketing and Engineering to Securities. Each change was met with a degree of success that ultimately turned into a decline. His income dropped from well over $100,000 in 1981, to $1,400 in 1986.

He had no reason to expect anything but success at anything he tried. His basic abilities shouldn't have changed any. For him the only obstacle should have been the time it took to learn the new product. He rationalized the drop in income knowing that any job change required starting over but he missed the greater picture.

As if the career crises and his divorce weren't enough to deal with he was also faced with a number of personal losses. His mother, with whom he had a very close and loving relationship and who he saw as indestructible, died in early 1984. His brother-in-law John Roup, another person he cared for very deeply died of lung cancer shortly after. The final blow was his sister Mary. She was diagnosed with cancer six months after her husband John's death and Tom was devastated when she succumbed. On top of that his relationship with Judith had changed. He was finding himself more and more isolated and on the fringes of what had once been his life. Everything was changing around him and he couldn't seem to gain control back. Confusion and fear had to have played a large part in his feelings during that period. He was someone who had spent his entire life solving problems. This was one he couldn't solve.

He became more irritable, more demanding and sometimes inappropriate in his response to a situation. One has to understand that under the best of circumstances Tom could be all of the above and the fact that he was a little more so was excused in view of the continuing pressures in his life, i.e. the job loss, the career change, the divorce, the family deaths, the loss of income, the visual problems. Those damn visual problems! The only thing Tom could focus on and relate to was the realization that reading was more difficult and he was having problems with more abstract things such as blue prints and drawings. He blamed the problems on his vision. For some reason it didn't seem normal anymore, but he couldn't explain what was abnormal about it. He could still see. It didn't make any sense.

When I was finally given access to his closets and drawers I found among other things, eight pairs of glasses all with slightly different prescriptions. He'd go to a doctor, get a new pair, wear them for a while, find they didn't help, throw them into a drawer, and find a different doctor. No doctor ever got to see him twice in order to begin to piece together that a problem existed and he was totally inarticulate about describing his symptoms except to say ...

"I can't see anything out of these damn glasses".

As his isolation increased there was no one who spent enough time with him to really observe the clues or see the patterns of behavior that were developing. The people who had become his friends in church knew something was wrong but they had no frame of reference for Tom before 1981. With the exception of Judith, those who had worked with him and who would have been in the position to see the changes were no longer in his life. Tom's children saw him very occasionally, short visits for which he managed to pull himself together.

Everyone on Tom's staff made a career change when Tom made his, and not necessarily by choice. Judith was no exception. She was now facing her own career crisis and even though they were living together, their life together was becoming very strained and more and more distant because of the personality problems Tom was now beginning to manifest and because they no longer enjoyed the intimacy working together had given them. Her new association with Kodak, which would result in her placement as one of their top national salespersons in their corporate division, kept her out of town for extended periods of time and was very demanding of her time and focus when home. She ran the apartment, made his deposits for him, paid the bills out of their joint accounts, took care of his correspondence when he asked, and moved in a circle of friends that did not always include him.

It is also of note that none of the other people in his life were there for me when we first started dating. I had none of his friendships, none of his history except for what he chose to share, no access to his papers or finances, and because we opted to keep our affair quiet in the church, I missed what friends there might have offered. Judith and I passed like ships in the night. We were introduced to each other but for the first year of my involvement with Tom we hardly saw each other and never had any conversation. This was due mostly because Tom orchestrated it that way. I had no reason or need to seek her out and considering the relationship they still enjoyed together I was just as happy to keep my distance.

It wasn't until we decided to get married that Judith and I had any contact and even then, the mood although friendly, was distant at best. It was a major mistake that we didn't spend more time together and become friends sooner. For my part, I succumbed to all the suspicions and petty dislikes that develop when an aura of mystery is maintained. I can't speak for Judith, but I don't imagine it was easier for her.

During that first year of our courtship, I became aware of what I dismissed as idiosyncratic behavior, however Tom's verbal skills, attitude and demeanor were so impressive that he was still head and shoulders above the crowds. Like everyone else I wrote off the inconsistencies in terms of the changes that had happened in his life over the past few years. We led a solitary life together those first months, months that were filled with the passion of new love and of getting to know each other. He had become very adept at compensating. There were always explanations for why he did things in a certain way. It wasn't until we started to formalize our wedding plans and he began to involve me in the workings of his life that I began to observe, see, and feel the horror that something was seriously wrong. By the time I started to realize the potential of what might be happening to Tom, I was too deeply involved in his being to walk away.

LET'S FACE THE MUSIC AND DANCE

There may be trouble ahead
But while there's moonlight,
  and music,
    and love, and romance,
Let's face the music and dance.

Before the fiddlers have fled,
Before they ask us to pay the bill,
  and while
    we still have a chance,
Let's face the music and dance.

Soon, we'll be without the moon
Humming a different tune
  and then ...

There may be teardrops to shed
So while there's moonlight,
  and music,
    and love, and romance,
Let's face the music and dance ...
  dance ...

Let's face the music and dance.

words and music by: Irving Berlin

CHAPTER THREE

Friends have told me that Tom was the luckiest son-of-a-gun they ever met. More than one person noted his ability to always land on his feet. There were times when he not only survived a major pitfall in his career but prevailed, much to the consternation of some and the amazement of others. Those comments were shared with me after those same friends realized the extent of Tom's illness and the Herculean effort my decision to keep him at home was going to take.

I don't know that luck in it's truest sense had much to do with anything in Tom's life. I think luck for Tom was his uncanny way of seeing life's problems in their rawest form, his ability to see the options clearly, and the audacity with which he grasped the moment. Luck doesn't happen when your eyes are closed. Tom was not someone who ever walked around with his eyes closed.

He knew his life with Judith was coming to an end. Eventually she would meet someone, and at some point they would sell the apartment and go their separate ways. On some obscure level he knew he needed someone he could trust to fill her place in his life, but he also wanted someone to love. The very day our eyes met he told me he wanted to be settled with someone he cared about. He had always been the one in control, always five steps ahead of everyone else in his life and in some ways always a loner. For too many years he had been wrapped up in his work. He never encouraged longevity in his other involvements with women until Judith, and until Judith I doubt if he ever really thought much about being loved. He was too busy. As Tom put it ...

"Love, who needed love? I had people whose lives depended on me."

It occurred to me that giving love might have been easier for him than expecting to be loved back, although I'm not sure that sort of speculation even matters. He was now recognizing the need for something more. Perhaps he was feeling an undefinable sense of no longer being in control. Perhaps he was too intelligent to ignore the changes that were taking place in him. Whatever it was, it laid the foundation for a commitment of self and soul to someone who was willing to give back in like measure. If luck was involved, it was in our crossing paths. The recognition of what we had to offer each other was something else.

─────────────────────────────

During our early days I was totally infatuated with our affair. He was the most handsome, witty and honest person I had ever met. When we weren't in bed doing all those things I would never write home to 'Mom' about, we were doing all those other things people in love do. I starting jogging with him, a major sacrifice for me since my idea of exercise at the time was opening the car door, and he learned to sit still for an occasional television sitcom, a major sacrifice for him since he felt television had been invented solely for the purpose of airing news shows and documentaries about World War II ... and we danced. We both had a collection of big band music and we'd dance for hours in his apartment. It was almost as good as sex with him.

When we ate out it was usually at one of three places; a local Beefsteak Charlie's, whose main attraction was the unlimited salad bar and where several waiters knew Tom and catered to his little idiosyncrasies, a Lebanese restaurant where he joked and talked about his days in the Middle East, and The Abbey Tavern, an Irish pub where he practiced his Irish brogue and where he could always count on them having a 'pint' ready for 'himself' the moment we entered the door. (I always loved it when he 'talked' Irish).

He always paid with plastic, giving the bill to me to figure out because the lighting was bad or he'd forgotten his glasses, or he'd simply hand his credit card to the waiter, tell them to give themselves a 'decent' tip and sign the slip. He rarely paid for anything with cash and I never saw him write a check.

When he needed cash, he either used the cash machine or asked his banker for help. One of a number of people in his bank would come to his aid. They'd write out the check, show him where to sign, process it and give him the money, all of this amidst a running barrage of jokes, vignettes and much laughter on everyone's part. People smiled when Tom entered the bank.

After we married, The people in the bank voiced their relief that someone was helping him. They had noticed changes in him over the past two years and had increased their level of help for him of their own accord. Initially he had used the "I've forgotten my glasses" routine, but they soon realized it was more than that. They noticed he couldn't follow the lines on the check, his handwriting became illegible and his signature had started to disintegrate. He was so good-natured it was difficult to find reasons not to help. They hoped he was going to be all right.

Judith later told me his writing, although never great, became illegible between 1985 and 1986. He never sent a note, a letter, or a card to me but then I never expected he would. I honestly felt that activity was never a part of his frame of reference anyway. "That's what God invented assistants for", he'd say. Even Judith failed to realize he had lost the ability to read handwriting. I found that out when he started handing me everything he received that wasn't typed to answer for him. He had me playing secretary while he covered up with a barrage of details about the person who'd sent the note. I'd get so engrossed in the stories that I'd neglect to notice he was using me to feed him information he should have been able to read himself.

He insisted on walking everywhere in Manhattan instead of taking cabs or subways. He was certainly aware that his earnings were not what they once were and he felt walking was a way of saving money, besides walking was healthier. I never did figure out how breathing carbon monoxide at curb level was healthier than breathing it on a bus but then I decided it was just another one of his little quirks. The reality however, was that he was losing his ability to remember addresses and phone numbers and figuring cash and tips in his head was becoming increasingly more frustrating for him. As for taking public transportation, his visual problems further complicated matters because he couldn't find the station signs quickly enough to be able to read them.

He showed no lack or loss in his reasoning or verbal abilities, at least as far as I was able to see. He had occasion to help me with a small legal problem in December of 1985 in which he negotiated a resolution to the situation and dictated a letter finalizing the transaction, all to my benefit. I can still hear him during that phone conversation. He had an authority in his voice that was hard to ignore.

I remember wondering where he had been all my life. It was nice having someone there to back me up again. So what if he had his tee shirt on backwards or inside out when we ran. Runners in New York always seemed to function best in rags anyway. Anyone who ran in one of those cute little stretchy coordinated ensembles that are so much in vogue now certainly wasn't a serious runner. I viewed Tom's appearance as just another demonstration of his lack of pretentiousness. He certainly maintained himself impeccably otherwise. His suits, mostly Savile Row, were organized according to season, his shirts according to color and sleeve length and his shoes polished before every wearing. He had an outfit for every occasion from jodhpurs and riding boots to white tie and tails. Who could possibly suspect he wasn't able to maneuver an overhead shirt or sweater properly or that he was misreading the clues that labels and seams offer to determine proper dressing.

In January 1986 he asked me to help him organize his desk. The desk was a hopeless mess of notes, correspondence, tax receipts, bank statements, and Visa slips. His appointment book was a shambles and the address portion was so written over it was impossible to decipher which were the valid addresses and which weren't. We spent two months bringing it all up to date. I typed the whole thing in bold print because of his vision complaints.

His earnings showed approximately four thousand dollars for the year but he explained he had only started working for John Hancock recently and had taken most of the year off. The previous year's tax return was somewhat better but not much. I also noted that his accountant hadn't taken any business loss for him and had charged him an arm and leg for what amounted to a very simple return. I took him to my accountant after figuring out what was declarable income and what wasn't.

I frankly didn't know the difference between an annuity, a CD, a Money Market account, or a retirement fund at the time never having had enough money to concern myself with such luxuries. Tom took the time to explain what it all meant and gave me what amounted to a crash course in investment counseling. Thanks to him I was finally able to understand the complexities of his unanswered correspondence and figure out the status of his standing accounts. I discovered that most of his funds were tied up in his retirement account and his apartment. He had very little coming in on a monthly basis with which to live. He had been living on the eighty thousand dollars he received in a severance award when his contract in the Middle East was broken. Five years had passed since that award was made. It didn't take me long to figure those funds had to be just about gone. They were.

He was in the process of taking Judith's name off their joint accounts now that we planned to marry, and adding mine. It was now apparent to all of us that the apartment they shared was going to be sold sooner or later. As for the apartment, he was extremely vague as to what was his investment and what was Judith's. I was worried about maintaining the apartment and any quality life style if his earnings didn't improve, and I was very concerned about handling a mortgage on my salary alone in order to buy Judith out. He and Judith were listed as co-owners of the apartment so half of that investment was legally hers. I was earning a decent salary by New York standards and could probably have carried a mortgage, but his maintenance charges each month were over six hundred dollars and it seemed beyond my resources. It never occurred to me that he would cash in his retirement fund. Who knew what the future would bring? It was the only cash that existed outside of my earnings. He asked me if I wanted a diamond for our engagement. I declined the offer.

We decided to sell his apartment and live in my mine. I had five rooms with a garage and was paying under three hundred dollars a month. A rent controlled apartment was like gold in New York. Tom had already accustomed himself to the commute from Staten Island to Manhattan every morning and I was only a ten minute drive to work.

The commute to Staten Island involved some organization with regard to which ferry Tom would catch coming home. No matter how we planned it he was always two to three boats behind schedule. We'd agree on a time but he either had a last minute call, or he mislaid his glasses, or he had an errand to run, or he couldn't reach me. He finally agreed to phone me the minute he was ready to leave Manhattan and I'd figure out which boat to aim at.

Having observed his behavior in his own home when it came time to leave for somewhere I could well understand why he was always late. There were times when we were practically out the door and he'd remember something he'd forgotten to do, or something he'd misplaced. The only thing to do was to pitch in and help or he'd obsess about it until whatever it was, was taken care of. We were either very early for appointments depending on how successful I was at circumventing 'Murphy's Law', or very late depending on how successful he was at finding obstacles. One such incident stands out in my memory. It happened while we were on our way to a dinner party.

We had just passed Marble Collegiate Church and were on our way uptown on Fifth Avenue when we observed a couple standing on the corner. The woman was in high heels and was shifting her weight from one foot to the other as if her feet hurt. She was complaining in a foreign language to her companion and seemed to be near tears. Both were staring at a map and shaking their heads. Tom moved away from me and interrupted them, asking if they needed help. Within a few minutes he determined they had just landed at Kennedy, they spoke only Polish, they had missed their only contact in this country and were, for all intents and purposes, unable to afford any hotel in Manhattan. Their friend had mixed up dates and wouldn't be in town until the following day. It was already 7 p.m. and they needed a place to spend the night. Two hours later they were settled in a room at the YMCA, the two of us having helped carry their luggage and Tom had a promise that he'd be called if they missed their contact the following day. We wished them luck, and hugs and kisses later we were finally on our way.

I don't even remember the dinner party ... I do remember the two of us pinching each other and giggling as we walked down the avenue arm in arm. Come to think of it, we were very late. We made a pit stop at the apartment to make love before we actually made it to the party as I recall.

"It must drive you nuts when I do things like this, Beverly."

"I think it will drive me nuts when you stop, Tom."

It was difficult for me to see that behavior as a fault. What did concern me was how easily everything else fell out of his brain once his attention was diverted. Had I not been there the dinner party would have faded into the ozone completely, and friends would have wondered, once more, what had happened to him.

In retrospect, it strikes me that this demonstration of his was simply an example of Tom's ability to focus so completely on a task and his ability to make that task the priority. As long as there were others maintaining the loose ends he was able to do what he did best: see the problem, figure out a solution and provide the means. Someone else was responsible for remembering the other stuff. After he lost his backup people, and until he found me, there were a lot of loose ends floating around in his life.

There was also something else that struck me about this man. He noticed people. In a few seconds he could discern if someone was in trouble and decide whether or not to act, and what's more, how to act. No one was ever invisible to him. He noticed waiters, and doormen, and the person in the change booth on the freeway, and the noticing was not born out of condescension but out of an innate sense of connection with the world around him. He also needed to feel useful. He had been used to feeling useful all his life. He had a lot of spare time to fill now. Reaching out to others was a way to fill that time.

There was a great deal going on in this man, and the puzzle was getting more and more involved. His life was both ordered and in complete disarray at the same time. The biggest problem for me was the difficulty with which I was able to get information to help clear it up.

The letters I had put into neat little stacks hadn't been read and were yet to be filed. The files were re-organized, so that I could find the information he needed, which must have driven Judith nuts because I did it without consulting her. Tom kept telling me she was handling their checking account, she was doing enough and he didn't want her bothered. He never wanted her to be bothered. In fact he seemed to be doing everything he could to keep us apart.

Then there was the driving. In early summer of 1985 we took my car to Westchester to spend the day with Rob Williams, the new minister at Marble. Rob was living there temporarily and Tom thought it would be nice to visit some of the old mansions in the area and finish off the day with a picnic by the Hudson River. Since Tom knew the area well he drove my car.

The roads in that area are very narrow and twisted and there were times when both Rob and myself were quite fearful with Tom behind the wheel. He was either heading into traffic or driving so far to the right that the car actually scraped the bushes and tree branches growing by the shoulder. Several times I yelled at him to pull to the right or left because we were so dangerously close to an accident. Tom denied he was driving poorly, claiming there was something wrong with his glasses. Once we were back on a major highway however, his driving seemed fine. I had noticed nothing unusual about his driving on the way there from New York, although I do remember feeling uneasy while we were still in the city limits.

Since Tom's car was garaged somewhere upstate, we used my car exclusively from that time on. There was no need for a car in New York City because of parking problems and we walked everywhere we went in the city anyway. On Staten Island it was natural for me to do the driving because I knew where everything was and he didn't. He never got behind the wheel again until January 1986 when he drove me home from the hospital after some minor surgery. It was in the evening and he was all over the road. I remembered the driving incident in Westchester of some months earlier. The roads there were very dim due to the density of the trees and overhanging branches. The sunlight gave off a strobe-like effect as it played through the leaves while we drove and I remember thinking it was very distracting. I knew that night blindness was often a factor as people got older and wondered if Tom wasn't experiencing the beginnings of a serious visual loss. I started questioning him about his eyesight and began to encourage him to see a doctor for a thorough exam. He set the appointment himself. The exam resulted in yet another pair of glasses.

We were living together in my apartment by then and the closeness allowed me to notice things I had missed before. Without really knowing it, more and more of my attention was being centered on Tom and my creative energy (if it can be called that) was by that time fully diverted towards him.

There were a number of letters from lawyers. A few from his patent lawyer concerning his claim on patent infringements from his former employer, and several letters from a lawyer in Houston requesting copies of his yearly physical exams. I asked him about the last letter and he told me it was about a shoulder injury he had some years ago. He was seeing an acupuncturist on a regular basis at the time so I didn't think too much of it. I helped him find his medical reports which were very routine and forwarded them. I received a letter back from his lawyer thanking me for the information and expressing relief that someone was helping Tom with his correspondence.

I maintained records of his earnings, his commission checks, his financial statements from his retirement fund, and any other money that was coming in. I was also filing his insurance forms for him since he had neglected to do that for almost a year. The policy he had while he was working with First Investors ended when he changed to John Hancock, and for some reason he neglected to opt for the comprehensive program. The result is that none of his doctors expenses for that year were covered. They amounted to over eight thousand dollars in tests alone.

With all of this rolling around in my head, May arrived and two significant things happened that made me realize that Tom's behavior was more than idiosyncratic.

First, I co-chaired a workshop for the 'Help Line' volunteers at Marble. Help Line is a suicide prevention hot line. The calls they receive range from those in the midst of a suicide attempt to those just trying to find out what to do and where to go for help. Much of the volunteer's time is spent referring callers to other agencies for help. My participation in the workshop was to widen those resources for the volunteers. My main objective was to familiarize them with the workings of my agency, The Office of Vocational Rehabilitation, which is open to all handicapped people of any economic level for evaluation and vocational planning. People in emotional upheaval qualified for our services. I especially wanted to target single parents and battered wives, who were a large group in the call-in category.

During the lunch break, a neuro-psychologist joined me and we talked in great depth about what my agency could offer some of his patients and of some of the interesting things we were beginning to involve ourselves in ... most notably the closed head trauma cases that we were now getting in droves. Since the seat belt and helmet laws were passed in New York, people were surviving what would otherwise have been fatal accidents.

Dr. L.'s specialty was Closed Head Trauma and it was a chance to pick his brain. We spoke about the inadequacy of treatment facilities available to deal with those patients and the peculiar problems so specific to that group. The testing tools and evaluations in use were, for the most part, irrelevant to their needs because they had been standardized on other populations. Their predictive validity was therefore unreliable and the behaviors and learning problems manifested by survivors of closed head trauma didn't fit into the scope of existing programs. One of the interesting observations that developed as a result of tracking the behavior and learning problems this population manifested was the high correlation between the erratic behaviors of the so called inner-city youth and survivors of closed head trauma. We were beginning to recognize that much of what was written off as the result of inertia, poor role models, and the welfare mentality was really the result of battering children. It was an interesting time in my agency. A lot was happening.

For example, we found a person who had been in a coma for weeks might recover with little residual deficits, whereas someone who experienced severe whip lash or a beating was often profoundly affected. Those patients lost their ability to concentrate, to retrieve information, and to integrate new information effectively. There were short term memory lapses, perceptual problems, and poor judgment. Patients experienced mood swings, irritability, depression, confusion, or inappropriate response to a situation.

Depending on what parts of the brain were affected, significant functions that involved sight, hearing, and/or speech might be impaired. The important consideration was that without treatment, which was dependent upon proper diagnosis, the problems would most likely worsen to the extent that the person could then be faced with loss of employment and family support as well as face physical and psychological deterioration. Adding to the difficulty in getting a speedy and appropriate diagnoses, was that symptoms could occur within a short time after the injury or appear months later depending on the support system available to the patient, and how gradually it was withdrawn. The symptoms were vague and complicated. Many neurologists and rehabilitation people were not familiar enough with the nuances and severity of injury possible from a blow to the head without the instance of coma, and pressure was on from insurance companies to prove that victims of such trauma were malingerers who were not severely injured.

What I didn't realize was that I was discussing all the symptoms Tom was manifesting and made no connection because I didn't know the details of that shoulder injury. I, along with those still close to Tom, was also very heavy into denial. I was as guilty of justifying the inconsistencies in Tom's functioning as everyone else had been.

The second thing that triggered a response happened when Arthur Caliandro, Judith, Tom and I found ourselves together at the apartment after a church event. Arthur had stayed behind to talk and we decided it was time to tell him of our marriage plans. During the chatting that went on and some of the reminiscing, Judith made a remark about Tom's terrible driving. It was an off handed comment and by itself nothing much, but bells started going off in my head. I heard a voice in my mind saying ...

... this is a championship trap and skeet marksman. He is one of the most responsible people I have ever met. It doesn't make sense. He's too responsible and too competent to be a lousy driver. Something else is wrong.

That night I was unable to sleep as little by little the bits and pieces started coming together and the picture I was getting was frightening.

* Fright ... a feeling that starts in the pit of the stomach. It begins as a small knot that twists and grows as it increases in size. Tendons and feelers unravel and curl their way up the spine, grinding in through the brain stem leaving you nothing but obsessive thoughts about the worst possible scenarios, as other feelers crawl past the lungs and finally grasp on to the heart squeezing harder and harder until all your life's blood has stopped. *

I started to consider the possibility of stroke, or tumor and began to query Tom about headaches, illness, high fever, dizziness, falls. Nothing ... Tom had been healthy as a horse. He couldn't remember when he'd had a cold. He told me he'd go to bed whenever he didn't feel well and stare at the ceiling until whatever it was got fed up and left. He refused to tolerate illness.

When I began to question him about specifics I discovered he was able to respond in great detail once the proper questions were asked, but if asked anything as general as, "Tell me what you feel is wrong", he was unable to respond because he wasn't able to retrieve the information he needed on his own. When I finally asked him if he had ever been in a car accident, the details of the rear end collision came out.

The afternoon at the Hot Line came to mind and I described some of the behaviors I had noticed over the months in relationship to the possibility that his problems might very well be connected with that accident. To the best of Tom's knowledge, he had noticed no problems prior to the accident and in fact dated all his difficulties from that time. He was very shaken. He knew things just weren't coming as easily as they once had but he had no idea what was happening. A familiar complaint from head trauma victims. What I didn't consider is that it was also a familiar complaint from early stage Alzheimer's and dementia victims. The dance was about to begin.

I told him I wanted him to have a thorough eye exam and this time I was going with him. He gave me the name of a doctor in Philadelphia who had treated him on and off for twenty years. The next day I called Dr. K., spoke with his nurse about what I thought was happening to Tom and set an appointment for the following day. Dr. K. phoned back as soon as his nurse explained why Tom was coming in and we spent over half an hour on the phone while I described Tom's symptoms and my observations. As it turned out, he was already concerned about Tom. He hadn't seen him in two years but he had noticed some problems in his last examination and had told Tom to get a neuro-ophthalmological work up. Tom didn't follow through for a number of reasons, not the least of which was his feelings about wasting money on doctors.

The next day, Dr. K. spent most of the morning with Tom. He noted holes in his left field of vision and he was past pointing, which meant there was a delay between what his eyes saw and when his brain registered the picture. This explained why he'd reach for a door handle several inches away from where it actually was, and why he was picking up my glass instead of his own at dinner. It also accounted for the driving problems. The doctor also felt that his response to directions was impaired. He suggested we see a neurologist because he felt the problem was not with Tom's vision but with how his brain was interpreting what it saw and heard.

We took the train back to New York, and called Arthur Caliandro at Marble to tell him what was going on. We needed the name of a good neurologist and hoped with his contacts we might get a referral. Arthur had been through two by-pass surgeries. His doctors were the best in the city. I reasoned the best had to know who the best were. The doctors my agency dealt with were not suitable, in my opinion.

Arthur phoned me the next morning with the name of a neurologist. He also told me to let him know if we weren't comfortable with that doctor because the man his cardiologist wanted us to see was out of town. Because time was important he felt this man would be a good substitute. I should have waited for the other doctor because Dr. P. turned out to be everything I loath in the medical profession. However, at the time, how was I to know? What seemed to matter was that we were able to get an appointment within the week, which also gave us time to call Tom's lawyer in Houston and advise him we thought there was a lot more going on with Tom's case than a simple shoulder injury.

According to the latest correspondence, Tom's lawyer was due in court that week and Tom wanted the case delayed until he could evaluate just what the cause of his problems really were. The correspondence that had gone on since 1981 in itself pointed to a major problem. Letters were unanswered for weeks at a time and when answered did not always address the issues. As I read through the letters, I could see the mounting frustration with the inadequacy of Tom's responses. It was no wonder that the lawyer expressed relief that Tom was finally getting some assistance. Tom had also given a deposition the previous year which again was undermined by the intricacies of the questions. Thankfully the case wasn't settled and the door was still open to re-evaluate the seriousness of the accident in terms of Tom's present condition.

The next morning I phoned Dr. L. and spent a considerable amount of time discussing Tom. He felt the behavior I was describing was in keeping with a closed head injury but he would have to see Tom and do a comprehensive test battery in order to make a determination or set up any course of treatment. I told him we were having a neurological work-up done and was cautioned about taking the results of that examination in stride. He also encouraged me to get an EEG, an MRI, and a spinal tap to exclude any other possible explanations for Tom's symptoms.

"Other possible explanations for Tom's symptoms."

How ominous those words sounded, how ominous the words that followed sounded; tumor, Alzheimer's Disease, encephalitis, stroke, cancer. It was almost anticlimactic hearing them finally spoken.

There it's been said, it's out in the air, words just spoken. I am not going to lose it at this stage of the game. Let's get those damn tests over as soon as possible, and please Lord, be there with us.

DANCING IN THE DARK

Dancing in the dark
Till the tune ends,
We're dancing in the dark,
And it soon ends.

We're waltzing in the wonder
of why we're here.
Time hurries by and were here
and gone.

Looking for the light
of a new love
To brighten up the night.
I have you love.
And we can face the music together.

Dancing in the dark

words by: Howard Dietz   music by: Arthur Schwartz

CHAPTER FOUR

In the fall of 1988 Tom and I visited his friend Bill Poe and his wife Jewel, in upstate Michigan. Tom had been Bill's boss and it was obvious from a previous meeting in New York three years earlier, that their relationship went much deeper than that of employer, employee. Bill was very affected by the changes in Tom since their last visit together. Tom was now 7 years into his symptoms and into the mid stages of dementia.

Tom's memory and verbal abilities were now obviously impaired. He had more difficulty retrieving words, thoughts and concepts. He was at the stage where he had to complete his comment without interruption or he forgot what he was talking about and questions had to be kept simple with simple choices or his mind just went blank. When those blanks happened I'd observe his eyes glazing over for a second or two before darting around the room to see if anyone had noticed his lapse. He was acutely aware that he was losing it. He couldn't have described what was happening to save his soul but he knew he wasn't anything like he had been a few years earlier. For me, it was the hardest time of his whole illness. There was very little he could still do for himself without help and yet he was still cognizant enough to be able to mourn the losses and feel inadequate at the same time. That he didn't lash out with anger was remarkable, but then he was still trying to rise above it all.

Those of us who witnessed those gaps in conversation would fill in until Tom could find his bearings and then we'd hand the conversation back to him. Filling in the gaps for Tom had become so much a part of my routine that I was almost unaware of how involved it all was. In many ways I had become a combination mind reader and straight man. That evening with Bill was one of those moments when I realized just how much Tom had lost and how much I was compensating for him. So much of my focus was centered on him and making sure he was never left out of anything or made to feel insignificant that I had almost ceased to exist myself.

[In the beginning I filled in a word here and there ... and then I ended his sentences ... and then I fed the story giving him the punch line ... and then we reached the time when it was just me talking while he watched, his only communication being a laugh at the appropriate moment ... and then the eyes began to wander ... and then one day I noticed the laugh was gone.]

At the time of this visit however, we were somewhere between ending sentences and starting his story for him. Tom could still engage in conversation as long as the material covered was old territory. He had ceased to be very interested in the news or recent happenings in the world because his memory just couldn't hold on to new information long enough to use it. He'd respond with the same level of emotion to any event that had recently happened as if he was hearing it for the first time. A news story could be repeated ten times in one day and he'd listen to the details with the same unflinching intent, and then we'd repeat the same conversation about it as many times. However, he could still pull events and information that happened twenty years ago from his memory bank if prompted properly.

Needless to say, it was easier on everyone to keep conversation focused on Tom's world, such as it was. I wrote Bill and his wife before our visit and described Tom's deficits so they'd have some notion of what to expect from him and how to help him over those little humps that got in his way. They were wonderful. Our time together went too quickly. It was the most attention Tom had gotten in a long time and something he really needed. The two of us had become so isolated that both of us were starving for contact with someone else. This was the closest thing we'd had to a social experience since leaving New York. I remember feeling vaguely depressed when the time came to return home. I remember Tom expressing much the same feelings.

The only dark spot in the whole weekend was Tom's constant interrupting of conversation to ask Bill one particular question.

"Is there any sort of work I can do?"

His question was both obsessive in nature and unrealistic. We all knew it. Bill was the first person from his past who understood what work had meant to Tom and who might have helped him find a job. He'd interrupt again and again to ask the same question over and over.

" Is there any sort of work I can do?"

Bill would direct his answer to Tom regardless of how often he was asked to do so. He kept emphasizing how necessary it was for Tom to get it more together before he could possibly return to work, an answer that did not satisfy Tom or put him off in the slightest. Bill noted that Tom's approach was very reminiscent of how he had operated in his prime.

"He was often like a dog on the scent. Once he got an idea in his head he'd keep at it until someone wore down and finally gave him the OK to go ahead. It was rare when he didn't get his way."

I remember nodding in agreement, having already learned about that particular aspect of Tom's personality from first hand experience. Bill laughed when I murmured an adage Tom often used ... "You're talking to Noah about the flood."

Bill finally reached out, after being asked the only question on Tom's mind, yet again. He laid his hand on Tom's and making sure he had Tom's total attention he said ...

"I want you to know this, Tom, there will *always* be a job for you when you're able to go back to work. That is my promise to you. That is something you never have to worry about. Your job right now is to get well and that is where all your energy should be going. Finding a job is never going to be a problem for you. There are too many of us in your debt. We all owe you a lot, Tom, and none of us are going to forget it."

Even Tom seemed to know that this was the final comment. He rarely mentioned work again after that visit.

On a grander level, that question carried much more significance than a simple request for work. It was as if Bill had suddenly been endowed with miraculous powers. All he had to do was tell Tom he could go back to work and the nightmare would end. A job was all Tom needed to prove to everyone he was all right again. Most of all he could prove it to himself. It was a demonstration of how desperately he missed his world and another attempt to avoid the future that was just looming over the horizon. Who could blame him? The future was a vast unknown to both of us, and it was already apparent to me that our lives were moving more and more into the past, a past I was not privy to and of which I desperately needed to learn.

If I could keep the past vivid and real enough we might be able to stave off the future for a while besides, I needed to hear the history as much as Tom did. Tom's behavior in his past was the only link I had with which to gauge the behaviors he was exhibiting now. How could I recognize what was left of the man fading before my eyes today if I didn't know what he had been like yesterday? I was also living all the years we didn't have together and wouldn't have together, vicariously. Thankfully Bill had more than a few stories to fill up the weekend and in spite of the difficulties presented by Tom's deterioration the weekend was filled with laughter. There were also a few tears. In some ways Bill got to say goodbye to Tom. Given the logistics of our lives, we all knew we'd probably never see each other again.

Ironically, Bill's first encounter with Tom ever was over a job interview. He had weathered the initial screening in seeking a spot in Tom's operation and was facing what we refer to in show business as a call back. He had spent the morning talking with various people and was wondering what was next on the agenda when he was informed Tom planned to meet him over lunch. He had heard about Tom but he had never met him. He already knew Tom's reputation through the grapevine and he knew the job hinged on Tom's appraisal of him.

Bill and one of Tom's colleagues were already seated and had ordered a drink when a white-haired gentleman entered the door. The man stopped to shake hands with the Maitre D', joked with him, patted him on the back and stopped to acknowledge a couple of others at various points as he made his way to their table. Bill noted . . .

"He was wearing expensive tailoring, he appeared to be someone very much at ease, someone very confident, and someone very much in charge."

Bill said he wasn't surprised when he stopped at their table and introduced himself as Tom Murphy. After exchanging a few basic amenities Tom turned to Bill and started asking questions. Bill recalled that the questions were very probing in nature and not like anything he had ever experienced before in a job interview. They weren't easy questions to answer. They were multi-layered and seemed to have more to do with conduct and finding out what sort of human being he was than about experience. He said he could easily have fallen into trying to second guess Tom's agenda but he chose to answer as honestly as he could instead. He found himself revealing himself. He had never had an interview quite like that before and has never encountered anything like it since. He realized now that Tom needed to know if he could be trusted. That is what set his staff apart from others, and that is probably what made he and his staff so invincible.

Almost as abruptly as he had entered, Tom left. He shook Bill's hand, leaned over to his colleague at the table, spoke a few words and was gone, working the room as he made his way to the door. Bill said he was then asked to return to the office for a few minutes and was left waiting again while phone calls were made. A few minutes later the gentleman returned shook Bill's hand and told him he was hired and he was to report to Tom his first day at work and Tom would take it from there.

As it turned out, Tom spent days keeping Bill with him and following him around while maintaining a continuous barrage of jokes, banter, light conversation and not so light conversation. Bill wasn't quite sure what his duties were since Tom never specified what his function was going to be. So Bill did what he was told to do and used the time to observe the sort of man Tom was. He watched how he operated, what turned him on, what made him angry, what sparked a particular glint in his eyes and what made them narrow and dark.

One day Tom poked his head in his office and told Bill they were going for a ride. Tom didn't talk much during the ride and Bill noticed that Tom's eyes were both narrow and dark. They drove a couple of hours to a branch office, parked and entered the building with Tom striding ahead and Bill still unaware of the purpose of the trip. Tom entered the Branch Office Manager's office without knocking and stopped so abruptly that Bill nearly crashed into him. The man behind the desk stood up at the interruption looking somewhat surprised. Tom, without any introduction and without any hesitation, spoke in a voice that was clear, controlled in volume, and with an edge that could slice through silk.

> * *Silk, for all of its softness and pliability is the strongest natural fiber known to man. The edge on a Saracen's sword was indeed an edge to fear, for the sharpness of it could cut through silk like butter.* *

He listed a number of things he had discussed with this person concerning his performance, his attitude, and most notably his false sense of security. He pointed out that there had been no discernible change and concluded with ...

"As of this moment, you are fired." ... and looking at his watch, he continued ... " You have thirty minutes to clear your desk and get out of here."

He then turned to Bill ...

"You're now in charge of this office. It's up to you to keep or get rid of whoever isn't pulling their weight and keep me informed."

"And that was how I met Tom Murphy."

It was my impression from Bill, that the regard currently felt between these two men was cultivated and nurtured during those first years of working together. What the jobs were or what the nature of the involvement was in terms of their respective positions and accomplishments is probably not as noteworthy as what actually ensued as a result of the above; good old fashioned loyalty, honesty from both directions, and the healthy utilization of talent.

On June 12, 1986 Tom and I entered the office of Dr. P., hot shot neurologist, publisher of papers, and study in arrogance. The doctor entered the office wearing a white coat, carrying a clip board in one hand and a gold Cross pen in the other. He barely acknowledged our presence and spent several minutes looking over the written material I'd provided. The material included a summary of Tom's work history, educational background, and a chronology of his symptoms dating from 1981 when the accident occurred with a detailed description of that accident.

When he finally looked up he proceeded to address most of his questions to me even though Tom was the patient and even though there was no indication that Tom was unable to speak for himself. Tom had handled the opening introductions with his usual bravado and had introduced me as his fiancee.

Dr. P. asked Tom what date it was. Tom didn't know the exact date. I didn't know the exact date either. Dr. P. looked at me and mouthed the words ...

"He doesn't know what date it is."

I began to feel very defensive for Tom. I also started to experience a vague sense of hostility. Not only did I not know the date but I wondered how many people asked at random on the street could have given the correct date. If Tom had missed the month and year the doctor's response might have meant something but he hadn't.

Dr. P. then repeated three numbers to Tom and told him at some point in the examination he would ask Tom to repeat those numbers backwards to him. Tom got them wrong. So had I for that matter.

Dr. P. spoke to me again.

"He can't remember three numbers backwards."

He said this to me as though Tom wasn't there, and more importantly he said it as though Tom couldn't understand what he was saying. He then took his clip board and gave it to Tom and asked him to draw a picture of a clock.

Tom took the clip board and started to draw. The line was wavered, the circle incomplete, the numbers clustered in the upper right hand area of the clock. The arms of the clock were the same length. The drawing had an almost Daliesque quality about it. Dr. P. looked at me and this time he held the drawing up for me to see while he pointed at it with his gold Cross pen and shook his head. Tom looked at me and I could feel his gaze. I know that I must have registered some reaction on my face because I was familiar with the Bender Gestalt test for brain damage and I couldn't deny that in spite of my early dislike of our doctor, the results of drawing that figure couldn't be dismissed.

The Bender Gestalt was meaningful to me. It was a test all our psychologists used in the clinical assessments they provided for our clients in my agency, and this seemingly boring statistic suddenly took on a life of its own. It was now in black and white. The clinical attitude I had been carrying around once the possibility of brain damage became a possibility for Tom started to crumble. All I could think about was that Tom was in serious trouble.

Dr. P. then asked Tom some simple arithmetic which he did correctly, but with difficulty. He made excuses during this part of the exam protesting that he could do higher math in his head. He couldn't understand why he was having problems with such simple questions. Tom looked at me with such sadness in his eyes. It was heartbreaking. How could so much fear take over our bodies in such a short time? Our eyes held this sadness while the madness continued.

The usual motor tests were conducted and Tom was set up for an MRI (Magnetic Resonance Image) of the brain, and an EEG. The doctor dismissed the possibility that the accident could have contributed to Tom's problems and ostensibly ended any further discussion regarding that accident. I told him I had set up neuro-psychological testing for Tom adding that I wanted to set up cognitive retraining for him. Dr. P. minimized any reason for doing so, stating he doubted it would help but added the testing might be useful in appraising the level of brain damage. Since I knew the MRI and EEG were necessary to rule out other possibilities, I urged Tom to agree to getting them over with. Tom on the other hand was not happy with Dr. P.

[That is an understatement and for the record, 'P' is not the doctor's real initial. I chose 'P' for the word Pedantic. I was torn between that and the initial 'I' for Insensitive, and as I write this the letter 'P' comes back to mind for the word Putz.]

I called the day after the tests and was simply told that Tom passed the MRI and failed the EEG. They gave us an appointment for June 25th almost a two week wait to get the details and ramifications of what those test results meant.

On our way to that appointment Tom checked the date to make sure he had it right this time and asked me the exact name of the hospital because he had also failed that question, and he had been practicing drawing clocks. He was going into battle and from what I observed he was not going to be caught off guard this time.

This time his clock was a completed circle with the numbers fairly well placed. He also got the date right and he managed to get the name of the hospital into his conversation on his own. He didn't get to feel too much on top of everything for long because he was then asked to write something. He printed ...

"Tom Murphy, I live in N U C".

He read the N U C as New York City, and this was noted in my direction with a raised eyebrow from the doctor. I was more than aware that Tom had obvious deficits but the way the examinations were conducted on both occasions I couldn't help but feel this doctor had an agenda and he was not kindly. Tom was a specimen to him and nothing more.

As an aside, I wonder about the validity of asking someone the official name of the hospital as a test of anything. New York is a city of short cuts and abbreviations. Half the people I worked with used shortened names for most of the major medical facilities in the surrounding area as did most of my friends outside of the field. The fact of the matter is I never told Tom the official name of the treatment facility in the first place. All he knew is that we had an appointment and I was going with him. To nit-pick on those issues was to me more than stupid although had other questions been asked it was now obvious that Tom would have had difficulties anyway.

I found that because of the high level of anxiety that accompanied the examination I was unable to answer some of the questions myself but I was also aware of some learning quirks in my history and could never have answered those questions spontaneously. I had a master's degree to prove just how relative they were to learning ability. I also felt that many of Tom's responses were more an indication of his learning quirks than anything else. I'd already begun to suspect that he had always compensated for some dyslexic problems based on information I'd wrestled out of his memory and in watching how he functioned. This was corroborated by Judith and others who had worked closely with him over the years.

His use of the English language could only be described as imaginative. He was noted for never using the expected word opting instead for the descriptive phrase, the somewhat archaic term, the word just slightly off target but in some ways more expressive of the situation. This is often the result of compensating for word finding problems. He said he never seemed to do as well on multiple choice tests as he did on those requiring content. The simpler the test, the more difficult a time he had with it probably because he skimmed the answers too fast. He was also someone who read in blocks, absorbing content but never focusing on individual words.

His handwriting and spelling were always poor, yet his verbal abilities were in the superior range. He always worked with a pocket dictating machine or the phone when not in his office. His notes such as they were, were cryptic and in a form of shorthand that only he and those close to him learned to understand. He never did his own drawings while he was in engineering school always having someone else do them for him. He could visualize the concept and what the finished problem should look like and he could read blue prints as well as anyone, but he couldn't master the physical act of putting it on paper. He in turn did all the math for the projects in his head. He said he was always in trouble with the nuns in his math classes as a child because he could never explain how he got his answers. He'd look at a problem and know the solution but then be unable to do the work at the black board or on paper. He was always being accused of cheating.

Add to this the probability that he was a hyperactive child with all the brilliance and horror associated with that and you have a rather unique individual with a rather unique brain to begin with. The doctor wasn't interested in any of this background.

It was my theory that the accident's initial impact was to sever the compensating mechanisms that had allowed Tom to rise above his deficits. All the little tricks that had become second nature for him were no longer computing in his brain. He was left with all the information floating around and no way to access it.

Our second visit with Dr. P. began with his stating he had Tom's test results. After Tom got past the clock drawing and the other tasks he had been asked to do, the doctor reclined on his examining table and spent the next few minutes leafing through a rather thick book. He wrote a few notes, shuffled through the book some more, and finally raised his head and looked at Tom.

"You passed the MRI and failed the EEG."

"What does that mean?"

"It means your problems aren't caused by psychosis. In other words you aren't imagining your problems. There's no sign of tumor, stroke, or blood clots in your brain nor is there any sign of atrophy. In other words, your MRI is clear, however, your EEG is not."

"What does that mean?"

"It simply means that it isn't normal."

He then told Tom he needed some blood work done and would he step outside to sign the necessary forms for his nurse. For some reason Tom just stood up and walked out of the office without asking why. I suppose it was the quickest way out of our doctor's presence. He later told me he knew the doctor had something else to say and he was not going to say it to him. He figured the only way he'd find out was to let the doctor talk to me.

I felt as though I was watching this in a fog. I was noting the impersonal way in which this evaluation was conducted and I had already decided this man was not going to be around Tom for much longer. If I had learned one thing from all my training and experience it was to flee, not just walk away from a doctor I didn't like or trust.

Dr. P. motioned to me to join him at the examining table after Tom left the room. The book he had been leafing through was open. He pointed to the heading that read Jakob-Creutzfeldt disease and told me in a whisper, to read the paragraph under that heading. All I remember is that the course of this disease ran from three months to two years maximum. It was the only thing I focused on.

"Why are you showing this to me?"

"Because you haven't married him yet and you should know."

"What is that supposed to mean?"

"It's going to get worse" ... I'm going to write out a prescription for an anticonvulsant."

"Why?"

"Because the convulsions are going to start".

[Tom had never had a convulsion at that point. Tom has never had a convulsion at this point.]

"I think we'll just wait on that."

My brain was racing, I was filled with fear and I was grasping for reason. I started to leave his office when I asked . . .

"Why are you telling me this and not him?" (motioning towards the other room where Tom was talking to the nurse). The good doctor stated he didn't think Tom could handle the news.

[So much for twenty years of Elisabeth Kubler-Ross, Bernie Siegel and Norman Cousins ... you inadequate piece of ... (bird lime came to mind).]

I stood up, walked out of the room, put my arm through Tom's and told him we were leaving. Tom had the order for blood work and maintaining as calm an attitude as possible, I led him down the elevator to the lab. While he was punctured, I called a nurse I knew at the hospital and briefly told her what had happened, adding that I couldn't believe it. I asked her to please join us because I was afraid of losing it and I was terribly afraid Tom would pick up on my state of mind before I had time to think it all through.

Before she got off the phone she pointed out that if Tom had that particular disease, given the fact that his symptoms had been going on for five years at that point, and the prognoses for this disease was three months to two years he would have been dead three years before we met. She also added that my general appraisal of Dr. P. was correct. He was considered a pedantic, insensitive, putz by those who worked with him. I decided to cling to this and do my own exploration of this disease before I told Tom anything.

Our friend met us just as Tom came out of the lab where he had been busy charming the ladies. I decided to spend the next day in the medical library in my office going through "The Merk Manual", a volume of medical definitions and diagnosis. My friend pulled Tom's test results off the computer for me, bypassing the need for any further contact with Dr. P., and provided the name of a neuro-ophthalmologist whom she felt would be more appropriate for Tom. Tom's only comment when I told him we were changing doctors, was "Thank God".

["Jakob-Creutzfeldt Disease; spongiform encephalitis, transmitted by brain or eye tissue or other forms of contact (urine) to humans, chimpanzees and monkeys. After many weeks or months, the disease pursues a downhill course ending in death in one to two years. It should be considered if, the dementia progresses rapidly or if myoclonus, extrapyramidal, or cerebellar findings appear."]

Tom had never had a tissue transplant and the monkey issue was out of the question. Tom once said the closest he got to the wildlife in his travels was to look at them from the inside of a Mercedes. I had noticed no discernible change in his behavior from the time I had met him which was a year and a half period at that time so the progress of the condition could hardly be called rapid.

Myoclonus are those little spasms and jerks many of us experience when drifting off to sleep. Under most circumstances they are considered normal. When the spasms become overt and chronic they are symptomatic of many illnesses including Parkinson's Disease and Alzheimer's Disease. I had specifically told Dr. P. I only observed some slight tremors before Tom fell asleep and nothing more.

["Dementia, often the first manifestation of illness. Spinal fluid normal but may harbor infectious agent. C. T. Brain scan may show cerebral or cerebellar atrophy".]

No spinal had been done at that point, and Tom's MRI was clear. The spinal that he ultimately had with another doctor was clear.

["EEG, local or generalized disorganization which progresses to a characteristic pattern of sharp waves and pikes against a slow background or a burst suppression pattern of low voltage activity".]

I had no one to interpret the EEG at that time. The next doctor we saw glossed over that point probably because they were colleagues. The doctor we consulted in Houston later confirmed the EEG did not have the patterns predictable for J/C Disease.

The routine blood and urine studies Dr. P. requested did not include a check for B12 level, nor did he test for metal poisoning which was certainly a consideration given Tom's many years in the mining and oil industry. I subsequently learned both tests are considered routine in possible dementia cases because they are both treatable conditions. Patients who develop an inability to absorb B12 can develop many of the symptoms Tom had manifested to that date, symptoms that can be reversed with injections of B12. The amount of recovery is of course dependent upon how soon the problem is detected.

Before our doctor even had the results from the blood work or a spinal tap in hand he went directly from the most simple possible answer to Tom's problems to one of the most rare obscure diseases on the planet. The only neurological disease more rare than Jakob-Creutzfeldt disease is Kuru, a progressive viral dementia acquired through ritual cannibalism, confined almost entirely to certain tribes in New Guinea. It's a damn good thing Tom never mentioned some of the more obscure places in the world he had worked during that initial evaluation.

At the very least this doctor wasted our time, and his cavalier report was to follow us throughout the time we remained in New York. It interfered with my being able to provide Tom with therapy through programs that wouldn't drain our existing resources, and his 'suspected' diagnosis cast doubt on the feasibility for cognitive retraining. For some practitioners, doubt was enough. It was easy to interpret tests to lean in that direction and it was difficult to totally disregard his report because he was such a prestigious neurologist. The only reason it didn't influence further medical care after our move from New York was simply because Tom outlived the diagnosis. One doctor laughed out loud when he read the report referring to the diagnosis as 'Ole Monkey Brains Disease'. It is so rare a disease that he was incredulous that it even came up as a possibility.

As we walked out of Dr. P.'s office for the last time I determined to take the steps one at a time. Tom had already completed several testing sessions with Dr. L. and a verbal report would be ready within the week. It was of some significance that his final session was on the same day we saw our new neurologist. We left Dr. L.'s office with the knowledge that Tom's level of brain damage was diffuse and severe. There were many pockets of problems for Tom and given the history of his learning process the pattern was not out of keeping with severe damage as a result of a closed head injury. Tom was anxious to begin cognitive retraining and appointments were set for treatment to begin. We weren't in the best of moods when we walked into Dr. N.'s office.

Dr. N. asked why we were changing neurologists. I told him I didn't agree with the diagnosis Dr. P. had thrown at us and I found him to be cold, unreceptive, and arrogant. Tom put it more succinctly. After blinking at Tom's rather colorful description Dr. N. agreed that based on the information at hand it probably was a bit premature to make any definitive diagnoses.

After reviewing Tom's background information and the results of the tests Dr. P. had conducted he ordered some visual tests and set a date for the spinal tap. He then leaned back and told us that it was his impression that Tom was suffering from an undiagnosed form of brain damage, undiagnosed because he doubted that a definitive diagnoses could be reached without a brain biopsy. Because Tom had never been in a coma and because the damage had appeared to be progressive, he doubted the accident was the cause, although it might have precipitated another process. In all probability Tom had some form of viral disease which might have run its course and finished it's damage considering that his dementia had apparently stabilized over the period I had known him. Either that or he had a form of Alzheimer's Disease. In that case, the prognosis was still in the air because there was no way to make any clear predictions as to longevity or process. He encouraged the cognitive re-training we had set up and was hopeful there would be improvement. He wished us both the best and sent us on our way.

We left the office in silence, although both of us had instinctively grabbed for a hand. I don't remember leaving the building. We had walked about three blocks back towards Tom's apartment when Tom stopped.

"You're very upset aren't you."

He always had this way of speaking in terms of statements. All I needed to hear was any word relating to emotion and I started to cry. He put his arm around me, turned me towards him ...

"They're telling me I'm going to die aren't they."

"They're telling us they really don't know what is going on, but the possibility is that you might die somewhere down the pike."

"We're all going to die sometime".

"Yes, But I wasn't planning on your splitting this early in our life together".

"Beverly ... listen to me. I've had one hell of a life and I am not afraid to die, but I want you to understand something. I have been afraid of very little in my life for that matter and fear has never been something that ruled my life. If it's in the cards for me to go now, then so be it, but ... and this is very important ... I am not someone who ever gives up."

We stood there in each other's arms for awhile and I let the tears flow unchecked until I could breath again. He let go of his grip, and forced me to look at him ...

"I can't hold you to a marriage in view of what seems to be happening, so if you want to get out of it, I'll understand."

"Just what do you think I am. I've waited all my life for you. You're the best there is. It's not within my nature to turn tail and split. Like it or not you're stuck with me for the duration, and the only way you're going to get rid of me is to kill me."

We spent the rest of the evening talking. We decided to get married immediately because we felt the two of us united would provide a stronger and more formidable front to what was ahead of us. We believed it was possible to turn things around by the sheer will of our combined natures.

We decided to have a quiet wedding within the next few days. Among other things I had comprehensive insurance coverage through my job and with very expensive treatment looming ahead of us Tom needed all the coverage he could get. We had planned to marry in October and the only reason we delayed that long was to accommodate my family. Had it not been for that reason we'd have already married. He asked me to describe the worst and the best possible scenarios.

"With Alzheimer's you will gradually lose your ability to remember, to take care of yourself, to feed, dress or clean yourself. Your speech will disintegrate as will your ability to identify your friends or family. In the end your brain will forget how to regulate your bodily functions and you will probably die of pneumonia. If your condition has stabilized, as it now appears, it is still doubtful that you will ever be able to work again without assistance. At this time you aren't really functioning at work. Your income, except for your investments is almost non-existent and from what I understand from the neuro-psychologist it might not get appreciably better.

"The chances are the two of us can pull together a company with me running it and you working with the ideas and concepts. If that isn't in the cards and you're unable to work at all, and your condition remains stabilized, you can still live your normal life expectancy out with my supporting you. Whatever investments you have will be set aside for your re-training, your care and your needs. With my salary and provided your situation doesn't worsen, we can live out a very decent life together.

"Given the fact that you know and understand the workings of New York and you haven't a clue as to how to find your way around Staten Island, and given the possibility that your condition may not improve I think we should seriously consider remaining in your place until I can buy Judith out, or we have to make a major move to be near a support system, such as family."

"Do you think it's going to get worse?"

"It hasn't during the time I've known you."

"What if it gets worse?"

"We can only worry about that if it happens. Tom, if I were the one facing this would you run out on me?"

"No."

"Well, I love you."

We talked in a matter of fact manner. I couldn't imagine that Tom would want or expect me to be anything less than open with my feelings or my knowledge. In the course of the evening I told him about Dr. P.'s report and both of us had a laugh at the absurdity of it all. He delighted in telling people from that moment on that one doctor had only given him six months to live and he had already outlived the bastard's time limit. The interpretation was a little convoluted but it was also necessary for Tom to have a focus to rail against, and Dr. P. was so very available and so very deserving of that purpose.

The next day I went to work in Staten Island and Tom went to see Rob Williams, our friend and minister at Marble Collegiate Church. I received a call from Rob after Tom left him. He was very shaken by the news and we talked at length about the possibilities. He also offered that given the sudden nature of the wedding plans that it might be in our best interest to invite everyone, all of the family, his and mine, and give them the opportunity to make it or not make it. He added that Tom agreed this was a good idea and the date had tentatively been set for July 10th. I agreed.

He also added that he and Tom had a long and very emotional talk about the marriage and what I had come to mean to him. Tom's biggest fear was that he wouldn't be able to provide for me the way he had for his family and former wife over the years, and his biggest regret was that he might not have the time to grow old with me. Rob said Tom was adamant about my getting everything of his if he died and he had encouraged Tom to get his affairs in order if that was how he felt. I told Rob I had a hard time thinking about that aspect of everything. Rob encouraged me to respect Tom's wishes and encourage him to take care of business.

"Tom loves you very much, he knows what life might be like for you if he continues to deteriorate and he doesn't want you left without a future."

After the heaving stopped, I told Rob that more than anything else we felt the need to face this together as one.

"I can't believe that God has brought us together just to wrench us apart. I've waited all my life for this man. I can't just walk away from him. I simply can't! There must be a reason for this. I know too much about where we might be headed to be doing this with my eyes closed, and believe me, martyrdom is not in style these days. I think I am the best person for Tom right now and whether anyone can believe this or not, he is the best for me. We decided it is within our power to make the marriage work in spite of the possibilities and whether we have three years or thirty, they're going to be the best years of our lives."

Rob gave me his blessing and made an appointment for us to see him together the following day. I got off the phone, told my boss I didn't feel well and went home. Tom and I spent the rest of the evening phoning family and our closest friends.

On July 4th., Arthur Caliandro called me at home. He was leaving on vacation and he didn't want to leave without speaking to me.

"Do you know what you're getting yourself into?"

"Yes".

"Have you considered that Tom's condition might worsen?"

"Arthur, if Tom and I'd had the joy of being married to each other for 25 years and this thing happened I'd be there for him. I'd be unable to walk away then and I'm unable to walk away now. What am I supposed to do, dump him and run?"

"No. Of course not."

"We made a commitment to each other and that hasn't changed. I'm hoping for a long life with this man but if it's not to be, then the time we have is going to be the best there is, for as long as there is".

Arthur gave us his blessing.

By July 10th. the dress had been bought, friends had taken over the running of the party, the church had been reserved and my entire family and most of Tom's had gathered. Reverend Rob Williams of Marble Collegiate Church and Reverend Jack Groverland, my brother-in-law from the Unity Church of Boulder, Colorado performed the ceremony. We exchanged vows promising among other things, to love each other in sickness and in health, till death us do part.

[And so that no one would mistake our intent to have a marriage filled with love and joy no matter what the future had in store for us, we sent the following marriage announcement to proclaim just that.]

HE and SHE

He's ritualistic in an obvious way.
She acts like a flake in a storm at full play.
While he polishes shoes every morning with care,
She blow dries and combs out her long whispy hair
leaving strands over every cranny and nook.
He grabs for a broom.
Gives her such a look.

As different as couples can possibly seem.
He thinks she's quite swell.
She thinks he's a dream.

He has books that would rival a library room.
She knows all the cartoons on the TV tube.
She'll leave rubbish standing for days in the hall.
He'll leap from his chair cause he's spied a dust ball.
While she sits by herself with a drink in her hand,
He dusts it away.
She watches it land.

More opposite lovers you never might meet.
She thinks he's a riot.
He thinks that she's neat.

He likes sensible lyrics and tunes that will last.
She knows all the old songs and loves things from the past.
He can dance up a storm on the ballroom floor.
She follows his lead, embellishing more as she
hums sentimental tunes in his ear.
They both laugh a lot.
They both sometimes tear.

They're much more alike than you might wish to think.
He likes older broads.
She goes for antiques.

74

CHEEK TO CHEEK

Heaven, I'm in heaven,
And my heart beats so that I can
        hardly speak,
And I seem to find the happiness I seek,
When we're out together dancing cheek to cheek.

Heaven, I'm in heaven
And the cares that hung around me through the
        week
Seem to vanish like a gambler's lucky streak
When we're out together dancing cheek to cheek.

Oh, I'd love to climb a mountain
And to reach the highest peak
But it doesn't thrill me half as much
        as dancing cheek to cheek
Oh I love to go out fishing in a river or a creek
But I don't enjoy it half as much
        as dancing cheek to cheek.

Dance with me, I want my arm about you
The charm about you, will carry me through to ...

Heaven, I'm in heaven
And my heart beats so that I can hardly speak.
And I seem to find the happiness I seek.
When we're out together
        dancing cheek to cheek

words and music by: Irving Berlin

CHAPTER FIVE

THOMAS AND BEVERLY MURPHY
JULY 10, 1986

... and they lived happily ever after!

Happiness by itself, is a fleeting thing and an unsatisfactory goal. It is elusive and unattainable if not experienced with the other extremes of the spectrum. It is a sand painting, intricate in its beauty but momentarily felt as the wind blows it all away. As long as you understand that it cannot last forever, it will be a continuing part of your experience. *

It was during the so called 'Cold War' years. The political climate between Russia and the United States was potentially volatile and the hype from the media and Washington made it difficult to imagine Americans over 'there' helping 'them'. The reality is that needs superseded politics and American technology and talent was as valuable as anyone else's to the Russians. A handful of American business men were in competition for projects in that scene as they were elsewhere in the world. Tom was one of those men.

He had been approached by the Soviets who were aware of his work on the Alaskan Pipeline and asked to come to Moscow to consult with officials involved in the construction of their new proposed gas line. It was his first trip there. He was given rooms in the main hotel in Moscow and access to phones and any other services he needed in order to conduct his business.

He remembered being ushered into his room, a room he described as adequate. He noticed there was a little metal knob situated near the ceiling upon which he decided to hang his coat thinking perhaps it was a listening device. He kicked himself for being paranoid but figured what the hell, why not. He was there without his entourage, it was still unfamiliar territory to him, and there was already an aura of suspicion attached to the whole project because he had been contacted by the CIA prior to his leaving and asked to submit to a 'debriefing' when he returned.

Tom told me he didn't view that as a request but more as an order, an order that was a part of his drill whenever he moved in and out of sensitive areas of the world. He once told me that if the CIA and the KGB based their recommendations on the basis of what they garnered from their 'sources', then our respective countries were in real trouble because it was people like Tom who were more often than not, the so called source.

However, the fact that he also carried security clearance in this country was significant. He explained that as being part of what business in the international scene was all about and it allowed him to travel in areas where others were restricted. He said that regardless of the aura surrounding his activities he was first and foremost in competition with other nations as well as major corporations for business. His explanation made sense considering the level and scope of the oil and mining projects he headed in the Middle East, South East Asia and South America. However, according to his records and the correspondence from various highly placed government officials in the world arena, one thing was certain, Tom was anything but a non player during a period of great change and upheaval in this world.

It was 1978, he was C.E.O. of Tiger Equipment Services, a subsidiary of Flying Tigers International, a company that had evolved out of the famous Flying Tigers of World War II. It was now a transport conglomerate reputed to have been deeply involved in the politics of South East Asia. It was obvious that Tom was part of the government team that toured the Pa Mong Delta and brain stormed what part our government was going to have in the very very rich oil fields there because he had the experience and the ability to contribute effectively in that arena. I also suspect that his activities often had an agenda not readily accessible to the public at large.

It was inconceivable that the Russians were any less aware of his status in the scheme of things in the world than we were of their people. The bottom line is that they needed help in the planning of their pipe line and Tom had the expertise.

His first morning in Moscow, as was his custom no matter where he was in the world, he put on his running suit and at 6 a.m. was out the front door of the hotel and down the street for his customary 45 minute run. The visit was destined to be all work and no fun. He said it was a fairly stark and lonely experience there since the Soviets were still unaccustomed to the wining and dining that generally followed business in the West. Tom added that they learned quickly however.

The second morning of his stay he left the lobby at the usual time and was about three blocks from the hotel when he noticed a large black car following him.

The third morning the same black car was outside waiting, and as he began his run he noticed the car was not only following him but there was now a man in a black coat and hat jogging along a block behind him. Tom ran about two blocks when he stopped, turned around and jogged back towards the man who was obviously out of breath, and who now signaled the car to stop. When Tom got close to him he said ...

"Hello, my name's Tom Murphy, what's yours? By the way, you could kill yourself trying to run in that coat and those shoes in this weather."

The man, who turned out to be a member of the secret police, burst out laughing. He told Tom he wasn't accustomed to doing road work that early in the morning, and it had taken him and his associates a while to figure out what in hell Mr. Murphy was up to running around Moscow at the crack of dawn. They had never seen an American businessman running just for his health before. Tom replied ...

"No, but I'll bet you've seen a few of us run for our lives before." The man laughed.

"Oh, that's only in American movies, Mr. Murphy."

Tom noted that George's English was not only excellent but rich with American idioms, as opposed to British expression. Tom invited George to join him for breakfast the following morning.

The next morning the car wasn't there but George was. During breakfast, George told Tom the maids in the hotel were very upset and had complained to the concierge who had complained to him. It seemed they had to get a step ladder every time they came in to clean Tom's room in order to remove 'the clothing' from the smoke detector device.

Tom noted the relationship between the hotel personnel and his KGB man, and that information about him seemed to flow with the speed of light. Oh well, he thought if they needed to watch they might as well get it first hand and he felt better having George by his side than in a car following him around. He told George he was beginning to get a stiff neck looking over his shoulder all the time and why didn't they just meet every morning instead and figure out where and when to reconnoiter without all the cloak and dagger stuff. George would become a friend, at least in so far as that was possible. If nothing else Tom at least had someone to dine and drink with.

Tom's moral to the story was: "Always, make friends with your KGB agent."

We decided to meet the enemy head on. We decided to live our life together to the fullest. We decided that hope, positive thought and humor were the most important necessities to our survival. We actively asked people to pray for us for strength, for guidance, and for a cure. Judith had Tom's name put on the prayer list at Marble. Friends in Westchester and Boulder included Tom's name in their weekly meditation groups. We received calls from Germany, England, Abu Dhabi, and numerous cities in this country. The friends were rallying and we impressed our needs upon them for as much moral support as they could spare. We read Norman Cousins' book, "Anatomy of an Illness". Someone sent the Simonton tapes and Bernie Siegel's book, "Love, Medicine, and Miracles" to us. We attended workshops with Dr. Siegel and listened to tapes by Dr. Peale on "Positive Thinking". We never missed Arthur's sermons on Sunday or tapes of my brother-in-law Jack's sermons in Boulder.

We read about vitamins, nutrition, and exercise. We used visualization techniques and reasoned that if it was possible to manifest healthy cells where malignant ones once were, then it was possible to manifest healthy brain cells where malfunctioning ones were. Tom, used his engineering to visualize a network repairing itself, I visualized blood pumping life into dried up cells.

We started each morning with a prayer, we ended every evening with a meditation. We had regard for the universe, we loved and respected each other and made a conscious effort to fill our days and nights with as much love, play, and laughter as possible. We were ready!

If all we'd had to concern ourselves with was Tom's illness, every waking hour of our energy and focus would have been filled to capacity. Nothing is ever simple!

My children had adjustments to make. With it becoming apparent that it was in Tom's best interests to live in Manhattan, there was the question of where my younger son was going to reside. He didn't want to move to Yonkers and live with his father which involved changing schools, and he didn't want to live in Manhattan with us. A reasonable solution was reached when my eldest son moved into my apartment on Staten Island so that his brother could continue his schedule without interruptions and live in his own home. I was still working on Staten Island, I'd be able to see them both every day and certainly be there for school needs. They were both welcome to stay in Manhattan with us whenever they wanted and since we were only a few blocks from Madison Square Garden, we were a likely crash place on concert nights. It seemed like a good plan.

Aside from the other problems between Tom and my boys; they smoked, he didn't; they liked their music loud, he needed quiet in order to concentrate when he read; they thought him arrogant and demanding, he saw them as immature; he was, they were; everything was just peachy keen.

Life for my sons had changed very little after the divorce from their father. Their dad and I had tried to maintain continuity in their lives, convoluted as it might have been at times, but one thing was basic; he was their dad and no one else was ever going to be their dad. My former gentleman friend had never involved himself in their lives and since marriage seemed less and less likely between us as the years passed, I didn't encourage it.

They resented Tom's attempts to establish his place in everything and they resented his world. It was everything their world wasn't. His attempts to oil the waters were basically inept because he wasn't able to shift gears quickly anymore. They didn't stop to realize that their world had once been his world. What they saw was a man of privilege getting in their face.

At least the feelings were out in the open. My children couldn't be anything but open, not with the mix of cultures flowing in their genes and the quickness and sarcasm that growing up in New York had brought to their learning process. Most of all they thought I was crazy to marry Tom in the first place knowing he had serious problems. They were very aware that Tom's children and former wife had had everything handed to them in life and it took little effort to see that those perks were not ever going to be a part of my life because of Tom's condition, if anything I would be the one carrying him instead of the other way around. I don't know who they were more angry at, Tom for being less than perfect, or me for taking on what they saw as a senseless burden. I elected to take the benign approach. It was my life and my decision, they'd just have to adjust. If they'd learned any thing from me, it was that adjustment was a part of growing up. Had time been on our side and had Tom been able to hold on longer things might have unfolded differently.

After six months of trying to give both my children and Tom their due, the personalities exploded. I felt my children were trying to force a choice between Tom and them. They had no way of assessing the depth of my relationship with Tom, they were still too young. From their point of view they were just trying to protect me. The end result was that communication broke down between us totally.

When the break happened, Tom urged me to let them be. Our problems went much deeper than just my remarrying and the needs from both sides, my children's and mine, were too deeply embedded in past behaviors to change easily. Distance for a while was probably the best solution. I felt they had the tools to survive and when the time was right for them they'd know how to reach me. Tom offered that they needed time to test themselves and evaluate their place in life. When the time was right for them, and he believed they were very capable of recognizing the priorities in their lives, they'd be back and it would then be on adult terms. The separation lasted almost two years.

They kept in touch with my mother during that period so I knew how they were and they learned over time what was happening to me. Needless to say it was not a happy period for me. I was facing the possibility of my husband's death and dealing with the emotional loss of my sons as well.

[Two years later Tom and I would find ourselves in a holistic treatment center in Phoenix where I started including my sons in my imagery exercises. I'd envision

Tom basking in a pure curative light and watch as that light passed through his body, starting at his head and penetrating downwards until his whole body glowed. I began to include both of my sons in that imagery, placing one on each side of Tom and including them both in the light. Two weeks after I started this exercise my youngest phoned having tracked us down at our motel in Phoenix after calling my mother. The next day I received a letter from his brother. Neither son was living anywhere near the other and both contacts were conciliatory in nature. Independently they both felt the urge to contact me and start the mending process between us all. Those two contacts would evolve to a point where my sons became a mainstay to both Tom and me. And Tom was right, it's been on an adult basis.]

As for Tom's side of the family, his children who were all adults, had a natural curiosity about where I'd come from and what I was all about. I tried to be as open and accommodating as possible and provided as much information to them as I had about Tom's situation. Knowing the potential of Tom's needs if he was actually facing Alzheimer's Disease, I very much needed to be liked by them. We would meet for the first time on the day of the wedding, a meeting I felt went very well considering our marriage announcement had been sudden by anyone's calculation.

Judith was unable to move out of the apartment immediately after the wedding because her new place wasn't available yet. She had expected the October date and our pushing up our marriage to July left her completely in the air. For two months after the wedding all three of us lived together. I was unable to bring any of my things in and set up a home for us and I quietly resented having to live out of a suitcase. We co-existed as best we could but it was very uncomfortable for all of us. It was of great interest to members of the church however and except for those close friends who understood our situation, we were a topic of conversation. That was probably the only real laugh of that whole period. People literally twinkled with curiosity. Little did they know how truly innocuous it all was.

The change of regime from Judith to me was accomplished with efficacy and dispatch. Tom and Judith closed their last existing joint checking account and she provided me with itemized copies of all the accounts they had shared dating back to 1982, so that I'd have as complete a record as possible. She and Tom formalized their respective investments in the co-op which allowed us to continue to live there for another two years. At that time we were to buy Judith out or sell the apartment. Judith would defer her share of the investment during that two year period and I would assume responsibility for the maintenance, insurance, and upkeep of the property for both Tom and her.

I listed Tom as beneficiary on my life insurance policies, provided the medical insurance for him and since he had no income except for interest from a small money market account, I was his sole support. I closed my personal checking account and transferred my remaining funds into our joint account. Tom in turn, named me as beneficiary on his retirement accounts.

What he didn't do was write a will, give me a General Power of Attorney so that I could assume legal control of our marital estate, or sign a Durable Power of Attorney for Health Care so that I could make necessary choices regarding his care, in case he became incapacitated or incompetent. He didn't make a video of his intent regarding my future status in his estate to prove his competency at the time of our marriage, nor did he specify the terms of a living will. Why do those things? We were in love, we were going to beat this thing. Besides, Tom thought a will was pointless because it could always be contested. He insisted that joint tenancy was the only protection for me he could count on. I accepted his judgment and hated dealing with the whole topic anyway. We weren't six months into a life together and the only thing that seemed to loom over us was what he wanted for me when he died. I hated the negative aspects of dealing with the thought of death when I felt the emphasis, the focus, had to be on life. To me, all the talk of beneficiary, wills, survivors was just admitting that death was going to win out. We were very stupid.

I was also dealing with the unarticulated feeling that I was coming into this marriage with less in terms of money and acquisitions than Tom. The combined worth of his share of the apartment and his retirement fund was considerable but none of it was accessible. On the other hand, I was coming into this marriage with a lifetime's accumulation of what were my possessions, my experience writing rehabilitation programs for others, my earning capacity, my intelligence, and my determination. I was prepared to take up the mantle where it had been dropped by Tom. I was determined to not only support him but I was prepared to integrate the best of what was left of Tom with all that was there of my own to offer. Tom made a point of offering our union up as a partnership in the best sense of the word. It's how I viewed our relationship then and it's how I view our relationship now.

When I asked him about his estate and what his wishes were regarding his family and me he replied ...

"I already provided for my children through my divorce settlement and they will inherit that as well as their mother's estate. What I have left is not a whole lot and if there's anything left when I die, it's yours. The arrangement I'm setting up for you is exactly the same arrangement I had with Judith. There is nothing new going on here."

All of that on perpetual hold, we got down to the real challenge. That of getting Tom back. We decided to concentrate on Tom's symptoms and ignore the possible diagnosis laid at our door. My aim was to set up a course of treatment relevant to a classic head trauma case, and since no doctors were really willing to go out on a limb and offer any definitive diagnosis I felt justified with that plan.

We got the detailed results of the testing Tom had done with his neuro-psychologist. Tom's level of deterioration was considerable. As was expected, he looked terrible on paper, but the reality was that he had knowledge and experience from which he could still draw and which was not reflected in testing. So much depended on how the questions were asked.

Standardized testing doesn't allow for such deviations. The results were indicative of brain damage, they were not, however, a definitive picture of his intelligence or his functioning ability. Tom still had pockets of information that surfaced inconsistently, but the fact that the information was still there and accessible belied the IQ scores and performance levels. Simply put, Tom could do things testing said was impossible.

There were also other realities to be discussed. Tom had no earnings coming in and the cost of running the apartment and maintaining any quality of life style was going to put us into debt. I felt that Tom should apply for Social Security Disability Insurance. I also knew that SSDI was not an automatic thing and it could take six months to two years to get approval, more if you didn't know what you were doing. It was important to start the application process soon. He'd then be eligible for Medicare benefits and because of his past earnings would probably be awarded the highest monthly payment possible. The greatest disadvantage was that Tom couldn't continue going to his office. He was working on commission only at the time so his going to the office, in itself, provided no income. His earnings by then actually consisted of friends of his who automatically renewed their IRAs every year. Tom had brought in little new business over the past two years.

Tom had to accept the fact that what was happening at his office was social and not work. This presented the biggest threat of all to Tom's well being. For Tom, life and work were synonymous. It was all he had known his whole life and the prospect of not having a place to go every day could be more damaging to him than facing the disability itself. Furthermore, SSDI would interpret his going to his office as work regardless of whether it generated salary or not and reject his application.

Tom had absolute faith in my interpretation of the situation and once faced with the reality that he only earned fourteen hundred dollars that year, he was able to appreciate the financial bind we were facing. Social Security seemed the only viable choice. He'd find other ways to fill up his time.

When I submitted Tom's application for SSDI, I presented a written case history, a detailed breakdown of his past work experience, his present work experience, and the relationship his disability had directly on his ability to perform those job functions anymore. I knew which medicals were necessary. I also knew what would be involved in appealing any decision against him since I had been involved in pleading cases for clients of mine whose benefits were wrongly discontinued. I tried to set the paper work in such a way as to preclude that event. I knew how slow the process could be and how arbitrary it could seem. I knew that many were eliminated simply because of an inability to understand and communicate in the bureaucratic jargon. Tom's application went in the beginning of August 1986 when he was 5 years into symptoms and entering the mid stages of dementia. He was notified of SSDI status with full benefits six months later.

Tom's vision was so impaired he was considered legally blind. Problems with focusing were manifested because his left field of vision had nearly disappeared from his brain. It was as if a void existed on his left side. If I asked him to move his head to the left, he would gradually pick up what I was pointing to but then immediately lose what was further to the left. This was complicated by the delay that occurred between what he saw and when his brain registered the visual image. As Tom put it ...

"No matter where I am, I ain't."

This would affect his scores dramatically on any test that involved visual interpretation. Paper and pencil tests were impossible for him and therefore the results of those tests were as invalid for him as they would have been for a blind person. They were not a valid interpretation of his intelligence level. You can't possibly imagine the ramifications of such a loss nor can you imagine how it affected every aspect of daily living. While the rest of us lived in a complete visual world, Tom only saw half a room, half a page, half a phone number, half a plate of food, at any given moment. Add to that the loss of numbers from his brain and imagine what making something as simple as a telephone call was like.

He couldn't remember a number long enough to dial it and he couldn't read the number because he only saw half of it. If I called the numbers out to him he could find them one by one on the handset, but even with help it was an arduous task.

In writing down a phone number, he'd write the first three numbers on the right side of the page. The next four numbers would crawl down the margin, sometimes in reverse order, or end up scrawled somewhere beneath the first three. There was also no guarantee that any of the numbers were in proper order because order no longer existed in his brain. His ability to write a legible note was just as impacted. Since there was no way to see what Tom saw through his eyes, there was no way of knowing if what was on the paper looked normal to him.

Since most of the addresses in Manhattan involve little but numbers it was suddenly understandable why he was having such difficulty finding his way around. However, once he got to a new address he could always return unassisted because landmarks were still remembered and recognized. He also retained where his friends lived and worked and since I was going most places with him and observed him finding those destinations without aid of a written address, I knew what was familiar to him and what wasn't.

I was beginning to realize just how battered his thought process was and how inadequate existing evaluations were to measure that thought process or the visual problems now manifested. Given the nature of the clock he had drawn that fateful day in Dr. P's office, I had doubts that Tom's visual world had any real relationship to the world I saw. And yet, he still seemed to be navigating it fairly well, so something was operating somewhere in his brain. I thought if I watched one more practitioner roll their eyes when Tom couldn't remember the date or draw a complete box, I would scream. Tom still had more in his brain than most of those people would accumulate in the rest of their lives. We were trapped in the midst of test scores that couldn't be applied to anything real in his life and faced with practitioners who, for the most part, had no sense of imagination or vision. On the most ignominious of levels, Tom had become the numbers on his test scores.

This was graphically demonstrated one day when Tom decided to meet a friend for lunch after his speech therapy appointment. He was very concerned about running late and must have asked the time several times, which she interpreted as anxiety on his part. He kept asking the time because he couldn't hold the numbers in his head and he didn't want to be late, but that was too simple an explanation. When she discovered his intent to go to his appointment on his own she called me at work. She couldn't understand how I could allow him to go anywhere in New York without a companion. My insisting he was going to be fine was too cavalier for her sensibilities. When Tom became adamant about leaving she wrote a note for him to carry and insisted he take a cab.

Needless to say he did not take the cab and when he caught up with me later in the day, having finished his appointment, he flipped her note at me. He thanked God that she hadn't pinned it to his lapel.

The note read ...

> "MY NAME IS TOM MURPHY. MY WIFE, BEVERLY, CAN BE REACHED AT THE FOLLOWING PHONE # ... IF I GET LOST, I AM GOING TO GRAND CENTRAL STATION."

"Can you imagine? She must think I'm an idiot."

What she didn't know was that getting to Grand Central Station was the easy part. He still had to find the office in the very large office building attached to the station.

If the professional helpers in his life weren't able to figure out that the lights hadn't all gone out at once, how could I expect friends and family to grasp that concept? Tom had severe limitations and he didn't need his life complicated further by others assuming limitations he didn't have. He was still functioning from what had been a normal brain with above normal learning ability. He had a lifetime of experience still floating around in his memory. He wasn't some organism that had just sprung up on the pavement untouched by human hands and limited by an IQ score, at least not yet. I don't think anything angered me more than others underestimating him or dismissing him.

If I felt protective of him I had a right to. He had difficulty expressing himself but he still understood what he was trying to say. He still understood when someone was condescending to him. He could still read body language better than anyone I'd ever met. There were times when things he said sounded out of proportion and on occasion almost silly. I'd watch people stare at each other and laugh as if he was some sort of buffoon. He most certainly noted the looks and the asides, as did I. In some ways I felt the slights more deeply than he did. There were occasions when I left his side long enough to confront those people with why he sounded so peculiar. There where times when Tom explained himself that he had suffered brain damage and he sometimes had trouble talking, and no, he wasn't drunk.

Its one of the problems people face who don't have visible disabilities. People reach out to those in wheelchairs or with canes or obvious deformities. People like Tom need the same understanding and acceptance but the assumption of illness isn't obvious. I can't tell you how many times we've been stopped by strangers, irate that I parked in a handicapped spot, even though Tom qualified for that privilege and the sticker attesting to that privilege was prominently displayed in our car. I can't tell you how many times those same people wish they had kept their mouth shut. I have no pride and they found out what instant Karma is!

The only numbers he remembered were ... his phone number, his address, his birthday, Christmas, New Year's Day, St. Patrick's Day and his social security number. He used his birthday for four digit codes, and St. Patrick's day for three digit codes on combinations and entry into bank accounts. We continued to use the same codes for all our accounts in order to maintain continuity in his life. Those numbers stayed in his memory for another three years and then they too were gone. (He would never remember my birthday, or our anniversary.)

Concepts were still accessible. He knew his money was invested, what interest was, why certain investments were more advantageous than others, when to negotiate a deal, when to withdraw, and when to cut his loss. All of the above was accomplished by him as long as I was able to provide the information he needed to make the decisions. I organized his statements so I could get him the information he requested at any time he asked.

Although it was a much slower process for him, he could still read. How he got any content out of what he was able to see on the printed page was amazing to me. Given his visual problems I have to assume that his peripheral vision was doing most of the work. I'd watch him leaf through the New York Times every day and be convinced he was just going through the motions, but then he'd drop something in conversation later that was almost word for word from the paper and right on target. If asked to read each word in a sentence however he got little if any content. The words just hung in space with no connection. This just supported my theory that Tom had never read individual words one by one anyway. His attention span would not permit him to enjoy anything as long or as complex as a book any longer, one of the great losses he had to deal with. He was now reduced to the New York Times and his trade magazines.

Given the problems with written communication, Social Security wanted to know if he could operate a dictating machine in their continuing attempt to prove he was still capable of work. He was no longer able to handle the sequence of operation on his pocket dictaphone and he was unable to see the buttons. When he demonstrated what he went through to make a phone call, dialing a number the claims examiner gave him, she was almost in tears by the time he finished. And ... he insisted on making that call without help. It took over five minutes for him to do it, but he did do it. That was the last call back he had to face with that agency.

On a more personal note, he could no longer change the channel on the television or find a station on the radio. In fact he couldn't even turn them on or off any more. He couldn't find the knob or figure out whether to push or pull or turn. The remote control was completely out of the question for him.

He'd push his food to the right side of his plate until it was pushed onto the table, whereas the left side of the plate was mostly untouched. I was not only turning his plate for him while he ate but he now allowed me to cut his meat for him. In restaurants he ordered stews and dishes that were already in bite size pieces to avoid the embarrassment of having me help. I'd also clear away all the unnecessary glassware, plates, candles, from the table as soon as we were seated in a restaurant so there'd be less for him to knock over. I began to look for better lit places to sit and we found ourselves frequenting the same restaurants because they became familiar with our routine and cleared the table as we sat down. Most of all, they cut his meat for him in the kitchen. We tried to pretend life was normal. How could any one who watched the two of us in action think for a moment that life for us was anything that marginally approached normal?

I refused to dwell on it. The main thing was to keep Tom focused and functioning. My discipline was to bend the environment to the patient not the other way around. I did for him what I did for countless others on my job ... I adapted.

I did know that the most important things for anyone dealing with brain damage was consistency and structure. Tom had already structured much of his life but I took care to set a schedule that was within his abilities and which would fill up his day while I was at work in Staten Island.

1. He'd read the paper every morning after I went to work.

2. He'd do the grocery shopping and take care of little errands that I couldn't do, thus freeing up more of my time in the evenings.

3. He'd take care of running and cleaning the apartment, something he was used to doing anyway. He liked to cook, he was extremely fastidious about his surroundings, and the apartment was laid out in such a way that it was very easy to maintain.

4. He'd go for cognitive retraining and speech therapy three times a week. This was in hopes of retraining his brain to pick up forgotten functions and to establish new connectors in his brain so that he could once again access information that was still there.

5. I set up a program of practice and study he could do on his own while I was at work. His neuro-psychologist provided paper and pencil exercises and we improvised physical therapy apparatus.

Tom was to complete four of the programs each day. With me not there to supervise, he quickly lost interest and each day the pages were fewer and fewer. The pages were also less and less complete. Other programs I set up were met with a similar response and I realized after a few weeks of trying to force the issue, that he was not gaining anything back. It was an exceedingly frustrating experience for him and he finally refused to do them anymore. Tom found it very difficult to see value in placing colored marbles in little triangles, or in circling letters, or in any of the other paper and pencil tasks that he was given. He was unable to translate those activities into anything meaningful in his life, anything that translated into 'work' and so he was totally unable to motivate himself. I had visions of Tom meandering around the apartment with nothing to do, no one to talk to, and the isolation only worsening with time.

I decided to relieve the pressure I was forcing on him, not that I had a choice. The deficits were there, they couldn't be ignored, I'd find a way to adapt some more.

1. I programmed the telephone so that all he had to do was punch a single digit to get my office, Judith, or Tommy (the maintenance man in our building). I posted those three numbers on the wall in large print.

2. We bought a white phone, one that was easy to see and find, and I put the black one in storage. It also had large numbers which were easier for him to see.

3. I set the answering machine to record after one ring on incoming calls, and glued a large yellow circle on the manual record button so that he could record his outgoing calls. I asked all our friends to remind him about the record

button if there was information they needed or appointments to set. It was amazing but he still somehow managed to get through to the people he wanted to talk to. I always reviewed the tape when I got home. This eliminated the need for him to take notes or remember appointments. It also eliminated missed dinner engagements and guests showing up unexpectedly.

4. We played a lot of Trivial Pursuit. I used the question cards to jog his memory and encouraged him to give as much detail in his answers as possible. I found that the questions often triggered stories about his life and his travels. He was a great raconteur and I learned the details of his stories so much so, that I was able to use them as a measure of his ability to speak. The day arrived when I realized the richness that had been so much a part of those stories was deteriorating. We stopped the exercise shortly after because it was now pointing out his deficits and it was no longer fun.

5. I went to my Area Director and asked for a transfer to our Manhattan office so I could be close to Tom in case of an emergency. Tom had locked himself out of the apartment on two separate occasions and one day I returned home to find the faucet running and the gas stove on. Thankfully he had remembered to strike the flint and the stove was lit. I had the pilot light permanently lit that day in spite of his protests.

Obviously he was now less attentive to what was going on around him. I had just married the man of my dreams and I was now in the position of having to explain that life for us was less than perfect. I had to give the details of our life that were necessary to impress upon my boss how essential that transfer was. It was not an easy thing for me to do, but there really wasn't a choice.

November 1986, the transfer was granted. This was no easy feat. Transfers were generally impossible because of budget cutbacks and personnel shortages. Fortunately, someone retired from a critical assignment and more fortunately, it was an assignment I was not only suited to but an assignment I desired. The obvious reasons aside, I believe my boss did what amounted to hand springs to get the transfer, and I will be ever grateful to him for his prayers and his effort. Things were beginning to fall into place.

My office was now a five minute walk from my home. We'd have breakfast together every morning, he'd walk me to work and go on to mass at St. Thomas Aquinas which was just up the street from my office. He'd go home, read the paper, phone me three or four times and at 11:45 his watch alarm would go off and he'd meet me for lunch. We'd have lunch together, slip into St. Thomas for a short prayer and he'd walk me back to the office.

He discovered a world of discount shopping which I introduced him to in our area, a world of hard milled soap for 39 cents a bar and end-lots for everything from snow shovels to underwear. He'd hang around the discount stores, do some errands, phone me three or four times and meet me after work. We'd run four miles every night, have dinner, watch the news, do a meditation, make love, and go to sleep.

[There is something to be said for structure. Never under-estimate the value of structure.]

Then there was the day he phoned me and asked me to meet him at home for lunch. I arrived to have him answer the door wearing nothing but his French regimental beret, a sword around his hips, and a grin on his face. He struck a pose and said ...

"Well, what do you think?"

"I see you've found something else to fill up your day Tom."

As I recall the incident, we never made it out of the foyer. Mother told me there would be days like this ... well not my mother ... but someone's mother.

[The only thing missing was 'a ring of rosies in his hair', but then ... that could always be arranged.]

OUR LOVE IS HERE TO STAY

It's very clear..
Our love is here to stay
Not for a year ...
But ever and a day.

The radio, and the telephone
and the movies that we know
May be passing fancies
and in time they go ...

But, oh, my, dear ...
Our love is here to stay
Together we're ...
Going a long, long, way

In time the Rockies may tumble,
Gibraltar, may crumble,
They're only made of clay
  but,
Our love is here..to..stay

words by: Ira Gershwin   *music by: George Gershwin*

CHAPTER SIX

After Tom had had his 'way' with me that very sunny summer afternoon, I asked what had possessed him. The whole experience had been one of surprise and unrestrained giddiness. He had spilled something on his shirt and in trying to change it was unable to get the clean shirt on. Rather than get all bent out of shape he said "screw it", and took everything else off. He'd stood there a moment stark naked wondering what to do next when he decided to call me. He figured he might as well take advantage of the moment, turn it into a happening instead of the disaster it seemed to be, and most of all avoid asking for help again. Besides, he was bored and he missed me. I had been out of his sight for almost three hours.

The soiled shirt was found in the laundry. The clean shirt was found with one of the sleeves inside out hanging on the corner of the bed. He was unable to figure out how to pull the sleeve back through to the right side. I could just imagine the frustration of his trying to get that shirt on, turning round and round while he groped for the elusive other sleeve, finally tangled up in the whole mess. I might have just ripped the thing into shreds had it been me. After finally giving up on getting it on, Tom had apparently tossed it in the air leaving it to float and land wherever it pleased. The rest of his clothes were laid neatly on the bed. Getting out of clothing was not the problem. It was getting them on.

Shirts were only a part of the problem. He also couldn't get his trousers on without my handing them to him in exactly the way needed to put them on. He could no longer handle the closing on his trousers nor could he get his belt through the loops. His ability to tie his tie involved several attempts. If he just let his body remember the motions and he finished the act without thinking about it he sometimes got it tied. It was done in a flurry of motion and with a tinge of madness. He knew if he didn't do it on the first try he wouldn't be able to do it at all. However even when he managed to complete it the thin end was usually longer than the fat end of the tie and his going out in public like that was really quite unthinkable for him. Tying it before hand so that all he had to do was slip it over his head didn't work either because he couldn't maneuver the shirt collar over the tie without help.

He couldn't attach the zipper on his down jacket anymore, nor could he manage the velcro strips I sewed on as a replacement for the zipper. I finally gave the coat to the homeless because Tom had it all cock-eyed and crooked every time he put it on. (So much for velcro as a solution.) He could put on his socks and his shoes but I had to hand him his shoes one by one or they went on the wrong feet. The shoes were now slip on shoes and his socks often ended up with the heel on his ankle. I had to tie his running shoes for him.

In order to get that sword around his waist, he had to improvise a series of steps that was quite intricate for him at the time. He had to place and step up on a chair in order to remove one of the Civil War swords hung over his wine cellar. He had to find a belt to hold it on his hips. He had to weave that belt through the hilt of the sword and tie that belt around his hips. The French Regimental beret was an afterthought and easily plucked off the hat rack in the foyer, an added touch of whimsy I couldn't help but notice. He knew how much I loved that hat on him. There is something to be said for tenacity, motivation and a profound sense of the silly.

Going anywhere with Tom those days meant always knowing where everything that wasn't attached to his body was. Anything could be laid down at any time or mistakenly thought to have been put in a pocket, when it had fallen on the street behind him or off his lap as he got out of a car. I learned to keep one eye ahead and one eye focused behind him and when I failed to do so something was invariably lost. I was beginning to feel like the 'Keeper of the Flame'. I felt as though I looked like a pack rat scurrying around, constantly gathering stuff.

In the face of all of this I still tried to believe the changes I saw weren't changes but my increasing awareness of his existing deficits. I also believed that the inactivity that was now a part of his life was adding to his problems and might also be reason for what I saw as continuing deterioration. Denial is a remarkable thing. I grasped on to anything that explained what was happening to him. However, looking back on those days, deep down I knew he was losing ground. No matter how I tried to compensate for him or rationalize what was happening the losses continued and each one was to be permanently branded on my brain.

I would remember and recall in minute detail the day he could no longer tie his tie, the first day he walked into the living room with his shoes on the wrong feet, the first day he lifted the telephone receiver upside down and couldn't figure where the voice was coming from. The hardest part was the expression on his face when those things happened. I came to refer to those events as *the little deaths*. *Little deaths* that were mourned completely in their own right when they happened and *little deaths* we faced together until Tom was blissfully let loose of his awareness of those passings. I wasn't as lucky as he, I got to see it all. What he had been and how he must feel took over me at times sometimes leaving little room for my own feelings. I was the one who got to watch and mourn the loss of every nuance, of every motion, of every task that allowed him to function independently on the most basic of levels and the final event, death, wasn't even in the picture yet.

How or why we didn't exist solely on rage during that time is remarkable. How could we not be angry at what was happening? What kept both of us going? I think we were both too busy getting through each day to think about it too much. I discovered that our life existed as a series of plateaus. We'd go along for a period of time and then notice something else was lost. Both of us grieved those losses in our own way, but we were also trying to shelter the other. We were so busy trying to boost each other up that we didn't have much time to feel what was happening. And since we were nearly always in each other's presence there wasn't much opportunity to let it all hang out elsewhere. And ... Tom refused to let it take over his life. He was as determined as I to look forward to a positive future. We were going to beat this thing and wallowing in depression was not part of the plan. However, as much as we verbalized our hopes there were still those moments when reality took over. There were times when Tom voiced his feelings of helplessness and rage over his illness and his fears about ruining my life as well.

"You're being cheated Beverly. Life with me should have been something else. Why are you still here? Why don't you just leave and get on with your life? I'm nothing but a burden."

"I love you, Tom. You said it yourself ... life has no guarantees. In spite of everything I'm still happier with you than without you, so I guess you're stuck with me."

He'd ask, I'd respond, we'd fall into each other's arms and we'd get on with life. "A jug of wine and thou" ... it was what most couples prayed for and we had it. We also had a lot of sex.

---

25 September 1990
Tokyo, Japan

Dear Beverly,

Your letter of 5 September was waiting for me when I returned home from Europe four days ago. I am sorry that Tom has started to slip. It must be very sad for yourself, let us hope that Tom is at peace with himself. Tom obviously has been extremely fortunate to have someone like yourself to take care of him under the present unfortunate circumstances. Even this, though, if I may be allowed to say it, is typical of Tom. He possessed the perpetual ability to fall on his feet no matter what.

I met Tom for the first time in May `1968. He was in London and was searching for a supplier of a big special container handling crane. He visited an exhibition where there were such firms with stands. He stopped at the stand of the firm I worked for. A colleague telephoned me to say that an American wanted to buy a big crane and if we were interested, he could be contacted at the Hilton Hotel.

This was the first experience for me to try to find Tom in a hotel room. I was to discover that Tom was a night owl and the only time you could be sure of finding him was around seven in the morning which was hardly the time an Englishman would dare phone someone. Tom, I was to find out, needed less sleep than most. He could and did survive on six hours, perhaps less a day. He had the ability though to take cat naps. In the middle of a meeting in his office, in a car with others around him, he would close his eyes and take forty winks. How he could do this with all the disturbance and noise around him remains a mystery but somehow he could switch off, sometimes to the annoyance of others because he was refreshed and they were not.

Later Tom was to become my boss. As a result I became almost as peripatetic as himself. He would think nothing of flying to London for a day nor would he think it strange to ask someone else to do the same. Once, when I was based in Singapore he suggested we meet in London, once there he said; "Let us go to L.A. and talk to the Chairman". So three of us flew to L.A. for a day with my having to return to London and then back to the Far East.

Shortly after one such whirlwind tour (I had been back in my Korean apartment for a few hours only) he phoned at 1 a.m., my time, and inquired if I could go to Anchorage the next day. I had to point out that for me it was already the next day! But, to Anchorage I went. I think in those days I was in a plane every third day but so was Tom as he was never at the same location for more than a day or two.

Despite Tom's wanderings, you could always find him. He would leave word where he was or was expected to be. When he was not on a plane he would be on the phone. He could use the phone to good effect and did not like to be in a position where he could not reach out for a handset. He did not like to wait at airports. If he had five minutes he would spend six of those phoning someone. Tom would expect a plane to wait for him and at times they would, though once at La Guardia we were denied boarding even though there were 3 minutes till official departure time. This at least gave him an excuse for his usual banter. There was another flight by the same airline within 30 minutes but this was not relevant to Tom!

'Once met, never forgotten', certainly applies to Tom. Not everyone liked Tom, some perhaps were jealous of his salesmanship, others might have found him rather exhausting to be with but most were charmed and amused by him. This would be true for those who saw him regularly including those working for him.

In London, the Hilton was his home. He kept a case full of clothes there permanently. All of the staff knew him ranging from the telephone operators to the doormen. One of the doormen, Jack, to this day asks me whenever I see him; "How is Mr. Murphy", and is genuinely sorry about Tom's present condition. It must be some ten years since he has seen him.

Tom retained a handful of relatively close friends upon whom he could rely, they remained friends even if there was no business between him and them. Tom needed friends but would not admit it to others, perhaps not to himself. He was not a man to be by himself. It was therefore an unpleasant shock for those who had known him for many years to see his health deteriorate and for him to cease being the 'Old Tom'. For this reason when we meet we remember him as he was.

Best wishes
John Dobson

Six months after our marriage I noticed Tom slurring some of his words and he was beginning to repeat himself. The cognitive retraining sessions with his neuro-psychologist were becoming strained. Tom had made initial progress in his sessions but the progress wasn't fast enough to suit him. He had already refused to do any of his homework unless I stood over him and I began to feel he expected me to somehow make him better. We went head to head on this issue with little discernible change in his attitude. He bitterly resented what he called busy work when what he wanted to do was go back to work.

His therapist encouraged me to find a comprehensive program for him that included cognitive retraining, speech, physical, vocational and psychological therapy and one that relieved me of the teacher status in his life. He felt my trying to do it all wasn't healthy for either of us. The problem is that while such programs were available for head trauma victims their cost was considerable. It was cash that wasn't available to us and insurance was not interested in cognitive retraining for Tom, given his medical report from Dr. P.

I went to my agency and asked if there was anything they could do in terms of evaluations and treatment. The bottom line was feasibility for employment. Unless there was a level of employment which could be realistically set for Tom, training was going to be denied. Helping him maintain independence within his home would qualify. They agreed to do the evaluations.

This man who was capable of flying on a minute's notice to Abu Dhabi, and then to London, and then to Anchorage and then to Houston and then ... went into a panic about finding his way from 29th Street and Broadway, to 33rd Street and 6th Avenue, four and a half blocks. We practiced over the weekend because I was still working in Staten Island and unable to accompany him. I received a call from the supervisor who had been handed his case, after his interview. She literally gushed about Tom.

"Beverly ... I can see why you fell in love with him ... he is so charming and so handsome and so sweet."

She then outlined her proposal for a comprehensive evaluation at the Rusk Institute at New York University Medical Center, one of the most prestigious rehabilitation centers in the world. Dates were set and I asked for the time off to go with him.

When Tom completed the occupational part of the evaluation the therapist came out into the hall where I was waiting ...

"He told me that he runs by himself everyday". This was said with a hint of sarcasm in her voice.

"He does".

"He can't".

"What do you mean he can't?"

"His vision is so impaired it can't be safe".

"He not only runs by himself, he also runs with me. He leads the way, we run evenings and daytime, through traffic and past pedestrians. I've observed no problems with his movement throughout such traffic and in fact he has pulled me out of the way of cars on a number of occasions. The problem is in his following me. He can't keep me in his view and I am constantly losing him in stores and on the street if I get more than a few feet in front of him. As long as he doesn't have to find a particular object or person, his peripheral vision takes over and he compensates and navigates rather well on his own."

"The testing says he can't do that. His perception is too impaired."

"I'm telling you, he can". (change of subject)

"He also tells me that he does the shopping and cooks dinner every night".

"He does most of the daily grocery shopping and as often as we eat in, he has cooked his fair share of the meals. Why?"

"He can't do simple math. How can he count change?"

"He gives the checker the money, and they give him his change. He doesn't expect to be cheated and he never is."

"How does he cook?"

"How does anyone cook? He makes stews, chili, baked beans, and turkey ... his favorite dishes, all from scratch. His vegetables might be chopped up a little funny but they're still eatable."

"According to the testing he doesn't know which task to do first."

"Maybe the problem is in the questions. Maybe what you need is a hands on test of his abilities. I've been trying to explain to you people that he does more than testing will show. There's a gap in his brain that impedes his response to direction. He can, for example button his shirts himself but if you tell him to button his shirt now, he won't be able to complete that task."

She went back into the room where Tom was waiting and asked him to unbutton his shirt. He became very anxious and his hands started to flutter. He managed to get two buttons undone before making excuses for himself. It was all very humiliating.

During the two months that it took Rusk to compile all the results and make an appointment to see us, we flew to Boulder Colorado and went skiing for two weeks ... something else they said Tom could no longer do.

The final results reflected previous tests and reports. As an aside, once the ball is rolling there is virtually no way to stop it. Whatever appears in a report will be regurgitated and spit out endlessly whether it is correct or not. What is of more interest is that much of the wording the reports reflected was based solely on information I had given them in the first place. I could have made up Tom's first report, and every word on that piece of paper would have been taken as gospel. Most practitioners don't have the time or the inclination to be original and if what they see before them makes a modicum of sense it's incorporated as fact.

As proof positive, Tom had not been tested for speech earlier so there was no base measure by which to compare. Speech therapy was recommended. He had not been tested for occupational therapy earlier, occupational therapy was recommended. The results of the neuro-psychiatric evaluation reflected the previous reports, including Dr. P's, and were very negative. Vocational training was not recommended. This translated into no sponsorship by my agency.

["Formal intellectual assessment reveals that Mr. Murphy's overall intellectual functioning has significantly deteriorated. His long-term fund of factual information remains within the average range for his age, but is significantly compromised in comparison to estimated premorbid abilities in the superior range. Concentration has deteriorated to the extent that Mr. Murphy is unable to reverse the order of even two spoken numerical digits."]

I just loved that last line. Dr. P. strikes again. I'm not denying that Tom was in profound trouble but you have to consider just how stupid that two number backwards thing really was. Dr. P. only asked Tom to remember and repeat three numbers backwards the previous year, which he couldn't do. How could anyone assume that he could remember two numbers. For all I knew Tom couldn't remember one number backwards. The whole concept of numbers was gone.

["On the Booklet Categories Test, a measure of visual-spatial reasoning which is highly sensitive to overall organic dysfunction, Mr. Murphy made almost twice as many errors as he had made on July 18, 1986 (when he already scored in the impaired range)."]

We subsequently found out that Rusk had used a longer version of the test which had twice as many questions as the test given the previous year, ergo twice as many errors. When I pointed the above out to the psychologist she became very annoyed with me and told me I was obviously very shaken by my husband's illness and my defensiveness was understandable. I walked away before I was brought up on assault charges. It was apparent to me that Dr. P.'s report was influential in leading them to seek the worse possible interpretation of the test results. I could have kicked myself for even giving them a copy of the report in the first place but by then his name was forever tied up with Tom's MRI report.

The doctor who handed us the final written results of the testing and who was supposed to go over those results with us, told us to make an appointment with the Millhauser Alzheimer Clinic for a definitive diagnoses and supportive therapy and walked out of his office leaving us there alone. When he didn't come back I went to find him. I was told he had other commitments but we could use his phone if we liked. I had a husband in shock, not to mention my own state of mind, I had to go home with him facing yet another death sentence and the doctor was unavailable to discuss the results. Are there words to express my feelings?

"What in hell would I want to use his phone for?"

"I'm sorry, but the doctor won't be back and I don't appreciate your attitude. You may leave if you wish or you may stay in his office for a while if you need the time."

[Time for what ... time to slash our wrists?]

"No, we'll be leaving and I want copies of the testing."

"I'm sorry, you'll have to get those from your vocational counselor at O.V.R. (Office of Vocational Rehabilitation)."

"I am sorry, but I am an O.V.R. counselor and you will give me a copy of those results right now. Legally you have no right to withhold that information from us. I know it and you know it, so let's just save us both a real bother and make copies right now. I am not leaving until I have them in my hands

"I'll have to speak with your agency about this."

"You do that, and while you're at it tell the doctor I want to speak to him also."

I went back into the office where Tom was waiting with the copies of the test results in my purse and no further contact with Rusk in my future plans.

"What in hell is happening? Where did the doctor go?"

"I think he's in hiding."

"Hiding? What in hell is wrong with him?"

"More I think than is wrong with you Tom. Let's get out of here."

"How do these guys function?"

"Beats me."

Rethinking that entire exchange with the staff I realize now how angry I was. We were being told that even hope was going to be denied us and no one seemed to have a clue as to how to help us deal with any of it. The doctors and the staff seemed annoyed that I would question a diagnosis that probably seemed obvious to them. I knew by then that Alzheimer's Disease meant there was no treatment, no cure, no prognosis, no parameters or pattern to the illness, and no sense of longevity. I had some vague idea of how all that might translate into care needs but not a clue as to the emotional toll I was facing. We were expected to leave quietly and go home and die. Why would I want to accept what they had to say to us? Why would either of us want to accept such a verdict? Why wouldn't we be angry and upset?.

I phoned Tom's neuro-psychologist when we got home. Dr. L. came over to our apartment and went over the results with us. He asked Tom how he felt about it all considering we were now dealing with the possibility of the dreaded "A" word. Tom responded after a long pause ...

"Well, I'll tell you one thing, it certainly dampened my ardor".

"See what I mean about his language Beverly? Who would normally use such a word as 'ardor'? Tom, you're something else."

Tom and I made love after he left our apartment. We were making love a lot those days. For us both it was a base from which we drew strength and cleared our minds. It put everything into perspective and defined what was really important in all of this. Us! We were important! It was a unique form of meditation that united our minds and our bodies. Oh, who am I trying to impress? It was the best fun either of us had ever had and at least one thing Tom could still do as well as before the nightmare started. We indulged ourselves to the point of gorging almost as if we were trying to build some sort of retirement account from which we could draw the memories later. We didn't know that when the time came, the time when physically making love was no longer possible, we would move into another level of closeness that made the physical act no longer necessary. As Tom's memories of those days faded, mine didn't. I can say with a glow in my heart and a touch of whimsy in my voice, that we had one heck of a time while it lasted.

On a more practical note, my office started scheduling me for every training program, workshop and seminar available on Closed Head Trauma, Alzheimer's Disease, Dementia, long term planning for the terminally ill, and anything else that could be applied to my situation. I was able to view all this with a somewhat detached clinical eye, taking the information I might need someday and divorcing myself from any feeling about what 'someday' might really mean. I was doing all right until the program on Alzheimer's, and the video switched from filmed studies of a Naval Captain at the height of his career to six years later showing the same man in the final stages of the disease. I remember standing up very abruptly, slamming my folder shut, feeling my throat closing, feeling tears welling in my eyes and almost shouting out loud as I slammed my chair away from behind me ...

"That's it ... I'm outta here". (So much for clinical demeanor.)

I was told that with a closed head trauma injury, Tom would gradually get better not worse. Literature exists that does not always support this.

I was told that if he had Alzheimer's, no matter what was done in the form of treatment or therapy he would not improve but steadily worsen. I checked off Tom's functioning on the chart I received that delineated the various stages of the disease. One thing was clear, once someone reached the last stage of the disease there was little that would remain functioning from the first stages. Tom had checks in all the categories including the last stage. He didn't seem to fit the pattern for Alzheimer's.

Wanting to prove Tom's illness was anything but Alzheimer's, I approached a speech therapist who was covered by my insurance and asked her to set up an evaluation for him. She was enthusiastic about working with him until she read Dr. P's report. She got as far as his diagnosis and stated that unless she had a definitive diagnoses of Closed Head Trauma she didn't feel she could justify training. She had difficulty looking in my eyes as she spoke. She tried to hug me as I prepared to leave her office. I was trying to figure out why she thought a 'moment' was called for or why she assumed I wanted or needed one from her, as I headed for the subway already plotting my next form of attack.

I approached another speech therapist and presented myself as Tom's private rehabilitation specialist instead of his wife. I sent her a formal referral letter on my letterhead. I included the speech evaluation from Rusk and none of the other medicals. He was set up for therapy almost immediately and the therapist was covered by our insurance.

Tom again made initial progress but the program was short term and it would be another six months before other training could be set up. Like it or not we were tied to insurance to pay for it. We tried to keep up the program on our own but without a formal setting and other people to talk to his speech began to slip again.

In the meantime, Tom was becoming more and more isolated. He was also becoming more irritable, more opinionated, more demanding, and more obstinate. I wrote the behavior off for what it was: frustration, loneliness, lack of focus, and boredom. His ability to communicate was also deteriorating. He wasn't listening to what others had to say. He'd break in while someone else was speaking and dominate the conversation whether he was on the topic or not. He'd be introduced to someone and it was as if he not only didn't see that person, but he only heard bits and pieces of what was being said. I noticed his brain was now playing tricks with his hearing as well as his sight. He began to drive people away.

At the same time I was trying to mobilize people we knew at Church to make efforts to phone him during the week. He desperately needed to maintain contact with the outside world. I tried to set up a lunch schedule with friends so that he could count on at least once or twice a week with someone other than me. Like it or not, I was fast becoming the only one in his life. Except for those lunches, church and an occasional dinner date, I was it.

Everyone was interested in helping, the problem was in finding the time. A few tried for a while but the reality was that everyone had a life and fitting Tom into it wasn't easy. How do you look forward to spending time with someone who is losing their ability to handle conversation? How do you face the horror that is happening to your friend knowing it had been totally unexpected in his life while knowing it could therefore be just as unexpected in your life? It was the ultimate test of friendship. It was so much easier to just pray for him, not that we didn't appreciate the prayers.

Tom told me of a friend at Marble who had suffered for several years with cancer. She was deeply loved by the people who knew her, including Tom. Tom could hardly speak of her without tears forming in his eyes. She fought the valiant battle for years doing everything she could to fight the disease. When she finally realized the battle was lost, she met with her friends at the church and talked to them about her disease, her fight, her desires, and her fears. She spoke to them about her death and how she had resolved the inevitability of her death. She spoke of her desire to remain in her apartment as long as possible. What she needed most was to be amongst her things and her friends. She asked her friends to help her. She needed volunteers to help her with the everyday chores she could no longer do by herself. She needed company as much as she needed help. People set up a schedule on a weekly basis. At the appointed time, that person would show up at her door and provide the function he or she volunteered for.

Tom gave his time as did numbers of others from Marble. He told me it was a painful thing to watch this vibrant human being deteriorate. Through it all she remained articulate in her thought process and was able to help a number of people deal with their own fears about death because of her insight and empathy for them, and her acute awareness of her own mortality. It was a profound experience for all of those who were with her during those last weeks. The people who involved themselves shared a sense of oneness with each other and carried that experience with them after she died.

The point of this is that in spite of the physical shock of her illness, the difference between the response she received from people as compared to the response Tom was facing revolved around her ability to express herself and to still reach out to others with compassion and insight. Tom's needs were just as great but he looked the picture of health. He was robust and agile and strong. He had always had a dominant personality and there was no expectation that would change in the slightest now. If anything his personality had become more so. His behavior made it very difficult for people to want to be around him.

> *Do you want to know what happens when the ability to communicate erodes? You are avoided like the plague, that's what happens. Who has the patience to help you maintain your train of thought? Who has the patience to ask the right questions that help you finish a sentence? Who has the patience to allow you to be larger than life in your proclamations because your judgment and ability to discern the nuances of polite conversation have eroded? Who? And even though your behavior at best, has always been on your terms, who wishes to tolerate it's being even more so now that you have no perks whatsoever to offer and all you have is your naked self... in need? Who?* *

If I allowed anger to surface at all during that period it was always directed towards those who didn't rise to the occasion. I suppose it could be characterized as displacement, but much of it was a legitimate response to our being and feeling abandoned. It was the first realization of how alone we were in all of this, and how alone I was. I had become his nurse, his therapist, his cook, his valet, his secretary, his companion, his priest, his friend ... his lover, all this and a full time job as well. Wife seemed to get lost somewhere in all the above.

I remember a brunch with friends in the spring of 1987. Tom was being his usual take-over self and had probably hogged the spotlight a tad too long. He was telling his favorite rendition of the six month death sentence he'd received from Dr. P. for the umpteenth time and how he planned to outlive The So and So, when a member of the group who some months earlier had been the recipient of Tom's rather heated views on politics, turned to me ...

"You must have been really disappointed when he didn't die".

[... and Merry Christmas to you too!]

And then there was the woman who approached me one Sunday and said ... "I really had some questions about why you married

Tom, but I see how you take care of him. You really must love him."

I guess it never occurred to me that people might question my motivation for marrying Tom. That was an eye opener.

I don't know what I expected from the people around us during that time. I don't know what I expected from family for that matter. I do know I wanted them all to jump on our bandwagon with understanding and support and unquestioned reverence for the challenge we were facing. I was not prepared for the reality checks that were constantly thrown in our faces. The reality is that our particular bandwagon was not anyone's idea of a place to spend time. Those who hung in there with us weren't friends anymore, they were saints. Those who fled were just human. I found myself constantly stepping back and forcing myself to let go of anger aimed at emptiness. How can you be angry at people who aren't capable to begin with? The answer to that question was a long time coming. Years. What finally got me past all of those expectations was the acknowledgment that Tom and I were each other's best friend. We made the decision to face this thing together and our reasons were valid ones for us. Why should I need or expect more from anyone else? The problem is, of course, I did.

In February of 1987, seven months after our marriage, we flew to Houston to see Tom's lawyers about the accident case which was finally showing activity. Tom saw a head trauma expert there who agreed with me that the initial cause of the problems Tom was now experiencing was most likely the accident. He agreed that Tom did not fit the pattern for Alzheimer's Disease and would most likely be dead if he had Jakob-Creutzfeldt Disease, adding that only a brain biopsy could determine a true diagnosis. He added that there really wasn't as much of a pattern to Alzheimer's Disease as I had assumed but agreed that Tom's scattered pattern was still unusual. The doctor told me about the work they were doing in that area of the country in terms of rehabilitation and seemed aware of the resistance we were getting to treatment in New York. He encouraged us to consider relocating. His rational was that since we couldn't get a definitive diagnosis it made sense to consider treatment for the head trauma Tom had received. If he improved we'd still have a future, if he didn't we'd have at least tried.

We planned to spend a day or two with his family before returning to New York. There was no denying Tom had changed radically since they last saw him. Seeing him only periodically meant they had no chance to ease into the changes that his illness manifested and even on good days Tom was a handful. I needed time to explain Tom's behaviors to them and that was not going to happen as long as Tom was physically present. It was still impossible to be candid with him standing by and I constantly found myself altering what I wanted to say about his illness in order to save Tom the humiliation of hearing the truth. This placed me in the awkward position of boosting him up in front of others while giving the impression that life was easier than it actually was, all to save Tom's feelings.

The evening we planned with the family took on the aura of a farce. The goal was to keep Tom occupied long enough with part of the family so that I could sneak off to another room and talk candidly with other members. However, Tom's need to have me in his sight was far superior to anything the family could counter with. Their distractions never worked for more than a few minutes and the reconnoitering resulted in no one getting the full story intact. Tom, of course, sensed we were all talking about him and there was no way that he wasn't going to be a part of those discussions. As fast as I deposited him in one room he was on my heels as I entered another.

[To those outside our very small loop, and this included anyone who had occasion to watch Tom and me together, the remark that surfaced most frequently was about Tom's obvious devotion to me. It was more than devotion, it was dependence. However, his dependence on me had nothing to do with my need to hover and control, even though it might have appeared that way. It had to do with my being the person he trusted most and his only remaining link to the world. He would not let me out of his sight. The reality was that I was the one who felt controlled even though Tom was the one doing all the complaining, and the hovering that was going on was as much from Tom's direction as it was from mine. How can you not hover when impending disaster is lurking around the corner the moment you let your guard down? We had entered into a conspiracy of silence in our attempts to cover up the full extent of what was happening to Tom. We were both increasingly isolated from the rest of the world and increasingly protective of each other at the same time. If those feelings of isolation were contributing to my feelings of entrapment in Tom's dilemma, they certainly contributed to Tom's problems and therefore his functioning, all of which reflected on and impacted me.

We needed a great deal from the people who entered our lives at that time. We didn't know exactly what was going on with Tom but I realized by then the best we could hope for was that his situation would stabilize. I was unable to even hope it would improve and if there were prayers floating around they were that it wouldn't worsen.

Tom and I both needed emotional support and he needed people to spend time with him. While I still had my job, Tom had nothing, and he desperately needed to feel useful. Most of all, he needed to be loved. His constant presence was stifling at times. We'd been married less than a year and except for my hours at work, I hadn't had a moment to myself. I really needed an hour or two away once in a while for my own sanity and I needed a support system. I felt the only port in this storm had to be his family. I looked to them to fill a bottomless void in our lives without ever really asking them if they were interested in taking the plunge with us. It never occurred to me to ask. I did, however, make assumptions that life would improve if we moved.]

* *The greatest enemies facing loved ones dealing with Alzheimer's Disease and other related dementias are stress, fear, depression, anxiety, and grief, all of which conspire to overwhelm whatever abilities still exist for that person in the early course of the illness. The struggle to maintain thought and function while dealing with confusion and grief is unique. It is now fairly common knowledge among the scientific community, the medical community, and the lay community, that if an Alzheimer's person can be maintained in a supportive environment relieved of stress, they will continue to function at their optimum level of ability, keeping in mind that the optimum level of ability is always at a lower level than it was prior to the onset of the disease and a level that will continue to deteriorate no matter how that environment is maintained.* *

My attempts to maintain Tom's environment placed both of us in situations neither of us would have dreamed of just a few short months earlier. And our *'conspiracy of silence'* only added an aura of craziness to our actions. For example, going to the bathroom had become a two person act within six months of our marriage and we were constantly playing hide and seek with who ever we were visiting or dining with in order to cover up. Among other things, Tom's aim wasn't as good as it once was. His sense of touch was also impaired and he was having trouble maneuvering his zipper. He had trouble finding the tab and once the tab was found he'd have to rely on rote body memory to close it because he couldn't make his mind follow through. Once he got it moving he'd flip it up and down a couple of times hoping it was closed when he stopped. The problem was that he often left it in the down position. He didn't want to face anyone with his fly unzipped and I was overtly conscious of what a mess could be made with his misguided aim. We therefore spent a great deal of time slipping away to bathrooms on the premise that there were some things no one needed to know just yet. In the beginning we actually thought the pretense worked and that it mattered. In retrospect I wonder if any of the gymnastics were worth the effort.

On top of the physical problems his illness presented there were the verbal problems. His biggest concern about leaving New York was whether or not he'd be able to get a job elsewhere. He had contacts in New York. He knew no one in Houston who mattered in his life any more except for family. He asked the question which was always on his mind, several times over that night, a question for which no one had an honest answer. I couldn't tell him the real answer to that question without sending him into a tail spin, and there was no way his family was going to be able to be any more straightforward that I. And so we sat there nodding and smiling and assuring him as he asked more than once ...

"What kind of work can I do?"

I was exhausted trying to maintain some aura of normalcy in front of his family and Tom wasn't helping much. I did manage to get questions in about housing and we spent much of the next day looking at property with hopes of finding something we could afford. We returned to New York with the intention of moving to Houston.

We had no idea what the co-op in New York would bring in terms of money and we had no idea what the accident case would settle for, if anything. We had no idea what was ahead of us on any level. Tom had spent his entire life embracing the future and for once in my life I was going to put aside fear. I informed my office I'd be leaving by the end of the year thereby taking my vested time towards my retirement, but setting myself up for a pension far below what it might have been had I been able to finish my work career with that job. We put the apartment on the market and we informed our friends and relatives we had decided to make the move to Houston.

The adrenaline that resulted from this decision gave Tom a new boost. He was happier, his speech seemed to improve, his demeanor improved. He now had a goal. Something to look forward to. As his demeanor improved so did my outlook. I was taking him home to his family. I felt great!

IT HAD TO BE YOU

It had to be you
It had to be you
I wandered around and finally found
somebody who

Could make me be true
Could make me feel blue
And even be glad, just to be sad
Thinking of you

Some others I've seen
Might never be mean
Might never be cross or try to be boss
But they wouldn't do
For nobody else gave me a thrill
With all your faults, dear I love you still

It had to be you
Wonderful you
It had to be you

words by: Gus Khan   *music by: Isham Jones*

CHAPTER SEVEN

When I was fourteen years old, the conductor of the Syracuse Symphony Orchestra phoned my mother and asked if he could come over to talk to me. He arrived carrying a reel to reel tape of what he planned to be the final number in a concert he was putting together. It was a medley from 'My Fair Lady', by Lerner and Lowe, and its playing time was approximately twenty three minutes. The concert was to be held at Lincoln Auditorium, the largest concert hall in Syracuse, and he wondered if I could choreograph a routine for my sisters and me to perform to that arrangement.

My sisters and I had been performing professionally in person and on radio and television for years. He had seen our work countless times. I didn't even relate to the thought that I was only fourteen years old. It seemed a perfectly normal request to me in spite of never having attempted such a project before.

I lived and breathed the entire experience. The ideas poured through my head. I remember waking one night having worked out a part of the routine in my dream. In the dark, in my bare feet and still in my nightgown, I went through the steps in order to imprint the movement on my brain so I'd remember it the next morning.

My mother rented a tape player for me and we hooked it up in our basement where my sisters and I practiced. In a space that measured 12' x 15', I choreographed a dance that filled a stage measuring 20' x 50'. We would only have two rehearsals with the orchestra the morning of the concert which left us with just a few hours to make necessary changes. The dance also involved a complex series of costume changes. We'd whirl off stage at the end of one song in the medley and re-appear seconds later in a complete change of costume. The thought occurred to us that the costume changes might get as much applause as the dance itself. They did.

The final number in the routine was "I Could Have Danced All Night". It consisted of non stop high flying leaps, acrobatics, spins, and kicks that lasted the entire length of that number and covered the entire stage. There was one point where Norma and I actually threw our youngest sister Sandy into the air catching her just before she flew off the stage.

When the performance was finished we were so out of breath from the physical strength it took to complete the routine that we could barely come on stage for our bows. The conductor had flowers for us and we made several bows before we were signaled to leave the stage ... however, the applause continued. We were still gasping for air when the conductor came back stage and asked if we could do it again. My sisters and I nodded at my mother who scooped up our costumes and ran behind stage to set up the changes while the conductor announced that since we didn't have an encore we'd repeat the entire performance.

The second time around went even better than the first. The kicks were higher, the leaps wider, the acrobatics done with more abandon. We were functioning on adrenaline only because I don't remember any of us being able to breath anymore. We might have been a little wild eyed, but it was the most exciting and exhilarating experience of my young life. I have experienced other highs in my lifetime but I don't think anything will quite reach that one.

People have asked me how I was able to deal with Tom's illness and all that transpired as our marriage unfolded. It seems that I have been blessed with an abnormal amount of stamina.

Had Tom stabilized during our first year of marriage as we had hoped, we could have lived the rest of our lives together with a fairly normal existence. I'd have continued working and supporting our daily needs and the money Tom had left would have covered the little perks that make life fun. However, by the time our first year of marriage had passed there was no longer any doubt that things were getting worse.

I was now more and more fearful of leaving Tom alone and his dependence on me had increased. He could still function as long as he had help, but on his own he was quite defenseless. There was very little he could do on his own for enjoyment. He was never one for 'hobbies' and the only sports he truly enjoyed were skiing and skeet both of which involved skills that were fast deteriorating. His ability to maintain even superficial contact with other people on his own was mangled because of misinterpreted cues and his inability to remember anything long enough to keep even cursory conversation going. His ability to fill up his time productively was also eroding.

His only source of new information was the newspaper and television. However, his ability to read was now greatly impaired and books were totally out of the question because his attention span had shrunk. Television was a new and previously disdained necessity in his life that was totally inaccessible if I wasn't there to put it on and change the channels for him.

He'd ritualistically pore through the New York Times every day. There'd be a rattling of paper that went on for an hour or more and shards and pages all over the apartment by the time he finished. He'd hand me torn pieces from the want ads when he was finished and I'd dutifully send his resumes out as he requested. I say dutifully, because he stood over me to make sure I did just that. It was very difficult to just 'yes' Tom. He had a sixth sense that honed in when anyone tried to put him off, and he was still able to recognize malarkey when he heard it. It was interesting that the jobs he found were within his former abilities. I knew, even if he didn't, that there were not going to be any jobs for Tom unless there was a miracle and the miracle we had in mind didn't seem to be in the making.

Remarkably, he still managed to glean information out of the news, but the information was terribly convoluted when he tried to relate it verbally. With help and proper questioning he could still get to the root of what he wanted to say. I realized that somehow it was all clearer in his brain but accessing it was arduous. For people who didn't have the time or patience the assumption that he was completely out of his mind was unfortunately helped along by what appeared to be bizarre notions he sometimes nurtured. He'd concoct elaborate details to support those notions and he was as adept at arguing his point as he had always been, but he made little sense. What triggered the notion was often based in fact, but his brain was now playing all sorts of tricks on him and the information that went in was not always computed correctly.

One occasion comes to mind. There was a woman in the congregation at Marble whom Tom treated very suspiciously whenever he saw her. She had been a part of the brunch group as long as I knew her so I wasn't paying much attention when he first started seeking her out on Sundays. I realized after a few weeks that he was always turning the conversation towards Reagan whenever he was around her pulling her into rather heated political discussion. It was as if he was trying to bait her in some way. Tom loved political controversy so at first I didn't think much of it.

However, one day he whispered to me that I should be very careful about what I said in front of her because she had the President's ear. It took me weeks before I figured out he thought she was Maureen Reagan. She did in fact resemble her slightly and who knows what she had said to him in passing that connected those particular dots in his head. He wouldn't let go of that notion no matter what I said to him or how I explained it. Fortunately, with me running interference from that time on I doubt that she had a clue as to what was going on. At least I hope not.

Sometimes I was able to get through to him, sometimes I wasn't. It all depended on how his brain was acting that moment. I was beginning to wonder if it was worth explaining anything to him anymore but then his understanding was complete when I did get through even if it only lasted for a few minutes. Realizing that he could no longer grasp the nuances of what was happening also made him feel more useless and embarrassed. It was a no win situation. He once murmured after one such encounter with an acquaintance that he must sound like a buffoon.

"No wonder people laugh at me. I must be the biggest bore in the world."

I was so acutely aware of his needs for human contact that I found myself filling his hours as much as possible with me. Outside of work, I went nowhere without him, and even at work he was still the dominant force in my life. Once a week I was at my official station, a place where he could neither accompany me or call me, six hours when he was completely on his own. The rest of the week was either spent together or within reach of a phone.

Duties required that I visit facilities twice a week to touch base with my clients and confer with their therapists. Unbeknownst to my office, Tom accompanied me on those visits. He'd wait in the reception room with his newspaper while I interviewed my clients and then he'd accompany me to my next appointment. I tried to keep my meetings under a half hour which was Tom's limit and which was still in the realm of professional involvement. Longer than that and he began to worry and ask for me. It worked out well until the day he went into a panic about my being longer than expected. My meeting was interrupted by the head of the agency who wanted to know why I had left a patient alone in the waiting room.

Leaving him alone at home wasn't better. His time was spent in a quasi state of crises phoning the only number he could now manage to dial. He hit the white button on his handset which direct dialed my desk. If I was in conference or with a client or out of the office, my secretary who knew of Tom's growing problems handled his calls. She became adept at helping him through the crises which most often related to his missing keys or wallet or glasses. Sometimes she just chatted with him. Oftentimes she was left on the hook while he went to search for his missing items. Knowing the phone off the hook meant there was no way for him to contact me in an emergency and no way for me to contact him she was then faced with tracking me down to advise me of the situation. I received more than one harried call from her. I'd run home, put the phone back on the hook and run back to work while she covered my back.

His calls were legion in number. Its a wonder I got any work done at all. The constant interruptions couldn't continue unnoticed by others and the time was fast approaching when I'd either have to quit or hire someone to stay with him. We couldn't afford to hire anyone and Tom rejected that possibility anyway. He put it simply ...

"I don't need a baby-sitter."

Put into those words, along with the tone of voice he used and the posture he assumed, I knew he'd make the life of anyone I dared bring in an absolute misery. At least, that is what I convinced myself. I also convinced myself there was no point in putting him with strangers as long as there was even a glimmer of recognition of me. There would be time for strangers later on.

However, what had started out as an altruistic attempt to help Tom fill his time productively was fast translating into increased isolation for the both of us. And it was all so subtle. It was all so complete. I didn't even realize how it was sucking me into the belief that I was the only one who could do it, a belief validated because I was the only one there to do it. I was the only person Tom had to talk to, and the flip side is that he was the only one I had to talk to. Except for church on Sunday, and the occasional visit from friends, the only other major social activity either of us had were the conversations with the waiters in our most frequented restaurants.

It didn't take a rocket scientist to figure eating out was probably our greatest expense. We spent an inordinate amount of money on eating out. The truth was, we were eating out two and three times a day before we even left New York. The truth also was, that the need for human contact was the reason and it was to fill my need as much as Tom's. How much time can two people spend together with no one else to talk to, without going bats? And given the amount of work involved in everyday conversation with him, any break with another human being was a necessary break.

We entered restaurants the way most people anticipate a trip to Europe and we milked the opportunity as much as two people could. We were every waiter's favorite couple and all it took was eye contact and being friendly. Waiters and staff are so accustomed to being treated as non people that acknowledgment is hardly ever disregarded. Those who got to know us didn't need to be asked twice to cut Tom's meat in the kitchen or make sure we got the quiet well lit table, and it was more than nice to have them and the managers stop by to chat, which they did once we became regulars. Because the conversations were short and predictable, Tom was able to maintain an aura of normalcy and I was able to fill in the gaps with some degree of panache. On that level his natural skill in cocktail party conversation was still functioning, nothing too deep, simple short statements, a laugh in the appropriate place and eye contact. It was the ideal milieu for what was left of his conversational skills and his ability to read body language. I also add, that once strangers were made aware that Tom's behaviors were the result of illness, most extended themselves happily for us, otherwise, they assumed he was either drunk or crazy and avoided us entirely or on occasion snickered in our direction.

I remember the Abby Tavern in Manhattan with particular affection. We'd often stop in there after our evening run, or for lunch, and our church brunch group gathered there every Sunday. On Sunday, since I walked faster than Tom, I often arrived with part of the group ahead of Tom, who liked to take a slower pace and talk as he walked. I remember with such warmth, the shout from the bartender as I'd walk in the door ...

"Where's himself? ... and will he be wanting his pint when he arrives?"

And I would answer ...

"Himself is just a block away and you'd better have his pint on the table or he's sure to be in a dither." And we'd all laugh with great ceremony and Tom would always get a proper greeting from Sean, the day manager, as he walked through the door with the rest of the group. There was an element of make believe to the whole tableau, but it made our day.

I hear other caregivers of Alzheimer's loved ones, now that I've become involved as an active participant in the support group system, describing the effects of what is now referred to as *"shadowing"*.   Shadowing is the constant presence of the Alzheimer's person. It is the first major change in behavior and the first major harbinger of the realities to come. Books mention that it happens, but no one really explains why it happens. I have come to equate it with the phenomena every mother experiences as her baby reaches toddlerhood.

I remember spending entire days working about the house with my first born son seemingly oblivious to my presence. I remember calling to him, talking to him, with little if any acknowledgment on his part to the point of wondering if he was hard of hearing, but let the phone ring, or a neighbor stop by to share a cup of coffee, or the maintenance man arrive to talk about a repair notice and this child would suddenly discover I not only existed but he needed my undivided attention in ways that transcended anything Dr. Spock could explain. It was activity just short of clinging to my leg and yanking on my skirt. Of course, I realized there was more going on than a need for attention, on some subliminal level, that other human being was a threat to his autonomy, his ownership of me, his life line in a sense.

I thought about my son as I faced the early years of my marriage to Tom and the development of that behavior in him. Sundays after brunch Tom and I'd go home with the Times, he'd sit on one end of the sofa and I on the other. He'd shred his portion of the paper while I did the crossword puzzle. We didn't even have to talk. Hours of activity with only occasional words passing between us and then the phone would ring. I'd spring to answer it, and he'd be in my steps before I'd even walked out of them.

Dr. John Townsend in his book *Hiding From Love*, talks about the fundamental human need that I suspect prompted this behavior. He describes this psychological need as "Emotional Object Constancy." In a mature person's condition, acquisition of emotional object constancy results in "... a state of feeling connected even when one is alone ... the result of responding to many experiences of constant reassurance by a primary caregiver." The child, who is by necessity attached to its mother, experiences a profound sense of loss when that mother's attention is diverted. Attachment, or "bondedness" however, is the crucial element of the child's development as a spiritual and emotional being, a being who learns to relate to the needs of others when his most vulnerable self is sufficiently assured of love.

The difference between my child and Tom, is that my child would move forward and out of the clinging phase of that necessary life experience into a more secure and self sufficient connection with me and the world around him, whereas Tom would pass backwards into yet another stage of infancy and dependency on the only person he could truly trust to care for him. I now know his sense of security was being bombarded with fears and awareness of losses, and I was his only constant. I was as important to his sense of himself as air and food and water. And if he had been asked about this, I doubt he could have expressed any of it in words, although he did do just that a couple years later under circumstances that allowed him to spontaneously relate those fears.

As for my being *"shadowed"*, or Tom's quest for an 'Object of Emotional Constancy', there wasn't a phone call I made or received at home without him standing right on top of me adding his commentary to what he gleaned from my end of the conversation, often becoming very irate when I didn't inject his comments into my conversation. There was no way to talk candidly with anyone about what he was going through or what I was going through. I was trying to keep a low profile at work so I couldn't talk there. Friends and my family had to read between the lines. The constant presence was unnerving. It gave the song, "Me and My Shadow", new meaning. There were times when I was so strung out by his constant presence that I just shrieked at him to leave me alone for a few minutes. One phone conversation in particular hangs in my memory. I put my hand over the receiver and just barked ...

"For God's sake Tom, will you put a lid on it, I'm trying to talk to my mother."

"Oh, I'm sorry. What are you talking about?"

"Tom, I'll tell you when I get off the phone. I can't handle two conversations at once."

"How much longer are you going to be."

"How do I know how long I'm going to be, I'm talking to my mother, it's long distance, I'll be off when I'm off."

I took a deep breath and tried a diversionary tactic.

" Why don't you pour us both a glass of wine. I'll be in the living room in a few minutes and we can take a break together."

The diversionary tactic sometimes worked in getting him off one subject ... but he always found another.

"Want to ... screw around?" Wiggling his finger in the air as he asked the question, the words spoken with a combination of seduction and deviltry, his eyes motioning towards the living room, the shrug of his shoulder adding just the right pizzazz to the picture, totally forgetting that I was still on the phone with my mother ...

"No Mom, he's not talking to you, he's talking to me. Never mind what he said. Let me get him into the other room. Maybe we can actually have a conversation then. Hold on I'll just be a minute."

I took a deep breath in an attempt to lower my anxiety level and rested the receiver on the desk.

"Tom honey, why don't you go get the wine. I'll be with you in five minutes."

I said that as gently as possible while walking him into the kitchen. It was a tactic I'd often used with clients who were unwilling to leave my office when their time was up. It worked with them because once they were deposited on to an elevator they were out of my life. With Tom it meant, he simply followed me back to where ever I was headed.

"I love you, Beverly."

I heard the words as I walked back to finish my phone call not realizing he was directly behind me.

"I love you too, Tom."

... picking up the phone as I spoke those words.

"Yes, Mom! I'm back."

... looking up to see Tom standing there again.

"... no Mom, I am not drinking too much."

Tom was difficult enough to handle sober. I can't imagine what dealing with him with a hangover might have been like. It only took one bout with a migraine to realize Tom's needs weren't going to go away because I didn't feel well.

If life was unique when we were alone it wasn't any easier in the presence of others. Every visit held the potential for trouble. I had to be constantly vigilant about his feelings, his needs, his lapses, and any time I let my guard down and indulged in my own needs for contact I was very quickly brought back to Tom's reality. If conversation excluded him for even a moment he became petulant and often very critical of me. If he was able to recognize any one thing quickly anymore, it was feeling left out.

I didn't realize it yet, but I had already given my life over to Tom's needs. I was existing on a detached plane that allowed me to function, think, and plan, but which allowed little if any room for me. We existed as Tom, and we existed as us, but I-by-myself was hardly there anymore. Perhaps he knew it instinctively before I even had a notion of what was going on but he made it very clear that it was obviously my responsibility to get him through the demise of his thinking process. It would be years before I reclaimed myself.

The only thing that got me through this period is that I knew his intent wasn't to blame me or take his frustrations out on me although that's what was happening. I already knew there was little to be achieved from behavior modification or talking things out, not that I didn't try. Telling him of the pressures I was feeling was always greeted with understanding but the next day it was as if the conversation had never taken place. With all my experience and training with a psychiatric population, I thought I had some understanding of what he was going through. I thought I had some understanding of how fickle the brain could be. I found there is a vast difference between living 50 empathetic minutes with a client who leaves when their session was over, and living the 24 hour a day experience with someone you are actually attached to. His constant needs were taking a toll. It was an extremely demanding and debilitating time for both of us. I had no idea how long and how debilitating it would become or that this was only the preliminaries.

As difficult as it might be to believe, even with all the craziness going on, the good moments still far outweighed the bad. While I scrambled to keep life as normal as possible Tom was able to spend his time and focus on what he did best. In our case it was telling me he loved me. We found ways to fill time as productively as possible and through some miracle I was able to step back and detach myself from the madness. Through some miracle I was still able to see the joy and the love and the tenderness. Through some miracle we were able to see the irony in the whole thing. We had met the love of our lives, and one of us couldn't even dress himself without help anymore.

God had to have one bent sense of humor. But then I always knew that anyway. Maybe there was a reason why *Lady Chatterly's Lover*, the *Book of Job* and Homer's *Odyssey* were among my favorite reading as a young adult. Here I stood with my Mellors, dressed in Job's plague of pestilence, weaving and unweaving the tapestry of our lives while ingrates banged on our door for attention. How could you not laugh at what was going on. The only thing missing was a screen credit reading, 'Produced by Mel Brooks'. We had one of two choices, we could laugh or we could cry and laughter seemed the better choice.

Our last talk with his lawyers in Houston had not been encouraging. They told us our chances of a settlement on Tom's accident case was going down the tubes. The defendants were taking the stance that Tom had Alzheimer's Disease or Jakob-Creutzfeldt Disease. With Dr. P.'s medical on record, all they had to do was wait. On the other hand, Tom was still an imposing figure on initial contact, and since questioning was to the point and short, requiring short answers, all of which allowed Tom to function at his best, there was no way to know which way a jury would go should it go to trial. Other similar cases had netted over a million dollars, then again other similar cases had netted nothing. Tom had yet to see their doctors. Our lawyers were doing everything in their power to push the process forward. It didn't sound promising. However, he had been fine before the accident. He was very much less than fine now.

After hearing the bad news he became obsessed about his money and whether there'd be enough to last his life out. He started contacting everyone he could remember who owed him money. He started murmuring about investments and loans he had made to people, most of which I couldn't decipher. Things started disappearing out of the apartment, some of them mine. He sold my art deco lamp to our realtor and the only reason I found out was that I walked into her carrying it down the street. He got twice what I had paid for it, so some of his skills were still working. It was returned. Hand woven Mohawk baskets my father had given me as a wedding present were gone. There was no way to calculate that personal loss. For all I know Tom thought they were trash baskets and left them in the trash room, which he had done before with other bins in the apartment. He was apparently finding ways to keep busy on his own.

He was due $945.00 on his 1985 tax return which hadn't been received. I had been doing the necessary paper work to follow up on this but I couldn't convince Tom of that to save my soul. He had been told everything had to be done in writing but he had always been at his best face to face and he insisted that personal contact was the only way to get things done. The fact that he would never see the same person twice at the IRS made no dent in his resolve. He could be relentless in his resolve.

The hold up was a result of two digits in his social security number having been transposed on a IRS form which required reams of letters to everyone concerned. The red tape was unbelievable. It took almost eighteen months to straighten it out. Tom would, after Herculean effort on my part, accept that everything that could be done was being done but that acceptance could last as long as three days or three minutes. He invariably remembered he was owed money and it would start anew. It was endless. There seemed to be no way to put him off the scent.

Rinnnngggggg ...

"Hello, Beverly."

"Hi Tom, what do you want?"

"I just got the mail, and my tax check wasn't in it."

... (Deep breath)

"Tom, the bank only sent the W2 last week, the IRS said it would be at least six to eight weeks before it's reflected in their records and another six to eight weeks before it translates into a check."

Realizing I was going into too much detail I stopped, took a breath, and started over.

"It's too early to expect the check."

"I want to go down there tomorrow morning and demand my money ..."

"Tom, how many times do we have to go over this. You'll have to wait, your check will be sent when ..."

"... with interest. They owe me interest."

"... as I was saying, (teeth now clenched), your check will be sent ... with interest."

I tried a diversionary tactic.

"... besides, I'm at work right now and I can't do anything about it until tomorrow. We'll talk about it later."

The diversion didn't work.

"You, know, if you were more aggressive, people wouldn't walk all over you. You have to let these people know who's boss. I'm a taxpayer."

Knowing how far that tactic got with me when my clients used it, I could well imagine how far Tom was going to get with the IRS using it.

"Beverly ..."

"Yes Tom, what?"

"Let's go there tomorrow ... they owe me interest too. You said tomorrow. I want to go there tomorrow."

[I don't know when it was that I started having personal conversations with God. I know I was very young. I was born with a sarcastic mind, and since sarcasm is missed unless shared with some greater audience, and since I knew most people would view me as a sassy child if I let my tongue wag too loose, God, was the name I gave to mine. While other kids were dealing with not eating meat on Fridays and harboring unclean thoughts, what ever that meant, I was having a running banter with the Ultimate Greater Audience. My Audience not only had an extraordinary sense of humor but an ability to recognize baloney as baloney at the snap of a finger. This relationship started out as little asides manifested as thoughts in my mind, thoughts that carried the full range of color my language permitted. I could be as caustic and as sarcastic as I needed, my only expectation being an imagined all knowing grin on the face of this Being now serving as my Personal Sounding Board. A Being who recognized my cleverness and quickness. A Being who found me funny. This relationship raised me above feeling victimized by others I perceived as nasty, unfeeling, insensitive, or boorish to me. This relationship allowed me to handle just about anything that was thrown my way.

As the years passed, the asides developed into full fledged dialogues that served to help me face my reality head on. As a result of those dialogues I was no longer permitted to fool myself, nor did I want to. They had a way of getting me to the truth of a situation, a trip that wasn't always pleasant, but they helped me understand the choices I made as my life unfolded and to accept the consequences of those choices. As a child I saw myself as a quiet, somewhat depressed child. As I rethink those years, I think I was fairly happy and content, and busy. I was born knowing I was all right. I was a survivor and I knew that in the core of my soul.]

I also knew as soon as I got Tom off the phone that day at work, it would only be a matter of time before the scene repeated itself. He would spot the mail, register that his check wasn't in it and pick up the phone, again. I was really ready to scream if I heard his voice one more time on the other end of that phone, and of course he phoned again. I found myself slipping into a familiar mode of behavior.

I'm going to scream, God. Watch me here, I am just about to lose it. (Holding the telephone an arm length away from my ear trying to avoid the sound of Tom's voice.)

You can't lose it, Beverly, you're at work and Tom doesn't have the notion of an idea that this is his umpteenth call. Why respond to the craziness?

I am tired. I have clients backed up to my neck and I haven't had an hour of peace for myself in months. I am so tired I could die.

As for peace, I've always seen that as a state of mind Beverly and not a place, and you're not going to die, at least not now. You might as well take charge of the situation.

Do I have a choice?

Not that I know of, unless of course you're ready to move on and let Tom be someone else's challenge.

That's a choice?

It's the only one floating around right now.

I took a deep breath and returned to the phone call still in progress with Tom ...

"I really can't talk to you about this right now honey, I'm really busy. You can't keep badgering people. It won't help."

"That's how I made all my money, that's how I got things done."

There is more than an element of truth in that statement, Lord. That is exactly how he got things done.

"That might have worked for you Tom but I'm the one doing this now and that's not how I work."

He tried his own diversionary tactic ...

"Do you want to come home for lunch ... and we could ..."

"Come for lunch ... and we could what?"

"You know ... perhaps we could ... you know ... screw around."

I could hear the finger wiggling in the air since he was unable to utter the word *screw* without adding the visuals. I had laughed the first time he did it. I always laughed when he did it. It had become a regular part of the Tom and Beverly act and something that never failed to elicit the response he wanted. It was also the only diversion that seemed to work consistently.

"Tom, if you weren't so damn cute I'd probably murder you. Then again, if you weren't so damn cute someone else would have beaten me to it years ago."

"That's true, that's true."

I could see the fluttering hand thing he did every time he uttered those words and of course there was also the twinkle in his eyes, something that always followed getting his own way. He just loved to get his own way. He almost did a little jig when he got his own way.

"I'll be home at lunch time. Wait for me at home."

I had to be very specific about everything including where we were to meet. Nothing could be assumed. If I didn't keep directions short and clear it might be hours before we'd connect. Lunch at home always had the promise of being quite magical, something Tom knew. He functioned just fine in certain ways. As for me, well, co-workers often wondered why I came back to work humming, when afternoons were not reputed to be my best time of the day.

In spite of my best efforts we made a total of four trips to the IRS. We'd enter the building at the crack of dawn because you had to be there by the crack of dawn to be seen that day. I'd take a number hoping it was low enough to get us into an interview before lunch and find us a seat. Tom would immediately start complaining about being made to wait. He always complained about waiting. It drove me up the walls, over the ceilings, and through the ventilating system. If his comments had been directed solely at me I might have handled it better but Tom always played to the greater audience. (Something else we had in common.) He'd throw comments at whoever was in hearing distance and wait for a reaction. Sometimes he'd have an entire conversation with a stranger before the light changed while waiting to cross the street. I grew to expect the little circle of empty seats around us at the IRS as people tried to disassociate themselves from his constant harangue about civil servants and how their behavior wouldn't be tolerated in private industry.

This would continue until our number was called and then he'd turn on the charm, a veritable beam of light as we approached the desk, Mister Personality charming everyone. He walked in an aura of good will and geniality, a spring in his step. Needless to say, they loved him. He'd have them doing computer printouts and making calls they made for no one. It was awesome. Who says civil servants are cold and unreceptive? However, the answer was always that he'd have to wait at least six weeks to see anything reflected but that didn't seem to matter. What mattered was the laughter, the hand shakes, the smiles from everyone when we left the desk.

It all had to do with control. Tom was less and less the one in charge of his life. He needed to get his way once in a while. Frankly speaking I think he needed to stir things up and this was without doubt, the best exercise his mind had had in a long time.

Then there was the acquaintance who had borrowed $900 from him prior to our marriage. He had been trying to recover the money for over a year with no success. By now it was a great deal easier to blow Tom away than it had been when the loan was made but that's just an intentionally snide observation. Tom was also trying to keep this bit of news from me now that we were married. However, I had noted their semi-frequent short conversations for over a year at that point and had also noticed he seemed annoyed when he left the conversation. When I asked what was going on he'd respond with comments about that person leaving town again, or having problems. (He could still be intentionally vague when he wanted.) I wondered what it was all about. Finally, he asked me to dial this person's phone number for him. In short, he was refused repayment and told the money had been a gift and he must have forgotten because of his memory problems. Tom's last comment was to insist he had never referred to it as a gift. A major mistake was made when this person hung up on him. Tom saw red.

We had used the term memory problems, when telling our friends what was happening to Tom. This person had been included in that group of people. I tried to differentiate between long term and short term memory and describe some of the details of what it all meant in terms of Tom's behavior and memory, but people don't absorb that sort of commentary. Unless they spent time with Tom they had no way of knowing his long term memory was still quite intact and however circuitous his immediate thinking process might appear, he was still meeting an amazing number of his goals. The assumption for many was that he had suddenly turned stupid.

He took his claim to Small Claims Court and won. (So much for memory problems although he did need help finding the witness chair.) He decided to waive the award he won after the first two payments were made. He had made his point. He was still in charge. *Himself* could still make the heavens move.

If nothing else, life was not boring for me.

In June 1987, we returned to Houston for more conferences with lawyers and doctors. Our decision to move was discussed in more depth with the family and it was agreed that they would look for a property for us and let us know if something came on the market in our price range. In mid-July such a house appeared and we flew out to see it. It was a two story house, built in 1916, so I guess I can safely characterize it as *old*. It was in the same suburb as Tom's children and within walking distance of the township business district. It was also a mess. The bathroom needed to be entirely rebuilt, walls and floors needed work, the outside stucco was cracked, the ceiling upstairs was acoustical tile that was water stained and falling down, a room on the back was little more than a shed, the plumbing and electrical work was ancient and we would discover it needed a new roof and then a new furnace, and then air conditioning. It was endless. There were also obvious changes that had to be made to accommodate Tom's present and potential physical needs, but the house had a certain charm. In other words, it was within our financial means.

Money was a concern to us both since we still had no real idea as to what we would have to live on if I couldn't work. I couldn't work unless there was always someone with Tom. Who that someone would be looked more and more like me since everyone else in the family was working. However, we'd be near family and I envisioned a door always open with people in and out and Tom occupied, even if I was still the primary time filler for him. We all got on well together, I believed in families sticking together and I felt Tom needed them as much as I believed they needed him.

We made an offer and returned to New York. In September, with a cash outlay of $50,000 which I sent family members to hold for us to be used for the purchase and renovations while we were back in New York, the property closed. We were now in a financial commitment, a financial commitment we couldn't back out of. We had cashed in part of Tom's retirement fund to provide that $50,000. It was the only cash we had at the time since we were now living on my salary and we were counting on the sale of the co-op in New York to provide what we would have to live on after our move. Walking away at that time would have left us with no cushion. I couldn't afford help for Tom while I worked and it was impossible to leave him alone on his own wandering around New York, so remaining in New York was out of the question.

We made arrangements to start the renovations and we returned to New York with the intention of wrapping up our life there. We were leaving one of the most beautifully appointed apartments that existed in New York City for a house in Houston that offered on the most generous of descriptions, shelter. And so started the saga of the house, a saga that gave new meaning to the phrase, *money pit*. Everything that was done to it resulted in new unforeseen nightmares to take care of.

Compounding the problem was the ever present need for Tom to have this project suit him when it was finished. His need to have things his own way were legendary. His friends and his family all had stories of those experiences with him. Even I, in our short time together, knew how particular he was about his surroundings. He called it order. His definition of 'order' spanned a lot of things. If it was an essential part of his history it was even more important for him now. A person's essence doesn't change a whole lot because their mind starts to die, if anything it seems to become more so. Tom had a real talent at that point for being very much *more so*.

Over the years he had collected antiques in his travels around the world. He learned to be as meticulous and as competent in those choices as he was at everything he did. He didn't just drink wine, he was an expert at choosing, evaluating, and caring for it. He was one of those rare individuals who could identify the vineyard and year of a choice vintage. He often said to me that he couldn't function unless his surroundings suited him.

A friend and colleague of Tom's shared the following story with me. It demonstrates Tom's particular needs in ways I could never capture:

Tom had come into her life as an independent contractor with her firm. He was going to be in charge of the leasing operation among other duties and as usual was working on a contract basis rather than an employee basis. He had been assigned one of the executive offices out of which he immediately had all of the furniture removed. The following day a moving company arrived with his own things, an English Partners desk, leather chairs and an assortment of tables, cabinets, paintings, and leather bound books. All of it traditional and all of it authentic. He told her he wanted the wall paper changed. He added that he could live with the carpeting since it was a neutral color and he was laying his own Persians on top anyway.

She advised him there wasn't any money in the budget for such an expenditure and added the office had been recently papered. She was sure he'd understand. Tom, not handling 'no' very well no matter how it was housed, although he was certainly adept at using it himself, immediately dictated a memo to her regarding the request for new wallpaper. She returned the memo to him and stated she was not going to authorize new wall paper.

One of Tom's people observed the encounter and offered that perhaps it wasn't worth the hoo-ha that was about to erupt and it might be easier in the long run to just authorize the new paper. She didn't feel she could justify it. She was also unfamiliar with Tom's penchant towards a good old fashioned argument and she had not a clue as to how determined he could be when it came to having his own way.

The next day Tom invited her to lunch and explained that although he understood her position his request was more than merely a selfish demand. He simply couldn't work in a room with that wall paper. He found it distracting and annoying and most of all it was in exceedingly poor taste, it was flocked!

She offered understanding of his needs but she didn't see how she could justify it especially since it was anticipated that most of Tom's time was going to be spent out of the office, most likely out of the country. Lunch ended amicably enough.

The next morning Tom called her into his office whereupon he showed her that the paper was curling up around the light switches. She noted that he must have taken a pen knife to pry the edges up. She pushed the corners down, told him it only needed a little glue and she would have the maintenance crew fix it. Tom put his fingers under the torn corners and with a circular motion that tore

the corners into two large holes, he turned to face her and said ...
"There, now it can't be fixed."

She said the two of them just stood there planted head to head
while they glared at each other. She remembered saying as evenly
as possible before storming out of the office ...

"That's it. That's the way you want it. That's the way it stays."

The next morning she arrived to find workmen in Tom's
office. They were removing the offensive wallpaper. New paper
rolls were on his desk along with a copy of a memo he had dictated
the previous evening which stated he was, at his own expense,
replacing the wall paper in his office.

She found Tom talking to a colleague. She waved the memo at
him and acknowledged he had won. Tom smiled at her. She said
she will never forget that smile nor the charm he turned on as he
said ... "Now I can do what I'm being paid to do ... work."

Tom was reimbursed for the wall paper. Considering the
amount of income he generated for that firm, it was a small thing.

There was no doubt in my mind that every change I ordered in
the house was necessary, and yes I was worried about the money. I
was not ordering top-of-the-line anything and I was not the one
making the decisions. The co-op in New York had yet to get a
nibble and it seemed the only activity we got from our realtor was
in lowering the price. Our house in Houston needed major work
which had to be completed by the sale of the co-op so that the move
could be made as smoothly as possible. There was no basement in
the house which meant everything would be cluttered in the middle
of the floor until it could all be put away.

Tom couldn't stand clutter. Tom was never able to stand clutter
for that matter. I knew that chaos could send Tom into a tailspin.
Order and structure in his life were vitally important if he was to
function at all. This was not a new phenomena in Tom's life since
one of his favorite comments was: "I am a Libra, and I need order
in my life." Clutter would disorient him terribly. The move could
be a very destructive time in his life at a time when time was not
expendable. He was being uprooted from everything he knew and
put into an area where he couldn't even take a walk by himself

because of his inability to find his way home, or remember his new address or phone number.

I counted on his no longer needing to go anywhere by himself because I'd be there, as would his family. We were all within a few blocks of each other. It was just a matter of making adjustments, easy adjustments if everyone co-operated.

Back in New York there was some unfinished business I needed to take care of before we left. I needed to make peace with Judith. I had to admit that I had displaced a great deal of my anger and fears at her doorstep and had grown to resent her very much. I resented that she'd had Tom at his best. I resented that she'd been given opportunities to grow and develop and become successful in ways that would no longer be open to me. I resented that she had her freedom and her life ahead of her free of the worries I was facing. I resented that she never called him and I felt that she, more than most, owed him. Most of all, I resented that Tom continued to speak of her as if she walked on water while I continued to scrape off wagon loads of Tom's frustrations and anger, much of it directed at me because I was the only one there.

Along with those feelings, there were also the fears that filled my being. Fears of the future, fears of losing Tom to a slow demeaning death, fears of giving up my job, fears of leaving my friends, my family ... my rent controlled apartment. So much for embracing the future.

Of course, Judith had been calling Tom and seeing him. I suppose Tom kept Judith's visits and calls from me for what he felt were valid reasons, and I suppose Judith felt her continuing involvement with him might be cause for trouble between us. It was not a simple situation. The bare fact is that all I noticed was who contacted him and who didn't. Every day when I returned from work I asked who called. He always responded "No one". However, I didn't fear that Tom might be unfaithful to me, what mattered was that he felt useful and loved. He needed a life with people he knew and I had no need to put up barriers to that life because of plebeian ego needs or some convoluted lack of trust. Once everyone understood that, life got a lot less complicated.

Once I knew that Judith hadn't abandoned him, the rest of the knot in my stomach disappeared and we were finally able to talk openly with each other. She once observed that I seemed to understand Tom in ways he needed without his having to ask or explain and that I was one of the few she had ever met to say no to him. I

remember saying, "Now if I can only get him to pay attention to it."
We both laughed. She knew in intimate detail how difficult he could
be. When I added that I thought Tom and I were a lot alike in some
ways, she responded with ...

"Yes ... I know."

I believe that was the first occasion when Judith and I actually
made eye contact. We both laughed as some element of knowledge
passed between us. What had started out as a glib attempt at
justifying why I was hanging in there with Tom, ended up as acknowledgment of commonality. Those three words attested to my
strength and the elements of our personalities that Tom and I
shared. Perhaps it was time for me to own that strength and stop
acting as if I had to apologize for living. Judith had offered me a
compliment born out of generosity and understanding and it was
time for me to accept it with grace. She did a great deal to help me
rally the friends and she has remained a close personal friend to me
throughout this whole experience. She was there for me during
times when I felt completely alone. We shared more than a laugh on
that occasion, I believe we also shared a bonding. We manage to
laugh every time we have contact.

I don't know if Tom ever told Judith how very proud he was of
her accomplishments. I suspect he showed it in how he related to
her, but just in case she never heard the words ... Tom held a
special place for her in his heart, and her success as a business
woman, as a friend, and as a human being were a constant source
of pride and satisfaction and comfort to him.

Tom had his session with the defendant's doctor in Houston. He
very carefully picked his wardrobe that day. He spent a great deal
of time talking to our lawyer about what to expect, the purpose, and
the risk. He had a quiet moment to himself before the examination
to collect his energy and he was so impressive during that
examination that our lawyer felt a settlement offer might be made.
Tom's stance and affability could still garner a great deal of
sympathy from a jury. He had always been able to pull it all
together when it mattered. Furthermore, our lawyers were able to
convince the judge that further delays were only an effort on the
part of the defendant to circumvent responsibility in a case that had
been pending for almost seven years. Now that the ramifications of

Tom's injury were known to be so much more serious than originally thought, to delay further would only increase his long term needs for treatment. The judge ordered a trial date. Tom was just elated by the news.

In December a settlement offer was made, Tom accepted. It wasn't as much as he had wished for but with the money from the co-op sale and the rest of our combined holdings, we were looking forward to about a $400,000 estate. Even with the purchase of the house in Houston there was enough money to take care of his needs, and he hoped enough to insure my future as well.

Through the remainder of the fall of 1987 we packed and organized our belongings. All of Tom's rehabilitation went on hold. He was so wound up about getting out of New York that he spoke of little else. However, as the boxes in the apartment increased, so did his level of confusion. By the time December rolled around he was having difficulty finding his way to the bedroom or the bathroom without help. His speech slipped dramatically. He was more often than not subject to panic attacks about going out on his own and in fact went no where alone the last month we lived in New York.

He dreaded the chaos of the move as much as I. I, on the other hand, hoped the set back was a temporary one having expected the reaction as a result of all those seminars I attended that year. I hoped to get him settled in as soon as possible and then hook him up with proper medical care and training.

Just let me move him through life as effortlessly as possible and please God, give me the guidance I need to help him and still remain intact myself.

142

NEVERTHELESS

Maybe I'm right and maybe I'm wrong
Maybe I'm weak and maybe I'm strong
          But,
Never-the-less I'm in love with you

Maybe I'll live a life of regret
Maybe I'll give much more than I get
          But
Never-the-less I'm in love with you

Sometimes I know at a glance
The terrible chances I'm taking
Right at the start
Then left with a heart that is breaking

Maybe I'll win and maybe I'll lose
Maybe I'm in for crying the Blues
          But,
Never-the-less I'm in love with you

words by: Bert Kalmer   *music by: Harry Ruby*

CHAPTER EIGHT

It was shortly after our marriage and we were walking down Third Avenue in New York when we were stopped by a man I'd never met before. Tom responded by throwing his arms around him and the two of them hugged. The greeting was much more demonstrative than those I'd seen between Tom and other friends. He told Tom that he and two of his buddies were presently living in a flat in New Jersey and all of them were working. He chatted about what they'd been doing, who was working where, and how things had changed since last they saw Tom. He thanked Tom for his help and said he just wanted him to know he was doing all right. He was one of the homeless men Tom had come to know while doing volunteer work at a local shelter.

Tom had become increasingly more concerned about the problem in New York. It was difficult to ignore it when it was all around. We lived at the corner of 29th. Street and Broadway in the midst of a commercial area that had once been known as 'Tin Pan Alley'. At the turn of the century the co-op in which we now lived, was called the Gelsy House, the then reigning hotel in New York, a hotel that once housed General Grant, Gilbert and Sullivan, Diamond Jim Brady, and a host of other notables of that time. The color of that era was long gone and it was now the center of the flower market and a flock of Pakistani and Mid Eastern wholesale houses all competing for parking. During the day the area was total chaos. At night it was desolate with only the homeless and the desperate roaming the streets picking through the rubbish and looking for a place to sleep. Marble Collegiate Church, which was at the other end of our block, allowed the homeless to set up their cardboard boxes within the iron grating around the perimeter of the Church at night. The heating vents located there gave protection and some warmth during the winter months to a fair number of people. Every morning the homeless removed the boxes and every night after dark the boxes reappeared. A few blocks in the other direction was Penn Station, another illustrious housing place for the homeless.

The area also held the core of the remaining landmark cast iron buildings still standing in New York, buildings that were being reclaimed and refurbished into very expensive co-ops. Many of the Yuppies moving into the area were organizing in hopes of removing these people to someone else's back yard. Tom held a different attitude. He was no longer traveling on business and decided to use the time he now found himself with to do something constructive. He decided to get involved. It's a statement that he was still able to see the misfortune of others, considering the problems he was facing with the changes occurring in his own life.

Tom answered a call for volunteers from the Madison Avenue Baptist Church which was a few blocks from where he lived. They ran a nightly shelter and volunteers worked with a certified social worker handing out bedding, towels, and soap to the people assigned to that particular facility. Volunteers worked at least one night a month and their tour of duty ran from 7:00 p.m. to 7:00 a.m. They were expected to sleep in the same room with the street people and be there to supervise. Tom took the Saturday night shift and often filled in when others couldn't make it.

The people assigned to that shelter were not supposed to be mentally ill or dangerous but sometimes an episode erupted and there were often disputes between them that had to be dealt with. Volunteers, for the most part, did the tasks assigned to them, they stuck close to each other and had little to do on a one to one basis with the people. It wasn't a comfortable or inviting situation.

Tom said he saw it as a life experience and a chance to see if he could make a difference. He had been told to have no expectations for these people because their situation was a chronic one and there was little someone like Tom could expect to do for them. There were social workers and other professionals trying to rehabilitate these people and the success rate was negligible. True to form, Tom ignored the advice. He spent time talking to them and got to know who they were and what jobs they had held and how they had gotten there. Over a period of time he got to know some of them fairly well.

One day he overheard the manager at the local supermarket complaining about finding reliable people to deliver groceries. Tom approached and asked if he'd consider some of the homeless men he had come to know. The manager was very reluctant which only made Tom more persistent. He said he'd screen them, make sure they were presentable and provide ID cards for them. On this basis the manager agreed to a few interviews.

Tom gathered a group that night at the shelter and outlined his proposal. He explained they'd work for a dollar a bag and tips. It wasn't much, but it would establish work history and perhaps some of them could pool resources and get a start out of it. What he didn't add was that it would also help them organize their time, one of the first steps to getting back to work. He got the resulting group of men clean clothes, had name tags made for them, helped them fill out employment forms, and went with them to the job interview. He listed himself as their reference. A number of the men got jobs. The gentleman who stopped Tom on the street had been one of them.

There was a sensibility that Tom had in dealing with the world at large. He viewed life as a continuing series of choices to be made and problems to be solved. When I asked him what defined success to him, he said he measured the degree to which he felt productive and content. It was an unusual answer since most of us define success by other measures. As he saw it, every choice in life had the same potential for failure as it had for success. What made the difference depended solely upon attitude. As a result of his positive attitude, Tom saw life as an adventure instead of a fearsome place.

As his friends described him to me using terms such as formidable, insightful, centered, it occurred to me how difficult it is to intimidate someone who has no fear of life. Tom had no fear of life, and how freeing that must have been for him. He also didn't expect or need to be loved by those who crossed his path, although, when love was expressed to him, as it was by that man we met on the street, or by his friends, or Judith, or myself, or his family, he embraced it with a mixture of wonderment and warmth. He was not someone who was cold to the experience. Those of us who ventured near him felt respected and cared about. And isn't being respected and cared about as good a definition of love as any? That being loved back wasn't the requisite in his involvement with the people in his life, is what I found so unique. Not attaching those strings to his actions gave him the freedom to be his own man. It also allowed him to give others that same freedom without judgment. Some people thrive on that freedom, and some don't.

Tom demonstrated a clear view of his world to me and I was lucky to have enough time with him to benefit from that view. I don't ever remember being at odds with him, except for the pressures his illness presented to us, which was another thing altogether. I remember a walk down 5th. Avenue after a Sunday brunch shortly before our move to Houston. There were probably eight of us just rag tagging along from a restaurant and we were all laughing at something Tom had said. It was a little convoluted, but one of those truisms of his I had come to appreciate, a political observation that drew in some incident from his past but which was glued in a very unique way to an incident very much in the news. A friend looked at me with a twinkle in his eyes still laughing from Tom's observation ...

"Do you believe that?"

And I replied ... "I believe everything he says."

"That could be very dangerous Beverly."

"I think that's why its called true love." And we all laughed some more.

Tom was well into the mid stage of his illness by the time this particular brunch occurred. With his language as fragmented as it was, he was still able to get his thoughts and his feelings across and the members of our brunch party recognized he still had his humor and his insight and he was still someone who was as passionate about the things he felt deeply about as he ever was.

It was too easy for people to turn off when Tom started groping for words or used words less than correct to get his meanings out, but the meanings were still there if people only took the time to listen. So many others who've lived with loved ones with dementia echo this. There is an element of creativity in the mind that makes unusual choices of words to express itself when aphasia, (the inability to find and use words productively,) enters the scene, and there is an essential need for creativity on the part of the listeners to make the leap to connect what seems an inappropriate choice of words, but which often turns out to be almost profound when the meaning is finally ferreted out. Many of us have found ourselves enriched as a result of being there with someone like Tom. It is not the bottomless pit everyone expects it to be.

How often friends and family were surprised at how responsive Tom was to a given situation when their expectation was quite different, and how relieved they were to find the old Tom still lurking about when their belief was that he no longer was. It was difficult for people to assume Tom's essence and dignity was still there in the face of what was becoming abnormal behaviors. It was difficult because it never occurred to most that his essence and dignity were still there and intact. They had never been told to expect that. They already expected something quite different.

> * *A person's value in society is stripped away very quickly when they start to lose cognitive skills. As soon as the social mores are tested by odd behaviors and slurred speech and confusion, one is treated as if they have brought some sort of plague into everyone's presence. One day they are whole and welcome, and the next day they are better off dead. It's as if the move from being productive human beings, to being people to be pitied, people in the process of losing their dignity, people who will become a burden, happens the moment Alzheimer's Disease is pinned to them. The trial, the sentence, and the execution all happen simultaneously. I am constantly bewildered by the assumptions made about this illness by people who view it from the outside. Its been said before, and I'll say it again, "The lights don't all go out at once".* *

Family dynamics don't generally improve because someone gets Alzheimer's Disease. If anything, family dynamics tend to follow the same paths they always followed, only more heightened and more complex. The stories I hear in support groups about families being torn apart by this illness are legion in number. Old rivalries between siblings surface, hurts perpetrated by parents, (whether real or imagined), justify actions taken, guilt and the avoidance of guilt run rampant, and realities of money and estates and the cost of long-term care motivate actions that can't always be retraced once started. Moreover, chances to heal old wounds are gone, chances to share old memories and bonds become elusive, and dealing with the role reversals that occur bring all kinds of emotional baggage to the forefront. Add to that a lack of understanding about how this illness operates or that there is even a glimmer of a chance of meaningful interaction with a parent who is becoming more and more a stranger, and you have a breeding ground for fear that can only leap frog into faulty assumptions and decisions, sometimes made too hastily. The end result of all of the above is a parent in need of love and a caregiver, whether it be a spouse, an adult child, a sibling, or a friend, who is left isolated and at risk.

Those who do try to *"help"* often end up feeling rejected, and dismissed for their effort. Instead of smiles they are greeted with crankiness and criticism. Initial overtures to help are often so tentative and awkward as family members try to understand how to help without demeaning a person who was in charge of their lives, all of their lives, that those efforts are often interpreted as insincere and rejected instead of embraced. The problem that faces the adult child in this circumstance is that the offer of help is often too vague. It doesn't translate into anything tangible and as children, who have been programmed to wait for permission from their parent in order to act, and structure from them regarding how to act, the choice to start entering the inner life of parents isn't easy.

If the well spouse is also a second wife or husband and not the parent of the adult children, well, there are a whole set of problems that can surface, problems which complicate inter-relationships on levels that often can't be resolved. The illness progresses too quickly and the caregiver is often too frantic and too stressed out to help adult children make the transition. In these situations the well spouse is even more likely to be wary of what is shared.

Furthermore, the well spouse, is often operating from a place in history when asking for help just wasn't done. There are many people out there relying on mind reading as a means of communication.

"Hi Mom. How's dad?"

"Fine".

"Do you need anything?"

"No everything is fine."

"Well, phone me if you need anything."

"Love you."

"Love you too."

Well everything isn't fine. Dad has entered into the incontinence stage of his illness and he isn't sleeping. So Mom is facing enormous changes in their life, changes she is not going to talk about easily with her son or daughter for a lot of reasons. She is also becoming sleep deprived from Dad's constant prowling around at night, something else she doesn't want to talk about because she's afraid of being forced into making a nursing home decision when she's not ready to. And on top of that, there is no one to shovel the walk, and Mom can't leave Dad alone in the house long enough to do it herself, and at her age she shouldn't be doing it anyway.

The above scenario is how and maybe why a conspiracy of silence develops. It also evolves out of a heightened sense of commitment and bonding that happens as the early stages of Alzheimer's Disease develop. Unfortunately, with two people working in concert to cover up as many loose ends as possible, the bonding necessary to the Alzheimer's loved one and the primary caregiver for their survival is often a bonding that tends to separate other family members from each other. However, I think the real culprit in the separation of family members is the constant overlay of mourning and grief that greets each and every loss of functioning which also heralds the demise of the relationships. No one realizes that everyone, parents and family members alike are in a constant state of grief with everyone trying to hang onto what is slipping away. The *little deaths* are constantly present with each individual family member trying to deal with something yet unnamed. The sad thing is that there is no expectation of the level of grief that permeates a family unit facing Alzheimer's Disease and there is no one to explain that this is a large part of what is going on in the dynamics. Family members are faced with a very difficult barrier to break through and if the family unit is to survive, that barrier must be broken down. So the question is this ...

How does an unsuspecting adult child develop a sensitivity to how this illness is going to impact every member in that family, or to the fact that there is still a chance for meaningful exchange no matter how debilitated their parent becomes, when there is literally nothing and no one out there to tell them otherwise? There are no role models, no helpers, no professionals, no one who has a handle on what is motivating family dynamics through an illness that lasts for years and an illness that takes over everyone's life.

On a wide scale, professionals and numerous ancillary service people who come under the heading of "helpers in our lives", have aided in turning our society from one that takes care of and regards it's elder population, to a society that has come to think of them as expendable. Facing the care needs of someone with Alzheimer's disease means facing the *"pain of loss"* and since so many of these helpers haven't personally made the connection between that kind of pain and grief, they take the band-aid approach to counseling families which is to avoid pain. Unfortunately, the only way families can avoid this kind of pain is to desensitize themselves to what they and their loved one is going through.

It is often too short a step to equate the loss of memory, cognitive skills, productivity, and control of hygiene needs in our elder people with a supposed 'loss of dignity'. And once they've lost their 'dignity', then what seems to follow is their loss of value. Why should anyone sacrifice their time and love for someone who no longer has any dignity or value? How can caring for a person with no dignity or value be anything but a burden?

The grief issues aren't even addressed because death is so far off in the future with an early diagnosis of Alzheimer's Disease. It doesn't even occur to the professionals that this is the pivotal issue and because most of them haven't faced their own fears of death and loss they are basically unequipped to recognize grieving in action. Their use of phrases like 'loss of dignity', 'the burden of caregiving', and 'the needless sacrifice', do more to lead unsuspecting family members to under rate their place in the lives of loved ones with Alzheimer's Disease than almost anything else the disease itself can do. They rob people of the right to expect anything but horror from this illness. The instances of what happens to families who buy into the dehumanizing of Alzheimer's individuals are endless. Attend any support group meeting. One example comes to my mind.

The wife of an Alzheimer's spouse was in tears in a support group I led for late stage people at my church. Her son had not only stopped visiting his father but he stopped letting their grandchild visit as well. This woman was nearly in despair over her feelings of abandonment and disappointment but she was also grieving for a grandchild she barely saw anymore. When she confronted her son with her feelings and told him how much his father and she missed their family the response she got was this ...

"Its too painful to see Dad that way anymore and I want my daughter to remember him as he was, not the way he is now. I can't stand watching him lose his dignity. When are you going to put him in a nursing home and be done with this? Dad would not want you doing this for him, he would never want to burden his family this way. He's already dead as far as I'm concerned and I am not going to witness any more of it."

   * *When did old age and illness become so difficult to face? When did we start to delegate the responsibility of care to others, elsewhere? When did growing old become something to shield our children from?* *

The media at large, doctors, professional helpers, and often caregivers themselves have contributed to the reprogramming of our attitudes towards our elder loved ones, perhaps without even knowing that they're doing it. What amazes me is that the concept of having lost one's dignity isn't applied to our children who also need total care and we would never refer to our child rearing as a burden. Nor is a loss of dignity used in the context of a young adult in a wheelchair anymore. Thirty years of advocacy for the rights of the handicapped have made that attitude so politically incorrect that anyone who considers such a thing would be thought of as insensitive beyond measure. And most of us applaud the parents and spouses who hang in there with a disabled young adult. But to our elderly frail and our Alzheimer's people, the supposed loss of dignity seems to have become a prelude to characterizing their care as a burden. The two seem to go hand in hand.

How often do group leaders and social workers, in their misguided attempt to offer solace to an overworked caregiver, tell them they are not expected to sacrifice their lives for someone else. The problems caregivers face aren't about sacrifice at all! The problems are about a lack of help, and grief over out-of-control family dynamics. They're about lack of information about where to turn for help, and lack of recognition that a break from it all is desperately needed and that the real reason for all the rampant emotionalism has more to do with grief than almost anything else. To tell a caregiver that they don't need to sacrifice their lives is to tell them their commitment to honor vows once made in earnest is regarded with no regard by others. Perhaps it is time to rethink some of the mindless jargon being used in reference to our elderly frail and the disservice such comments do to their caregivers.

A man I met who does case management for home care families told me that even though most people want to remain in their homes, nursing home placement is really the only eventuality for someone with Alzheimer's Disease. I asked him if he was going to be so cavalier about going into a nursing home when it was his turn. I also asked him how old he was. Tom was only 51 when his road to nursing home care began. And then there was the professional lecturer I once heard speak, one of many touting the same clichés. He had a very entertaining talk that captured attention but what he had to say made my blood boil. I remember sitting there seething over the untruths and misleading images he promoted.

- Our parents did not work their whole lives so that their money could be spent on keeping them alive. They are outliving our ability to take care of them.

- You find an adult child taking care of a parent with Alzheimer's Disease and you find the unfavored child, the one who was overweight, unpopular, who is still overcompensating for feelings of inadequacy and a lack of love from that parent. A child who is still trying to gain favor and a sense of self, a martyr.

- I can't imagine my mother-in-law wanting me to help clean her after she became incontinent. It would be much too embarrassing for her. None of our parents want to become a burden to their children.

And everyone was sitting there taking notes! Well maybe not everyone. There were a few of us in that audience who weren't swayed by the talk. One man, a caregiver with a mother also in the late stages of Alzheimer's, sought me out to remark ...

"Me thinks he doth protest too much. He's trying too hard to cover up his own guilt! I don't feel any guilt! I'm tired and I could use a good nights sleep. But the one thing I don't feel is guilty about keeping my mother home!"

I agreed, because in spite of the neatly packaged talk, the words that were not spoken, the symbolic language we all use to express our unconscious selves, spoke louder to those of us cognizant of who we are as caregivers, than what was actually spoken to the rest of the audience. And had the subliminal message that was really lying beneath the packaged talk surfaced, he might not have gotten the applause he received when he finished.

- I don't want my wife to spend her share of my mother-in-law's estate on care costs, when the money can be spent down, and Medicaid can foot the bill.

- I don't want my wife to be the one stuck with her mother's care when there are other family members to take on the responsibility. My wife's wish to keep her mother in our home is overblown and unrealistic and most of all I don't want my life style changed by care needs.

- I certainly am not going to change her diapers or wash her. No way, not now, not ever!

As for becoming a burden to our children, the truth is none of us want to be a burden to anyone, especially if burden is defined by long-term care. But unfortunately, we don't always have a choice in the matter.

Perhaps, in this case, the right decision was made to place the mother-in-law in nursing home care, but I think it was made for all the wrong reasons. What bothered me was that the real reasons weren't owned up to, reasons that were just as valid as the spoken ones in the talk, no matter how unpalatable they might seem. If the care of a relative can only be viewed as a potential burden and the potentially burdened relative just doesn't want to take on the task then they shouldn't. But to cloud decisions in what I see as shallow attempts to bury guilt, is to do a disservice to those listening to the words and I don't believe it does much for the one speaking the words either. There is something to be said for being honest about what you can and can't do when faced with a life changing decision. I think it makes living with the decision easier which then leaves room to make the best of it.

Unfortunately, it's not just the professional helpers who repeat the same tired clichés over and over. The media represents this disease with the same ignorance and misconceptions. Dramas demean the victims of Alzheimer's Disease by blowing them away with mercy killings as if that's actually a viable solution to long-term care. They demonstrate their screaming lack of information about the illness and the humanity that can still be involved in the lives of the Alzheimer's person and their caregiver, even until death. They make up symptoms in order to move a story line along regardless of the harm it does by misinforming the public. Will I ever forget the "*L.A. Law*" character who turned into Ralph Kramden, complete with an authentic N.Y.C. Transit Authority uniform who then launched into verbatim dialogue from the "*Honeymooners*" every time his Alzheimer's Disease 'kicked in'. "*Pickett Fences*" had a character who was elected mayor after being diagnosed with Alzheimer's Disease who then had the tenacity to locate an adult sized hobby horse to ride in his office, clad in just a Depends brief and a Native American breast plate when his Alzheimer's Disease 'kicked in'. He was shot in a mercy killing by a son embarrassed by his father's loss of dignity with the entire town justifying the son's deed.

The producers who sink to that level of inanity do so for two reasons only, sensationalism for profit, and they are just too damn lazy to check their facts. They apparently haven't figured out how to use a phone, or that the Alzheimer's Association has one. It's not because information isn't available. Sadly, they miss the real point which is that there is drama enough in the real story of Alzheimer's Disease. What they do instead is to send a message that Alzheimer's people are ditzy/cute/comic figures who are open game for ridicule because they are conveniently nonvocal in condemning this sort of portrayal.

News shows are worse. They rarely report on the positives in the bonding that happen when families hang together through this illness. They only seem to report on which caregiver has gone over the deep end and killed or abandoned their loved one in a vacant football stadium somewhere. And they have a crushing ignorance of the stress that would drive a person to do such a thing. It's not reported as an act resulting from a lack of respite care, or lack of help navigating a system that is designed to drive people crazy, or lack of funds for care, or diapers, or food, or as the terrible human cost this illness imposes on family units. It's simply murder with a *capital M,* with exchanged soulful looks between anchors who haven't a clue. The unreported, unrelenting needs of full time care of a demented adult aren't worthy of real exploration because that information might be too graphic for the general public and everyone seems to want to keep their heads buried in the sand. It's so much easier to place blame on the caregiver instead of public apathy. Besides shouldn't all these people be in nursing homes?

And let us not forget the courts and the lawyers who have found a new lucrative field in the estates of those who have family members languishing in the quagmire of family dynamics. In situations where skilled mediators and family counselors are needed to help clarify group and individual needs and to facilitate cohesion amongst the various members, families are left to a system of lawyering based on fostering distrust amongst all the interested parties. A system where opposing teams are assembled and where lines of battle are drawn that are impossible to penetrate, a system of legalities based on the premise that to divide and conquer is the only game in town. The more involved and hideous the game becomes, the more deeply divided the family becomes. And, when the smoke clears, the lawyers have all done their jobs, the court officials have all done their jobs, the appointed *helpers* have all done their jobs, and a whole lot of money has passed hands, and there are nothing but victims left bleeding in place of what used to be a family.

And so I repeat my earlier question. How does an unsuspecting adult child develop a sensitivity to how this illness is going to impact every member in that family, or that there is still a chance for meaningful exchange no matter how debilitated their parent becomes, when there is literally nothing and no one out there to tell them otherwise?

There are really only two paths adult children can follow when facing Alzheimer's Disease in a parent. One is to find fault, feel rejected, place blame elsewhere, be critical of the caregiver, detest the thought of having to do things in care that seem beyond imagination, and to avoid contact with the person who needs the contact most, the Alzheimer's parent. The other is to get past the unfilled needs, the fears of death being something other than a natural process in all our lives, and simply love the person as they are. That means giving up being right, it means giving up control, it means giving up dreams of a future with that person, and it means embracing them as they are unconditionally. To love for no apparent reason whatsoever -- a selfless act that requires great commitment, patience, and a tremendous amount of creativity.

In an age when commitment is thought of as just another word for sacrifice, and sacrifice carries with it all the intrinsic implications of martyrdom, it's easy to see why flight might be the first reaction when facing the increasing needs of a parent with Dementia. But know this, those who do flee miss the only envelope of awareness left in the person they profess to love. They miss the chance to make a bond, a bond that will probably last the lifetime of their memory, and they miss a chance to discover their own strength. They might think they're missing the petulance, the deterioration, and the trouble, but what escapes them forever is the sweetness and the moments of contact, heart to heart and soul to soul contact, because they weren't present to share them. Instead both sides feel cheated, angry, abused, and rejected.

We are all born with the inalienable, inherent, universal attribute of our dignity as human beings which lasts from the moment we are born until the moment we die. That attribute is not diminished by whether or not we can dress, feed, or toilet ourselves or perform our cognitive functions in an acceptable manner. None of those things have anything to do with our dignity. Whether or not the caring for another human being becomes a 'burden' when all those skills begin to deteriorate, is really a result of the choice that is made by the caregiver and the other family members. The care needs won't change, but the attitudes of caregivers and family members can. The only true statement is that a person's dignity is ultimately reflected through the eyes of the people around them. *

In other words, family members have to make their choices and draw their conclusions without much help. The amazing thing is that vast numbers of family members keep their Alzheimer's loved ones home in the face of tremendous odds and in spite of criticism, deprivation, and lack of family help. The majority speak of strength, of unmissed moments and on occasion, joy. Some of them also die before their loved one from a lack of love themselves.

Tom was operating out of frustration and hurt from the moment he knew something was wrong with him and of course, the move to Houston did not alter that. If anything it enhanced it. After all, what could be more frustrating to someone whose entire life had been born out of his facility with the language, to have that facility fail him and know it? What could be more frustrating to someone who still knew there was a process involved in doing something as simple as getting dressed but who could no longer do even the simplest element of that task and know it? What was it like for someone who now only felt fear when he left his house, because the half mile square community he now lived in always looked un-familiar, but still remembered the far corners of the world as being just an airplane ticket away? How did it feel to fear his credibility as a human being fade?

Was he cranky? He sure was. Was he unappreciative? He sure was. Did he make unrealistic demands, was he contradictory, was he emotionally fragile? He was all of that. He was losing it, and contrary to much of what has been written about this illness, he knew very well that he was changing. I saw the tears, I felt his frustration, I watched him fail in bits and pieces and there was nothing I could do to stave it off. When he became unable to express his fears and his frustrations I almost thanked God for letting Tom off the hook and even then I couldn't be sure he didn't still have understanding of what was happening to him. To this day, I can't say he doesn't know who I am or where he is. Just because he can't say the words doesn't mean there isn't yet a part of him that relates to my being here with him, to my still being here.

Did we find ourselves participating in a conspiracy of silence to protect his family from the realities of our life? Of course we did. We also protected my family and we protected friends and we protected each other. Were we all in the throes of grieving without even knowing it? Absolutely. There weren't words in our vocabularies to express the losses we were all facing. I can't imagine what Tom's family felt as they saw their father deteriorating before their eyes and I was too deeply wrapped up in my own grief to be able to relate to theirs. Did communication between our families and us fail to develop in an orderly fashion? Of course it did. That was almost preordained by circumstances already out of control. And when the conspiracy of silence was finally broken, well that didn't help either. His children were exposed to Tom's needs in the raw and there was no where for any of us, them or me, to channel our frustration and fear and loss because none of us had had the chance to bond and trust and love each other.

What happened in this family was a tragedy. We were all out there on our own trying to stuff normal behaviors into totally abnormal situations. While some of Tom's children seemed to step back, ostensibly out of the immediate circle as a way of dealing with all the changes, others chose a focus in order to deal with the shock of what their father was becoming. They focused on what thousands of other family members focus on as the inevitability of this illness becomes apparent and control of the situation starts to slip through the fingers like so much sand. They focused on the estate, the one last thing that had any element of control left to it.

They involved the court by moving to have their father declared incompetent and themselves named as guardians. A move we were obviously forced to counter. They named me as a threat to the estate which had the ring of possibility to it since I was the second wife and had married Tom knowing he was ill. A move I was forced to answer. What resulted was a machine set in motion that couldn't be stopped by any of us once it was started. The court system is a formidable object that took over all our lives.

Once lawyers got involved and once Tom had been declared a ward of the court, all communication between family members and us stopped cold, because the divide and conquer phase of this particular version of the Crusades was now set in motion. The lines had been drawn. The only fair appraisal is that the Court became the enemy, at least for Tom and me. We found ourselves in the middle of a farce. A farce where people who had no place in our lives were suddenly in control of our lives. Judges, lawyers, court appointees, social workers, guardians, *friends of the court,* bank trustees, case managers, all jumping up and down as if they were actually doing something other than sucking money out of the estate and interfering with what was left of our lives. It became a matter of jockeying for position, planning battle strategy and determining which army could get more creative in terms of taking and holding ground. It took on a life of its own and ultimately had nothing to do with Tom's needs or anyone else's. It was a total waste. A waste of time, a waste of energy, a gross waste of money and a needless waste of what should have remained of a relationship between grown children and a father. It would be years before any of the happenings were put into perspective and communication re-initiated between us.

Did it impact on Tom. It sure did. Did Tom have any awareness of what was happening? He sure did.

========

However, just because things were deteriorating in terms of Tom's and my relationship with the family as the move to Houston was made, didn't mean that anything else in our lives would go smoothly. Needless to say, the house wasn't completed by the move. The walls were up and the doors widened to accommodate a wheelchair as I had requested, the kitchen was almost completed and the upstairs bathroom was done, but, the floors had been untouched and with six rooms of furniture, one hundred and eighty boxes of belongings, no shelves in the closets and no basement, the chaos was unfathomable. Trying to do the project long distance from New York was an impossible dream. The bathrooms ended up with vanities instead of the pedestal sinks I had asked for and were as cramped for space as I anticipated. The downstairs bathroom had no shower but there was a closet in its place. I considered having the shower built then but decided to wait until I actually needed it for Tom instead. Thank goodness I saved that money.

Tom hated the fact that every room in the house had been painted white. He had always hated white walls. He did nothing but carp about it for weeks. I painted the interior of the house myself. In order to maintain some level of continuity in Tom's frame of reference I used the same colors that were in the apartment in New York hoping familiarity would help his adjustment.

To make matters more interesting, he insisted on *helping* which was a life experience in itself considering his visual problems and his difficulty in following directions. Just having him help me move the coffee table across the room was an ordeal because he tended to do everything opposite to my direction, not that you could consistently count on that. The one room he helped paint had paint on the windows, the floor, the ceiling, and the molding before he lost interest. It was like watching a Laurel and Hardy routine. The only thing missing was 'the getting hit in the head by the swinging ladder', bit. However he didn't miss 'the stepping into the paint tray and tracking the paint around the room' bit. I decided on wall to wall carpeting for that room and made obvious repairs after he went to sleep.

This was a man who had never done house maintenance in his entire life because he had no talent for it. He could conceptualize the building of a hover craft capable of carrying four semi's fully loaded with pipe across the Yukon River in Alaska, but he was totally inept with a screw driver. Since he was the one to tell me this bit of news I had to wonder why he was so determined to do these things now. His reply was simple ...

"Because there's nothing I can do anymore and I'm so bored I could die. I can't even figure out how to load my own gun." A comment that was made more real by my having found him sitting in the living room with a gun in his lap, a gun that was unloaded because he couldn't find the ammo. The way our luck was going he'd probably have shot me thinking he was aiming at himself.

I asked family members to take the guns out of the house and continued to try to keep Tom included in as much of the work as I could. The problem was that furniture couldn't go up against the walls until the walls and floors were finished, and the boxes couldn't be emptied until the furniture was up against the walls. He couldn't follow any direction in order to help and he could devise nothing to fill up his time on his own that didn't translate into more work for me. If he was out of my sight for more than a few minutes trouble was sure to surface somewhere.

The *trouble* included, but was not limited to, the constant turning off of water because Tom couldn't figure out how to shut the taps off. Handles, which at least give some clue as to on/off direction, would have made that task a little easier for Tom and for myself, as opposed to ball knobs which give no such help. However, that was one example of how difficult it was to get directions straight long distance during the early renovations. The water taps became a constant source of irritation for both of us. Tom couldn't get a drink of water by himself because he became so confused by the knobs that he'd end up calling out for help or be so embarrassed he'd just walk away and sulk in the back room until I heard the water running, usually full blast. He never seemed able to get a normal mix of hot and cold and more often then not, it was steaming hot water that was pouring out. I tried adjusting the temperature gauge, but the pipes were so old that it was impossible to get a hot enough mix for the shower if the temperature was made safe in the other faucets. I won't go into the times he accidentally turned the spigot on to the counter, grabbing at anything that moved in order to stop the flow, only to have it flood the counter, the floor and him. The truth is I couldn't figure out how to shut off the damn taps myself because there were no two knobs in the house that turned in the same direction.

As Tom succumbed to the stress we ultimately faced in Houston, his compulsive need to move and fiddle with things increased and for some reason, running water held a particular sort of fascination for him. He'd spin a faucet as he passed a sink and move on through the house stopping only to spin another faucet somewhere else. There were times when I found myself running from the kitchen to the bathroom to the upstairs bathroom, doing nothing but turning off water. Those water taps came to symbolize the insanity our life was fast becoming and every time I had to rush to Tom's aid or fumble with them myself, I found myself uttering a series of invectives and diatribes, some of it in a rather creative fashion aimed at what was in reality, merely plumbing. I'd like to say it helped. It didn't. However, no matter what significance the faucets came to play in our daily lives, they were only a part of the continuing picture of what was going on with Tom.

There were also the glasses and dishes Tom left precariously on the edges of counters that fell and broke and had to be swept up or he walked through the debris. There were the pitchers of spilled juice, the tracking it through the house, the requests to open a bottle of beer because he couldn't figure out how to do it on his own and he couldn't find the bottle opener in the drawer, the bottle then being placed on its side so that the beer poured out. The only saving factor in the whole mess was the pile of unemptied boxes filling the downstairs which inadvertently created walkways that restricted his movement somewhat. And, no matter how much I explained the need to get all the stuff away he continued to feel very left out of everything and bitterly resented the time I spent working on the house as lost time with him, but someone had to do it.

The saga of the house would continue for months before the aggravation of tracking down workers who seemed more intent on lunch than in working, the constant drain of money and emotional resources, and the unrelenting noise and clutter ended.

February of 1988, two months after the move to Houston, Tom and I escaped to Boulder, Colorado, to visit my sister and to remove ourselves from the noise, aggravation, clutter, mess, and damnation that had become our lives. Tom's functioning had reached an all time low. He was more easily confused if conversation wasn't kept simple and it took more time to help him express his thoughts and make his meaning clear. The confusion in the house with the noise and everything out of place had a profound effect on him and he became more agitated and more demanding.

What we desperately needed was a chance to step back from everything a bit and think. A break wasn't just a whim at that point it was a matter of survival. Aside from anything else, I needed desperately to touch base with someone who knew I wasn't crazy. I hadn't had anyone to talk openly to in months. Tom wanted to see if he could still ski and so opting for the great outdoors instead of staying with friends in New York, we headed for Boulder, Colorado and my sister Norma. It turned out to be pivotal in our lives and in some ways the beginning recognition of the journey the two of us had truly embarked upon.

Tom could still ski downhill as long as he didn't have to follow me. However, he couldn't get his boots or his skis on without help. I had the good sense to leave all our equipment home and rented what we needed at the resorts. I can't imagine what trying to move all that stuff and Tom through an airport would have been like. Well, actually, I can. He couldn't concentrate long enough to hold on to his own skis, goggles, poles, or gloves nor could he maneuver getting on the bus that took us to the beginner slope without help. The sight of me, carrying two sets of skis, two sets of poles, gloves and goggles while I tried to keep Tom in tow, constantly calling to him to stay with me or move along, often dropping one or more of the above items while I coaxed him from the lodge to the bus, was beyond description.

Please Lord, let him hate it. Please let me go home.

The lift had to be stopped in order for him to get on. He couldn't judge the distance or the timing as the seat came around the belt. The lift had to be stopped at the top in order for him to get off safely and I had to talk to him through the ride, keeping his attention as much as possible. Midway up the lift I realized he had no idea how high we were. My voice reflected the panic I was experiencing as the ride up the mountain progressed.

"We aren't any where near the top of the hill, don't move, I'll tell you when to get off ... no Tom not yet, wait, we're not there yet, the man will stop it for you ... wait Tom ... sit still ... please sit still. I have your poles, I'll give them to you when the lift stops ... not yet, just a while longer ... we're almost there ... wait ... the man is stopping the lift ... O.K. ... here are your poles, take your time, O.K. ... go! Go!!!! I'm right behind you."

We went down the slope twice when Tom turned to me ...

"I don't think I'll ever ski again, Beverly. I'm afraid. I've never been afraid of anything in my entire life. Beverly, please get me out of here."

He had tears in his eyes. This guaranteed that mine weren't far behind. We drove back to the hotel and made love.

[Never underestimate the power of good ole' fashioned *fun*, and if there was one thing Tom understood unequivocally it was how to have this particular form of *fun*. He had a way of muttering little things in my ear and doing little things with his hands that signaled fun was about to begin. He had an uncanny way of dropping failure out of his hands while picking up strength, sometimes in mid-stride. It was as if he decided, "well, I can't do that anymore, but I sure as hell can still do this." He did what he could still do very well.]

We spent the night watching the Miss Universe Pageant, a experience heretofore, Tom had managed to miss, but one which I enlightened him about. He didn't know such a thing existed. He was almost mesmerized by the experience. We laughed a lot that evening.

[And people thought I had little to add to his life!]

The next day we opted to spend the day at the Unity Church with my sister, Norma, and her husband, Jack, who was the minister. As soon as Tom was with people who gave him the time he needed to get his words out and who accepted his difficulties and showed patience he improved. It took such little effort to be kind to him. All things considered and knowing from this vantage point where things were headed with his illness, life was still relatively serene and normal if he was given half a chance. He went to lunch with Jack, and I hung out with my sister.

Norma had been trying to convince me to look into a holistic clinic in Arizona for Tom, for months. It had recently started working with brain injured adults. Sharon, a woman in her church had just returned from there with her daughter who had been severely injured in a car accident. She was just raving about the results of their stay.

Initially I had been resistant to suggesting that Tom even consider such a program. I'd witnessed the deterioration that had happened in him since our marriage and I was losing heart. It was very difficult for me to see what holistic treatment could do for him when his verbal skills were so impaired.

[How can you manifest wellness when the organ you need most to accomplish that feat is your brain and it's no longer functioning correctly?]

The fact that I was already planning for wheelchairs and projected bathing needs was an outward expression of what I wasn't yet ready to verbalize. We still didn't have a definitive diagnosis, but Tom's continuing deterioration was obvious. I was calling it *Some Sort of Dementia,* Tom was still calling it *Brain Damage.* Neither of us were able to use the "A" word, not in our minds, not from our mouths, not to each other. He wasn't eligible for experimental Alzheimer's treatment because he didn't have the diagnosis, so we were out there entirely on our own and at the mercy of our own devices. However, regardless of how we characterized his illness, there was virtually no treatment to be suggested by traditional medicine and with nothing tangible being offered we felt holistic treatment was the only game left in town. Tom was someone who preferred acupuncturists and chiropractors to doctors anyway. Considering his belief in prayer and his fierce desire to live his life in the best way possible, he was probably more ready for the experience of holistic healing than I was.

The Association for Research and Enlightenment Clinic in Phoenix worked with people from all walks of religious belief and much of their emphasis was on positive thinking and attitudes as being essential to wellness. They used a holistic approach to treating illness and I knew Tom would have no problems with that part of the program. I also knew we could both benefit from some therapy and some attention. As for me, some months earlier I had asked God for guidance. I decided we had been given the opportunity to explore a different approach to Tom's problems and I would leave the decision up to Tom.

I told him what I thought were valid reasons for applying to the program and before Norma could find their phone number, Sharon unexpectedly walked through the door. Norma had been trying to reach her all morning with no luck. She had stopped by the church hoping to catch up with us before we returned to Houston. She was very anxious to pass her experience on to us.

Her teenage daughter had been so severely injured in a car accident that her doctors didn't believe she'd live and if she did her brain injury was so profound, it was doubtful she'd ever have a normal life. She survived the initial trauma but her speech was greatly impaired and she couldn't walk, dress or feed herself. She was also extremely depressed and unmotivated. The doctors told the family she would probably worsen and die. The very best they could hope for was to face the rest of their lives caring for her. They released her from the hospital and sent her home to face long term custodial care.

As a last resort, Sharon took her daughter to the brain injury program at the A.R.E. Clinic in Phoenix. They lived in a group home with other patients and for two weeks every waking moment was filled with physical therapy sessions and consultations. Their diets were taken care of and their activities prescribed. They participated in both individual and group sessions that were designed to treat the mind, spirit and body and all of the participants were asked to make the choice of facing life head on.

Within a few days her daughter's attitude improved. Along with that improvement came others. Her ability to coordinate her basic movements improved, her balance improved, her speech improved, her thought process improved. Her physical therapy programs increased her strength and stamina and within two weeks she was able to make her own bed, dress herself and communicate more easily with staff and fellow patients.

Upon her return to Boulder her doctors were so amazed at the improvement that they ordered a complete rehabilitation evaluation and treatment program. She credited the clinic with having taught her how to improve her concentration and her coping mechanisms. Most of all, she learned that she had the power to take charge of her life. Sharon told us her daughter is happier and more content with herself these days. That was in 1987. Since then and as of 1991, she not only finished high school, graduating with her class, but she is presently working as a fashion model.

Tom became more and more enthusiastic as Sharon talked. She talked specifically to him, answering all of his questions no matter how long it took him to get them out. It was wonderful the way she urged and helped him pull his thoughts together. He was more animated and happy than I had seen him in a long time. She felt Tom's speech pattern was reminiscent of her daughter's during the early part of her rehabilitation. She also told us who to call at the clinic and what to expect when we got there. Tom decided he wanted to go there ... immediately!

I called and asked for Eileen Black, the head of the Brain Injury program. I gave her as much of Tom's history and the progression of his illness as was possible over the phone, holding back nothing. I described the car accident and the subsequent deficits. I also told her about the continuing deterioration and that doctors felt it was probably Alzheimer's Disease. I agreed to send copies of his medicals as soon as we returned to Houston. She and her assistant, Carol Banozick, spent over an hour talking to Tom directly so they'd have a first hand picture of where his functioning was and just what his level of awareness might be in every day conversation. They also intended to start including him in their daily meditations and needed a sense of him in order to do so. Tom was so taken aback by that bit of news that tears came to his eyes. That strangers were that concerned for him and that motivated towards his state of health was almost too much to expect. When Eileen asked him if he thought he might want to attend, he took a deep breath and in a faltering attempt to cover his embarrassment over the unexpected display of emotion he said ...

"I would stand on my head and whistle Dixie if I thought it could help me."

I remember him laughing, I remember the light in his eyes, I remember the hope I saw for the first time in a long time. He ended his conversation by saying ...

"You'll know who I am when I get there, because I will be the one making the most noise."

He would be true to his threat.

I decided to concentrate on getting Tom set up with a good neurologist in Houston, which we had not yet done since I'd been hoping he'd improve a bit before setting any appointments. However, his medicals needed to be updated, which was required by Dr. McGarey in Phoenix, and I also felt it was important to get a base measure of Tom's functioning before we left.

Just to give an inkling of how stubborn Tom could be, after setting his sights on Phoenix, he refused to even discuss seeing another doctor. I spent two weeks trying to convince him that he had to see Dr. B. before we left town because the clinic needed an update of his condition. I can't count the times I explained and re-explained why we had to see yet another doctor. I finally got him to agree to see him once and once only. The day of the appointment arrived and we were halfway to the medical center when Tom changed his mind about going.

"I don't need to hear I'm not right again. I'm not going."

"Tom we have to go and we're going whether you want to or not."

"All right I'll go. But I am not waiting."

That was a threat he knew would pull my chain big time and he kept his promise. We weren't in the office more than 10 minutes before he went into his tirade and stormed out of the door. I didn't know whether to chase after him, knowing he hadn't a clue as to how to get back to the car considering the maze of corridors we had come through to find the office, or try to make a new appointment. I was desperate about getting the appointment over with and burst into tears out of sheer frustration. Thank God, the nurse realized what was happening and she helped me head him off at the elevator. We were all in a run by the time we caught up to him. If he had made it on the elevator it could have taken hours to find him. Between us we cajoled him and gradually got him to return to the office where the doctor, who had been summoned when the commotion started, was waiting. He caught Tom with a hand shake as we entered the office.

"Are you always this impatient Tom?"

"Time is money Doctor."

"I apologize for being late, but I'm here now and what can I do for you?"

"Don't make me wait."

The doctor smiled as he ushered Tom in the examining room. He asked me to wait by the door while he started his examination. He told Tom to undress for a general physical and when Tom removed his trousers the doctor remarked ...

"God, I could kill for those legs. On second thought, my wife would kill for those legs."

At which point Tom laughed.

"Are you a runner?"

"But of course. I run half an hour every day."

"Do you run by yourself?"

"God, no. I'd never find my way home. You'd have to start looking for me in Canada."

At which point the doctor laughed.

"Which direction is Canada, Tom?"

"Depends on where you are. From Alaska it's one direction."

"Is this Alaska?"

"Of course not. I worked in Alaska."

"Where are you now Tom."

At which point Tom smirked ... "Beats me."

"You have trouble finding your way around, Tom."

"If it wasn't for Beverly I'd never leave the house."

Dr. B. continued his examination, gradually getting information from Tom while engaging him in conversation. He ordered a new EEG and MRI and agreed to forward the results of the exam and his tests to Dr. McGarey in Phoenix. He had little to offer about Tom's condition except that Jakob-Creutzfeld Disease was ridiculous, because aside from anything else, Tom had already outlived the diagnosis. He seemed to be stifling a smile during that portion of the discussion. He told us he was anxious to see us when we returned and he greeted my description of the program in Phoenix with the same attitude he might have shown had I said we were going to Lourdes. However, he seemed to genuinely mean it when he said ...

"And good luck at the clinic. Be sure and call for an appointment when you return."

He was someone who held the power to do a lot of damage to our resolve to take back our lives, and he chose not to.

Thank you, Lord!

Tom decided he liked the new doctor and continued to be almost euphoric during the weeks prior to the trip to Phoenix. He seemed to be getting himself ready. He was a firm believer in "The Power of Positive Thinking" having had a long relationship with Dr. Norman Vincent Peale's ideas, and he kept affirming over and over that he expected to get well. We'd both been looking for a catalyst. The clinic was it. All Tom needed was a means of focusing his innate power and his pervasive authority.

172

THE WAY YOU LOOK TONIGHT

Someday, when I'm awfully low
And the world is cold,
I will feel a glow just thinking of you,
And the way you look tonight.

Oh but you're lovely,
With your smile so warm,
And your cheeks so soft,
There is nothing for me but to love you,
And the way you look tonight.

With each word your tenderness grows,
Tearing my fear apart,
And that laugh that wrinkles your nose,
Touches my foolish heart.

Lovely, never never change,
Keep that breathless charm,
Won't you please arrange it
Cause I love you
Just the way you look tonight.

words by: Dorothy Fields   *music by: Jerome Kern 1936*

CHAPTER NINE

THOMAS MURPHY   **DIVISION OF NEUROLOGY**
DATE OF EXAMINATION: March 18, 1988   **L.P.B.,M.D.**

PRESENT ILLNESS: This is a first Neurology Division visit for Mr. Murphy ... At the present time, his most prominent difficulty is with speech. He has difficulty both with word production and with proper use of words. In addition, his comprehension is imperfect. His comprehension remains considerably better than his expression. In 1986 he saw Dr. P. and Dr. N. At that time, Dr. P. was suspicious that he had a spongiform encephalopathy. Between 1986, at which time his EEG was "abnormal", although the report appears to have been only mildly abnormal, and now, he has had continued deterioration. It has not been that prominent and is perhaps not as rapid as in the past ...

PHYSICAL EXAMINATION: The sensory examination appears intact. The most remarkable thing about his examination is his mental state. There is as well, however, masked facies and a Parkinsonian stare. There is little in the way of cogwheeling although there is some in the neck. There is a marked disturbance of speech present. It is present in ordinary conversational speech. He tends to ramble although short sentences are clear and coherent. Paraphasic errors appear in his spontaneous speech. He is unable to repeat even simple nursery rhymes properly and in general his speech breaks down and is preservative ...

IMPRESSIONS: Progressive dementing illness. Could this be Pick's Disease? The course seems much too long for Jakob-Creutzfeldt Disease particularly the Heidenhain variant and one would suspect that the EEG should have been characteristic. The possibility that this merely represents a variation on Alzheimer's Disease cannot be entirely dismissed but I feel that he has something much rarer than that. We will repeat his MRI scan and EEG ... We will talk with him again once the results are available.

Thursday, April 21, 1988 Tom and I arrived in Phoenix, Arizona. We were met at the airport by the clinic van and driven to Oak House, our home for the next seventeen days. We were shown to our room, told we'd be sharing a bathroom with two other people and to make ourselves comfortable. Right! We unpacked our bags and looked with a deep sense of dismay upon the twin beds staring back at us. We stood there silently for a couple of minutes, Tom finally breaking the silence.

"Oh hell, we'll ... f.f.figure ... ..s.s.something out."

I remember reaching for his hand. Tom suggested we go for a walk and take a look around the place. We ventured out of our room to see a number of people milling about. No one seemed to want to make eye contact. I know I didn't. We almost bumped into a chair in the dining room before I realized someone was sitting in it. She was extremely thin, her face without expression and her skin coloring or lack of it had a grayish tinge to it. She showed little response to our blundering into her. Her name was Susan.

We were to learn that she had been diagnosed with terminal cancer. She had had all the chemotherapy she could tolerate as well as several operations. To complicate her life even more she had rheumatoid arthritis to deal with, her husband had recently died and she was facing the prospect of yet another surgery which might prolong her life but would not cure her. She had come to hate her doctor, she felt she was dominated by everyone in the world but herself, and she was having difficulty understanding any of it. She did know that she wasn't ready to give up, at least not yet.

Dr. McGarey arrived at 6:00 p.m. that evening and for the first time all of us drew together and sat down to dinner. During the meal Dr. McGarey acknowledged our fears and spoke of the need for positive thinking and laughter. He emphasized the essential need for laughter, punctuating the comment with a barrage of jokes. He was no Bob Hope, but he was very sweet and all of us needed something to break down the lead walls each of us had carried into that dining room. So we laughed while venturing to sneak a quick peek at each other, hoping to find a new friend if not a cohort in this rather scary adventure. Without exception, all of us were treading on unknown territory. Some of us were there in active defiance of traditional medical treatment and some of us were there in hopes of enhancing it. The commonality is that all of us were praying for a miracle.

He went on to talk about how each of us were different in our respective needs but for some reason we had gathered together in this place, at this time, for the common good of us all. It wouldn't be an easy journey, he said. Some of our expectations would be met. Some of our expectations might be changed. Wellness wasn't necessarily a state of the body or the mind as much as it was a state of being, and perhaps we all weren't so different in our needs after all. He hoped we'd be able to face our demons and conquer them.

He had seen countless others do so. We were embarking on a voyage that would test our stamina and our spirit but he was confident we were equal to the task or we wouldn't have come.

The next seventeen days were outlined. We were handed our itineraries and told to move to the living room and seat ourselves in a circle. Other members of Dr. McGarey's staff then joined us. They introduced themselves and explained their function in the program and as always happens when a circle is set we were asked to introduce ourselves and explain what had brought us to the clinic. There were a total of thirteen people in Tom's treatment group and an additional five of us so called 'helpers'.

Two other women besides Susan were there with cancer. Vicki was in her late twenties with young children. She wore a scarf around her head to cover the results of her most recent treatment. Her cancer had metastasized and was now, as she put it, crawling all over her body. Her delivery was matter of fact and detailed but devoid of much emotion as though she had finally tired of talking about it. Her husband held her hand throughout her talk. He volunteered that they had come because there was nothing else left to try. They both looked weary. Scott, her husband, had tears in his eyes while Vicki spoke.

Hilda then told her story. She was a woman about Tom's age and she was accompanied by her husband Amos. She had survived W.W.II in Germany, had met her 'young American flyer' after the war, married him and settled in the Southwest. She above all the rest in the group seemed to be the most in control of herself. She had been doing all the 'right' things. She was keeping a special diet, she was meditating regularly, she was maintaining a positive attitude, she was taking charge. She had been fighting the disease for years and had already pushed the odds far beyond what her doctors had told her to expect. She had experienced a recent set back and was there to give herself another boost.

Cassie had an unnamed disease that was literally eating the tissue inside her face. She was in her early twenties and she was in constant pain. She had come from Alaska and had weaned herself off her pain killers prior to her trip to Phoenix. Her doctors were not only dead set against her taking herself off her medication but they had referred to her intentions to attend the program at the A.R.E. Clinic as a 'Trip to Disneyland'. She ignored them. During the first few days of the program she was never without an ice pack which she held on her face. She was the only one to be excused from the group meetings because her pain was so intense. She also had the most raucous sense of humor I had heard since leaving New York and her asides were so hilarious that people tripped over each other in efforts to sit next to her.

Chucky was a hyperactive child of seven who was literally bouncing off the walls. He was with his mother Barbara who looked to be at the end of her string. Chucky's antics had been so out of control and so exhausting during that first day that when it was Barbara's turn to speak she started to cry. She just sat there with her face buried in her hands sobbing and then the sobbing stopped. Her body started to shake and as often happens under extreme stress she began to laugh loud hysterical peals of laughter. The laughs were then replaced with chokes and snorts and when she was finally able to speak, what she said was ...

"There was the time when I went into my back yard and hid from him in some bushes ... but ... he found me."

We all laughed, I had tears in my eyes as I laughed. I remember thinking ...

God! I know those bushes.

I had memories of my own. Memories of that private phone conversation I was still trying to have without Tom glued to my shoulder. I had finally bought a remote control phone when we moved to Texas because Tom had the habit of pacing while he talked. He had consequently broken five phones by pulling them off the table dragging them across the floor until they finally wrapped themselves around a piece of furniture. I had tried everything short of nailing the phone to the table. The remote control phone allowed Tom to wander anywhere in the house without restriction. The only drawback was finding it when he was finished, but then that was the very least of our problems.

There were days when our neighbors would note a somewhat peculiar phenomena in our house. They'd see me come out our front door talking on the phone, walk down the stairs, around the side of the house, in the back door, through the house, out the front door, down the steps and around the house again, continuing the cycle until my conversation was completed. All the while with Tom in hot pursuit, the pace sometimes just short of 'a jog'.

There was no time that I was ever by myself, not even in the bathroom. As soon as Tom missed my presence he'd begin pacing through the house calling my name as though I had suddenly vanished.

"Beverly, where are you?"

"I'm in the bathroom, Tom."

"Where?"

"I'm in the bathroom, Tom."

"I can't find you."

"That's because I'm in the bathroom, Tom!"

"What are you doing?"

Each response on my part getting louder until I finally told him, 'what', I was doing in the bathroom. I'd hear him respond ...

"Oh!" ... and before I could count to ten the pacing would resume and he'd start calling for me all over again. How could our neighbors not love us, we were the best entertainment to hit their parts in years.

Yes! I was familiar with those bushes. There were times when I wished with all my heart there was some place where I could hide in for just a while. Not long! ... but for awhile.

As the night wore on everyone had their turn to talk, including Tom. I tried to seat us in the circle with everyone else, but he had planted himself along the back wall and he wasn't budging. When his turn came, he tried to explain his problem and his reasons for coming to the program by himself but he wasn't making much sense. He was having trouble finding words and he wasn't finishing his thoughts very well. I helped fill in some of the gaps but it was an arduous experience. It was extremely difficult for him, it was heartbreaking for me, and it was hell for everyone else in the group because his problem didn't stop him from making comments during everyone else's turn, most of which were vaguely related to the point at hand. He behaved like someone trying to translate a foreign language and who was missing all the key words. It was a long and exhausting evening.

Tom was to admit during another of our group sessions that it was his intense desire to flee after that first evening. He said he had never felt so out of his element in his entire life.

"What in hell have I gotten myself into? God! Will you look at all these sick people."

It was a comment that made all of us laugh, but it was nervous laughter, as each one of us admitted to the same feelings. We were all experiencing a collective horror of the unknown as we entered the dining room that first night.

During the next seventeen days we would experience the whole range of human emotion together. We would live together, eat together, meditate and pray together, share our fears, our joys, our anger, our love, and our gains, together. It became an infectious experience. As one started to improve so did others. All of us during that time together got better. Some of us were cured. In some ways perhaps all of us were.

The first day of the program started at 6:00 am. We gathered in the back yard for morning exercises, showered, dressed, and went into the living room for the morning meditation. We ate breakfast and lined up for the van ride to the clinic where assignments had been made with physicians for physical examinations and review of reports. From that point on everyone followed their own itinerary. Breakfast was to be the time when all of us brought each other up to date on progress, and the time when we would discuss our dreams. Tom announced, loudly, that he never dreamed.

Tom was not only taking part in the general program but he was having their full neurology program as well. He'd be seeing an osteopath for adjustments every day, he'd have several deep muscle massages every week, and he'd be involved in the Physical Medicine Center which conducted all psychotherapy sessions, biofeedback sessions, and the stress reduction program. We'd be having counseling separately and together throughout the program. Our day started at 6 am and ended at 11:30 p.m.

Oliver Sacks writes in his book, <u>Awakenings</u>: "It is insufficient to consider disease in purely mechanical or chemical terms; that it must be considered equally in biological or metaphysical terms." He goes on to say, "One sees that beautiful and ultimate metaphysical truth, which has been stated by poets and physicians and metaphysicians in all ages ... that love is the *alpha* and *omega* of being; and that the work of healing, or rendering whole, is, first and last, the business of love."

But it wasn't just a matter of loving ourselves and others, it was a matter of finding *love* in the *agape* sense of the word. Unconditional love, not love with strings attached or love in purely passionate terms. *'The business of love'*, is not an easy road for most, and it is a particularly lonely and difficult one for the family members and friends of those facing serious illness challenges. For the clinic to simply talk about attitudes and empowerment as being essential to wellness would have been superficial. What they did was challenge me with an obligation to make my motivations about Tom clear of fantasy. Provisions were set in place to help me look into myself, to evaluate my choice to be with Tom during this illness and to prepare myself mentally for whatever was in store for us both. For the first time, the question, 'What if', was raised.

They also emphasized that I couldn't do it all alone and they urged me to take care of myself if it was my desire to continue to be a help to Tom. That meant getting myself into a focus that gave me meaning outside of Tom and for my own mental health I needed a break once in a while. It was time for me to start asking for help when I could and, if necessary, to hire an aide to continue his exercises with him. They suggested I keep the structure of the clinic as closely as possible to our home routine, and they emphasized my attitude was crucial towards Tom's problems if Tom was to find peace, strength or wellness. This was not to burden me with the responsibility of making Tom well, however. This was to help me understand that walking this walk with Tom had to be for the right reasons. It had to be about unconditional love or not at all. I had to start taking care of myself, both physically and mentally.

As a first step I decided to have a complete physical examination while I was there considering that I hadn't been to a doctor in over five years. I was in perfect shape except for my pap smear, which bounced. I started treatment while I was in Phoenix and was advised to follow up with a doctor as soon as I returned to Texas. As for hiring help, and coordinating family involvement, that was something that was going to have to wait until we returned to Houston.

A large part of Tom's day was to be spent at the Neurological Treatment Center where he would follow a very structured program. The treatment was based in part on re-patterning exercises reportedly developed by "The Institutes", a well known center for treatment of cerebral palsy and mental retardation in Philadelphia.

As I understood it, the belief was held that a baby must move naturally through the stages of learning. It must learn to turn over, to crawl, to creep, to walk, and then run in sequence. When any of those steps were skipped or learned out of order, or not learned at all as with brain injured or mentally retarded children, the learning process was undermined which made it more difficult for the brain to accept further stages of development. Consequently, speech, balance, memory, thought process, any number of functions could be effected. It was thought that with the use of re-patterning techniques, children with learning disabilities could go back and learn the proper sequence of steps and thus improve their ability to coordinate basic movements, organize speech, and thought processes more easily.

The program at the A.R.E. Clinic incorporated re-patterning techniques in their neurology program in an attempt to see if adults might also benefit. The program was offered under the umbrella of holistic treatment and their patients were not only exposed to the tasks endemic to re-patterning but to the holistic approach of treating the whole body, mind, and spirit. This was the program our friend's daughter in Colorado had gone through.

The clinic staff decided to treat Tom's symptoms and not get hung up on his many diagnostic possibilities. They were unique in that regard. They weren't afraid to let patients hope and they weren't afraid to let them try. Our doctor in Houston was to remark on how reasonable that attitude was especially since Tom was as much at a disadvantage without a diagnosis as he was with one. Without a definitive diagnosis, he wasn't eligible for any research programs and our doctor felt most treatment facilities were much too hung up on categorizing those who had one.

Tom would be taught to crawl again, to creep, and to walk. Through every step of the process he would be questioned and prodded. His memory was picked, his motivation questioned and examined, his belief system defined, his wants, his fears, his regrets, his hates, his loves drawn out so that he could look himself in the face and decide if he was someone he wanted to live with.

Tom was willing to do it all, however, had he not trusted the staff I doubt that we'd have stayed. He took a liking to all of them but he and Eileen Black hit a special oneness almost immediately.

He would refer to her ever after as 'Black', having always had the penchant of referring to his staff members by their last names. Hers would be the only name he'd be able to remember on his own although he knew who everyone else was and recognized their names when mentioned.

However, his liking of her didn't mean that he'd follow her directions blindly. He questioned everything she asked him to do, at every turn, and at every instance. She was often hard pressed to find the words that finally made sense to him and then, and only then, would he deign to cooperate. (This aspect of his personality would never change ... ever.) It was also a treat to watch someone else deal with the Murphy persona for a change. At least I knew it wasn't just aimed at me.

His initial evaluation wasn't good. He was unable to identify simple objects by touch, objects such as a screwdriver, scissors, key, or tooth-brush. He knew what the objects were once seen, and he could explain how they were used but his touch gave him no clues and he was unable to draw the name of each object from his memory.

When given flash cards to read, the words grouped into categories of furniture, vehicles, etc., he couldn't read one word correctly. However, the problem was more involved than an inability to read. The problem was with the flash cards. His brain couldn't recognize the concept of what a flash card was for. He got so lost in the shape and size and its being held up in front of his eyes that he missed seeing the words. The holes in his vision compounded the problem and we all wondered if he even saw the letters as words or the letters as letters for that matter. With the help of Eileen, and her colleague Carol Banozich, I was beginning to examine Tom's world with more attention.

They also found that his eyes wouldn't converge. He could follow a light with each eye individually, but was unable to follow with both eyes. This would seriously affect his ability to focus on anything.

When asked to crawl on his stomach along a floor mat, he was unable to follow the directions. He couldn't stay on the mat nor could he go from one end of the mat to the other without stopping every few feet, needing constant prodding. The yellow line down the middle of the mat provided nothing but trouble for him. We discovered that lines were no longer straight in Tom's brain, nor did corners meet. Tom saw curves and waves and followed them right off the mat. When Eileen and Carol turned the mat over to the solid side, he was able to crawl from one end to the other as long as one of them keep repeating over and over that he was doing fine and to keep moving. If her voice stopped, he stopped.

We noticed that he moved his right side automatically but his left leg and arm seemed sluggish and forward movement was generally slow as he tried to think through each movement of those limbs individually. Eileen told him he wasn't moving his left leg properly. Without stopping, and without missing a beat, he responded ...

"That's why I'm here, Black."

We were to discover that Tom's entire left side was affected. It was as if a string had tightened from his middle toe to his head. He had lost flexibility on that side with a limited range of motion in both limbs, and he no longer had full range of motion with his neck and head. The right side of his body seemed normal.

He was asked to lie on his stomach and switch his head, arms, and legs like a jumping jack toy. (He was asked to face his right hand and leg which were raised, his left arm and leg straight, then switch sides so that his head turned to face the left hand and leg, which were now raised, the right arm and leg straight.) He couldn't get on to his stomach. It took several minutes for him to figure out how to just lie down on the mat. It took three of us to help him complete the motion of switching sides, each of us in charge of legs, arms or head. His body would stiffen and we'd be faced with the task of manipulating each limb slowly in concert with the others in order to keep the movement continuous. We were able to complete the change of sides four times when he pushed us away and sat up.

"I don't know where I am in relationship to anything! If this is the way my life is to be, I don't want to live."

I stood there with tears streaming down my face feeling once again without hope. Tom and I weren't the only ones facing that reality. Eileen and Carol had anticipated Tom's arrival in the program with such hope themselves, especially after the phone conversations he'd had with them, that they too were taken aback by his profound impairments. Eileen would later confide in me that she felt so helpless after Tom's pronouncement that she almost burst into tears herself somehow believing she was failing him. She honestly didn't know which of us in that room she was trying to convince, herself included, as she tried to instill in Tom the necessity of a positive attitude.

"You mustn't give up before trying, Tom. So much depends on you and your attitude and we need your help in this as much as you want ours. None of us can do this alone. This has to be a team effort."

Tom evidently picked up on that nuance of the message in spite of his disappointment and fears because later that evening he *insisted* that I get 'Black' on the phone. He needed to talk to her and was persuasive enough to be given her home phone number. He told her not to feel bad, that he knew and appreciated what she was doing for him and that she mustn't give up on him. She and I were both excited the next day when we realized that instead of facing a tragedy we were facing a triumph. Tom had not only thought out the incident but had made a positive decision about his stay in the program.

The preliminary evaluation continued. None of it was encouraging. He could no longer count in sequence for more than two or three numbers before skipping ahead or starting over. He could raise his arm when asked, but he was unable to distinguish left from right and if asked to identify which limb was being touched, he could not. It was as if his brain had disassociated itself from his body and his sense of touch was of no more use to him in giving him the proper clues. I had a clearer understanding of why he was having so much difficulty dressing, and shaving, and everything else that allowed him to function as an independent person. Arms, legs and fingers can't respond to directions if the brain can't find them in the first place.

Eileen and Carol decided to put him on a patterning machine for at least an hour each day. He'd lie on his back, his arms and legs strapped to appendages that automatically simulated walking, with right arm in opposition to the left leg etc. The purpose of the machine was to stimulate left brain - right brain cross over. Meditation tapes were played while he was on the machine and the treatment was given in a darkened room. Sometimes Carol or Eileen would stay and talk softly with him, sometimes they just played soft music. They found he wouldn't tolerate any of the self awareness tapes they normally used.

I came to observe his first session. He had some difficulty getting himself on the machine. Our trying to help him only made matters worse because he couldn't follow direction and would stiffen in mid motion. He finally got himself set, the machine was started and a self-awareness tape was played. Eileen, Carol and I moved to the back room to confer while Tom hopefully, went into a meditation letting the machine do it's job. I could hear the tape droning in the background

"... I am a good person, I am a strong person, I am the best person I know. I can do anything I decide to do. I can reach deep down inside of me and pull my strength out. I can choose to make myself healthy. I am in charge of my life ..."

The tape had not been on for more than a minute when Tom began to bellow. We all ran in to see what was the matter thinking perhaps he had somehow caught himself in the mechanism. Instead he just yelled ...

"Will you turn that damn thing off?"

Eileen went over to him and said in her soft Scottish brogue ...

"Why, what's the matter Tom, it's only a tape to improve self image."

"If there is one thing, with w..w..hich I have never ha...ad a problem ... Black, it is ... my s.s.self ... image."

Eileen turned the tape off and spent the rest of the hour talking softly to him while I filled Carol in on what I thought made Tom tick. Tom made Tom tick.

Back at Oak House, dinner meant continued discussion of individual progress followed by our evening sessions in the living room which dealt with the interpretation of dreams and which taught us about visualization and its importance in our treatment. We also talked about finding our life path and facing our 'Judge' and we learned to feel our own energy and that our energy effected those about us.

We had group therapy every few nights, sessions that were often highly emotional. John, the therapist, had been trained in the Gestalt method, a form of treatment that is especially effective in short term programs and with groups. It gets to the core of a situation quickly so that it can be dealt with. We did role playing and other exercises associated with that method. It was very difficult to not be involved in what was happening to the people in that room, what was subsequently happening to all of us.

It was during one of those sessions that Tom explained why he was so afraid to let me out of his sight. John was talking about the importance of physical exercise when Tom interrupted.

"I run every day."

"That's good Tom. I'll bet that when you start, your body aches, but after a while you don't even feel it ... you forget about it."

"She's doing it now." (Pointing at me.)

"Beverly's running?"

"She sure is, I don't want to lose her before I die. I'd lose my partner, lose my life, and I don't want to be here if she's not with me ... I mean, you don't want your partner to die who's been doing all the work. Most men can't make a cup of coffee without help, and if she dies I'd have to start all over alone."

"Besides that you love her don't you, Tom."

"Damn right. We don't go anywhere alone. We go two by two or we don't go."

"So she is a significant part of your life."

"If I miss her for five minutes I'm afraid she's run away."

"Does she have reason to, Tom?"

"She sure does. She has a pretty tough job ... can you imagine ... months ... with me?"

People in the group laughed. They had watched the 'Tom and Beverly' act in progress. We not only went everywhere together but we showered together, we went to the rest room together, we dressed and walked, ran and sat together. The only time he was out of my sight was during his program and I was outside the door and often called in to participate with him or observe the video tapes that were made. Of course, they soon realized he needed help in doing most of the basics of life but they were also aware that there was no break for me. He could be very cute but he could also be very difficult. People asked me how I stood it all ... the needs, the closeness, the obsessiveness of it all, but then, on that occasion they saw him reach over and take my hand and tell me he loved me. That answered the question, at least for those people.

The weekend at the clinic was filled with music therapy, color therapy, dance therapy, and art therapy. Whatever means available to help people open up, deal with their fears and dissipate them was offered. Like it or not we were getting a crash course in self awareness and self acceptance

Tom's disability often made it difficult for him to participate. For example, he couldn't follow the aerobics in the morning so he used the time to practice his 'walk' while the rest of us did our exercises as a group. He was unable to participate in the art therapy session because he couldn't draw. It was too abstract a task and his left field void interfered. He took part in everything else as best he could.

He really seemed to enjoy the dance and color therapy session. Piles of colored fabric had been placed about the back yard. We were expected to choose a colored drape to play with while moving with the music. I felt extraordinarily silly as did most of us but as the morning wore on we all became less and less inhibited. I watched Tom, I always watched Tom. He pulled out a new color each time the music changed and went into his dance.

It was not my imagination that his 'dance' was like a strut or march. No matter what music was played he seemed to assume the persona of a Roman Senator, or King, or Chief. There was no mistaking his sense of himself, Tom was holding court. I will never forget the image of him moving across the yard, his left hand grasping a purple cloth over his right shoulder, the end of it dragging behind him as if a train, his gaze over the heads of us all, his walk purposeful and definite, and how those who were in his way moved out of his way as he glided past.

Dr. McGarey questioned Tom about his feelings during that exercise and Tom was quite at a loss to reply. He had difficulty with the abstract nature of the question and didn't understand what the doctor was trying to draw out of him. Dr. McGarey finally asked others in the group to give their impressions of Tom's 'walk' and to explain why they moved out of his way. It was an interesting session for everyone. At one point Dr. McGarey asked Tom if he viewed himself as a strong person, Tom responded ... "Hell, yes."

[Does the sun rise?]

In 1972, Bell Equipment Corp. was purchased by James Ling. Ling was one of the 'Wonder-boys' in his day. He had come from nowhere, he had built a conglomerate out of nothing, he controlled vast corporations and was capable of playing hardball with the best of them. He had bested a fair number by the time he purchased Bell Equipment and was already something of a legend in his field. Tom became C.E.O. of Bell and a member of the Board of Directors when this purchase went through.

Jim O'Leary, one of Tom's friends, told me that Ling hadn't met Tom prior to Bell's purchase, but Tom's reputation had preceded him as it always did. Tom's responsibilities in the new hierarchy included periodic reports to Ling personally but that first meeting was not to be set up for a time due to the logistics of the changeover.

Ling secretly assigned one of his men, whose sole purpose was to watch Tom. Obviously the secret didn't last for long and Tom, if he noted it, gave it the attention it deserved ... none! As the time neared for Tom to finally confer with Ling, O'Leary was approached by the 'secret agent' who voiced his concerns about that meeting. O'Leary said ...

"I doubt that Tom has anything to be worried about."

"It's not Tom that concerns me."

"Well, who are you concerned about?"

"It's Ling. I'm afraid that Tom's going to give him an inferiority complex."

Sunday evening, the fourth night of the program, Dr. McGarey talked to us about embracing the treatment we were receiving with love. As long as we continued to think of treatment of any sort, be it chemotherapy, surgery, diet or a simple castor oil pack as being bothersome or hateful, it's chances of working were diminished. We were being faced with diets that were difficult to deal with, and treatments and approaches that were foreign to many of us and in some ways emotionally threatening. He made the point, that as long as we approached treatment as a necessary evil instead of a positive and curative thing then we were resisting taking charge of the illness. It was the taking charge that could make the difference.

That night, I gave Tom his massage as usual. I then placed his castor oil pack over his abdomen, put on some meditative music to listen to prior to our going to sleep and was about to crawl into bed with him when he started to bellow out loud ...

"I....JUST...LOVE......MY...CASTOR..OIL......PACK...."

[The 'pack' was a holistic treatment required of everyone in the program. It reportedly removed toxins from the system, had a soothing effect on the neurological system, and it was an integral part of the A.R.E. Clinic program. It was the subject of some complaint and some giddiness as everyone tried to figure out the best time to use it and the easiest way to clean it off after the treatment was finished. Castor oil is not easy to get off the skin and if not washed off will attach itself to clothing and sheets. Given the full nature of each day's itinerary it seemed to be the last thing everyone did before going to bed. Some of us were still dealing with it at midnight each night.]

As Tom's voice finished bellowing, the cry was picked up by others in the house and before the night finally came to an end there had been a great deal of laughter. That night was to mark a turning point in Tom's treatment.

I am walking down the street. It is a street in New York, near where I live. There are often homeless people around my apartment and although I am aware of them, I don't often pay attention to them because, in doing so, they ask for money. I find a man lying in a doorway. He is obviously in bad shape. He is hurt and he can't speak. I think perhaps he has been beaten up and when I get closer I have the feeling that I have known him from somewhere.

I manage to get someone to call an ambulance and I stay with him until the paramedics arrive. They take one look at the man and refuse to help him. They want to leave but I won't let them. I take their names, their license numbers, I take the names of witnesses around me and finally I bully them into taking him to the hospital and to make sure he gets there I go with them.

At the hospital the same thing happens. The doctor there refuses to admit him.

"The man is a bum, he is of no use to anybody anymore, he is better off dead."

I warn the doctor that I am not someone to fool with. They are not to put him on the street again, and they are to wait until I return. I go upstairs to the top floor and I demand to see the administrator. The man is quite sarcastic to me. He will not agree to admit this man.
"The man has no insurance, he is a nobody!"
I tell the administrator:
"I am his insurance. I will assume all responsibility for this man ... You see ... he used to be somebody."

═══════════════════════

When Tom awoke that Monday morning he announced he'd had a dream. I picked up my journal and wrote as he spoke. There was some stammering and some repetition but it is above, essentially as he told it. It was the most complete telling of a story he had given in over a year. After he related the dream to the others at breakfast, Dr. McGarey asked Tom what he thought the dream was about. Tom responded ...

"Me. I am that man. The only one who can help me is Tom Murphy."

His eyes filled with tears and through those tears he said ...

"I'm going to get well."

From that point on Tom attacked his therapy with a vengeance. By the end of the seventeen days he had progressed to the point where he could now recognize every item he was given to identify by touch. This was not because of familiarity with the objects but because his concentration had improved and signals to his brain were being read more correctly. His ability to find the words had improved as had his speech and expression in general.

He was able to read every flash card without hesitation. He could now follow a light with both his eyes and his convergence had improved slightly. The eye exercise took about five minutes to complete and what had started out as arduous and time consuming was now completed without any interruption in the flow.

He could now crawl from one end of the mat to the other without going off even with the yellow line side of the mat up. He still dragged his left leg somewhat, but this had also improved and there was more flexibility on his left side. He was now able to get on his stomach by himself, and he could roll over without any assistance. He still needed some assistance in coordinating his legs, arms, and head, when switching position from one side to the other, but he could now manage the changes in position with only light touch on my part, and some of his movement was totally spontaneous.

He was beginning to identify his body parts by touch. He had a walking exercise which he could do on his own in the yard without any supervision which helped him force left brain-right brain crossover, and he was able to count to over thirty without interruption.

One day, about mid way through our stay in Phoenix I realized that we were actually having a conversation ... not me trying to finish thoughts hung in space, but a real conversation. I had taken him to see "Moonstruck". It was the first movie we had ventured into in months. Normally, the noise, the crowd, the darkness all conspired to rob him of his concentration and we'd end up leaving long before the picture ended. The theater was packed but I managed to get us aisle seats so that we could make our exit without too much bother to others. About twenty minutes into the film, Tom started to laugh out loud. A loud boisterous laugh. His laugh. It was a scene in which most of the characters, all of whom were just a tad bizarre, had gathered into the kitchen, and their interactions were hilarious. I looked at Tom as if he had just landed from outer space.

"You're laughing."

"Yeah!"

"Why? What's funny about it?" I couldn't believe he had gotten the joke.

He pointed at the screen and very softly said ...

"I know those people." ... and leaning in closer to my ear he said, "... in fact, ... we are those people." That comment followed by a broad smile and yet another laugh, this one shared with me.

I was taken aback by the almost profound interpretation of our life, while tears predictably filled my eyes. We were about to recover much of our social life. We could talk about what we saw on television, and what I read in the newspaper, and who we met on the street, and at the clinic. You don't know how much those things are missed until they are gone, and they were back along with that trademark spring in his step. To be able to laugh with him was probably the best part of this transformation because it was Tom's humor as much as anything else that had drawn me to him in the first place. I don't mean to imply that we lived happily ever after on a cloud of bliss, he could still be as stubborn as ever, but it was more in terms of his own personality and less in terms of a trapped organism.

He affected everyone he touched at the clinic. His personality and his determination turned a potentially depressing experience into a happening that very few will forget who worked with us. He made such progress that he was often asked to demonstrate his accomplishments after tapes of initial evaluation were shown and he became a source of encouragement for many people considering the program there. He was also known to present more than one reality check in the process. One such incident springs to mind.

One day during the last of our stay in Phoenix, Lindsay Wagner arrived. The whole place was abuzz and I, who always got a kick out of meeting celebrities, was really looking forward to meeting her. She had been a supporter of holistic treatment for years and was considering making a documentary about the clinic. During her tour she was introduced to Tom who, experiencing the stress of an unexpected crowd of people in his therapy room, went into a familiar mode. Noise and activity took over and he was unable to focus on who was talking to him, what was being said, and who to respond to. When Ms. Wagner was introduced to Tom he not only didn't respond to the introduction, he couldn't find her in his visual field, even though she was standing right in front of him. It was extremely awkward, with several people repeating on top of each other's voices who she was. She tried to say hello to him in order to get his attention but her voice was lost in the noise of everyone else's. During a momentary lull, Tom, still trying to find who they were talking about asked . . .

"Who? Where? I don't see anyone."

Someone, trying to jog his memory of this famous person standing in front of him finally offered, with a combination of panic and embarrassment in the voice . . .

"You know Lindsay Wagner, the television star, ... you know ... The Bionic Woman." (A characterization Ms. Wagner would probably have liked to remain in her body of work rather than surface as a definition of who she was.)

Tom turned towards the voice and said ... "The Bionic What?"

All of us, including Lindsay, were stifling a giggle. The whole situation was too, too priceless. The fact is, as I explained to everyone standing there, Tom hadn't forgotten who she was, he really didn't know who she was. He didn't know who Robert Redford was either, having had a similar experience with him on a plane headed for Alaska some years earlier.

I can't help but wonder what Redford thought when Tom wondered why so many people in the plane wanted to take pictures of the back of his head, obviously missing that the pictures were being aimed at Robert Redford. And I can't help but wonder what sort of amazement traveled through Redford's mind when Tom asked him who he was after Redford apologized for the intrusion.

"Oh, they're taking pictures of you. Are you someone?"

"Well yes, my name is Robert Redford. I'm on my way to Alaska. My movie is opening there."

"Oh, you're an actor? Have you done anything I might have seen?"

Redford's most recent movie was *All The President's Men*. Tom announced he had read the book but he rarely went to movies and launched into his favorite subject which was politics. The ensuing conversation resulting in Redford inviting Tom to his resort in Utah to ski with him and Tom arranging for him to get a tour of the pipe line.

[For the record, Tom also didn't know that *Singing In The Rain* had been a movie long before it was a Broadway play. When Tom talked about movie musicals, the dancers he was referring to were Fred Astair and George Raft. Everything that happened after that time period was out of his frame of reference. And it wasn't because he looked down on the entertainment industry, it was because he had a life that isolated him from the world apart from his work.]

Nearing the end of our stay in Phoenix, Tom's biofeedback therapist asked me to sit in on one of his final sessions. Tom was hooked up to a machine that beeped in varying degrees of loudness and speed depending on the level of relaxation attained. The therapist generally spoke throughout the session directing the patient to relax, first the eye lids, the face muscles, the neck muscles, shoulder muscles, etc., through the entire body. As the body began to relax the beeping sound would lower in timber and in speed. The sound gave the patient a measure of how they were doing. The patient could feel the bodily changes, come to recognize them, and bring about that physical state at will. There would reach the point when the patient could actually take control of the sound level of the machine and move it up or down at will.

During my sessions I was able to maintain a fairly low steady sound after ten minutes, but this was after a number of sessions. Tom was hooked up to the machine and the therapist began:

"I want you to relax Tom."

I then saw Tom close his eyes and I heard the beep go steadily lower and slower until it finally went silent. It stayed silent until fifteen minutes had passed and the therapist said ...

"Your session is over Tom."

At that point the machine started a faint but steady rhythmic sound until it was turned off and Tom was unhooked. The therapist asked me if I found that experience amazing. He felt this was not something Tom had learned in his care but rather an ability that Tom always had. Tom's ability to sleep in any circumstance came to mind. Apparently those cat naps that he was famous for weren't just cat naps. Tom could manifest REM sleep at will.

His personal counselor was to assure me that Tom was one of the more centered people he had ever met. When he had been handed Tom's case he remembered thinking this was going to be someone with wagon loads of detritus. He thought, no wonder he's sick. With his history, his stress level, his family losses etc., etc., there was no doubt that aspects of his illness were probably stress related. Instead, he found Tom to be extremely effective in getting rid of unwanted baggage. He did not carry grudges, he did not hold on to disappointments, he seemed to have found a way to deal with those things effectively and keep them in perspective. He said he could well understand why Tom was so effective in business, he didn't cloud his thinking with unnecessary junk. The sessions he had with Tom were open, honest, and to the point at hand in spite of Tom's deficits. He assured me that Tom had no fears of his mortality and he was very much at peace with himself in terms of how he had conducted his life. If Tom was fearful of anything it was that I would be all right if he died first. Tom felt I should be made aware of that and he had given permission to share the counseling sessions with me.

Tom no longer sat in the back row during the evening sessions but in fact sought the circle moving his chair each evening until he was seated directly opposite the therapist. He stayed in that position in the circle until the last session when he actually sat in the therapist's chair and had to be asked to move. He moved next to him. His behavior during that last session reminded me of pictures I had of Tom during his South East Asian Tour as a representative for the State Department and as a consultant in the re-development of the Mekong Basin after the Vietnam War. He had conducted a seminar on a proposed dam site in the Pa Mong. Watching Tom that last night in Oak House was like watching a replay of those photographs. The body language was the same.

He had changed from a listless sitting back posture with fixed vacuous eyes, which was very evident during those first days in the program, to a body that leaned into the discussion. His arms and hands moved with motion and purpose. He sat in a confident manner, his foot over his knee, his stance open, and ready for battle. His eyes were now focused and sharp, his speech was more fluid, his ideas more complete.

When I started writing this book, I listened to the tapes that were made during the evening sessions at the clinic. I heard the changes in Tom's voice and comprehension as those seventeen days passed. He sounded so damn hopeful, so happy. I suppose there are those who feel the changes had rational explanations. Tom was getting a lot of positive attention and feedback. He was being told he was still in charge of his life, and encouraged at every turn by people he respected. And so he was able to rise to his optimum level of functioning, a level devoid of depression, and fear, and aggravation, and loneliness, but a level which would eventually be compromised by his illness no matter what he did. At the very least, we were given some time back. Or, he actually had a shot at turning it all around as a result of all those positive things. From this perspective, if anyone feels the need to ask if I thought the experience was worth it. I can only say, I would go back in a New York Second if I had it to do over.

[A New York Second is the time it takes the driver behind you to beep his horn after the light turns green.]

There were changes in everyone.

Vicki seemed to have rid herself of a great burden. Her husband started to refer to their children as his children and although we all noticed that change Vicki seemed not to react. He received a job offer while we were there which meant they'd have to move, something that could be devastating for her. She insisted he take the job. During that time her color returned and she seemed more content and peaceful. She and her husband usually sat as near as possible to Cassie and they'd dissolve in laughter through most of the evening. I never heard from them again after the program ended but I will never forget the sound of her laughter and the joy that was so much a part of her those last days we shared together.

Hilda went into remission. During those seventeen days we became friends and she and Tom spoke German together and laughed a lot. The third day of the program she broke out in color, her clothes, her skin, her eyes. There was no mistaking the color and spark in Hilda's expression and countenance. She seemed to radiate light. She died a year after the end of the program. Her husband said she had done extremely well until a few days before her death. I will never forget her peace or her eloquence, or his.

Cassie stopped leaving the evening sessions mid-way through the first week and no longer carried the ice pack with her. She was pain free by the end of the seventeen days and the infection inside her face was beginning to clear up, the tissue taking on a healthy look. She decided to relocate to Arizona.

Chucky's behavior improved dramatically as long as he kept on schedule with his castor oil packs and stuck to his diet which eliminated all sugar, artificial sweeteners, color, and starch. We were to find out that there was a direct correlation between his behavior and his mother's ability to resist sneaking out for pizza and soda. When she dove off the diet, so did Chucky. It got so we knew which days had been good days for her and which days had not by Chucky's behavior. We all felt that Barbara was the one who really needed the program.

[Sometimes the magic works, sometimes it doesn't.]

That last night of the program, the subject of assertiveness was dealt with. It was of little surprise that assertiveness was a problem for most people there. With the program drawing to a close we were now facing the return home. We were leaving a supportive and loving community for home and relationships that were unchanged. How were we going to deal with it all? How would we handle the response to our new attitudes about ourselves and the changes that had happened to each of us ? Tom's attitude was offered as an example of how to make yourself heard. It was agreed by everyone that Tom was not someone you ignored for long. Tom offered that you simply have to mean what you say. "If people don't like what I have to say, they can screw it."

Susan stood and spoke. She openly expressed her fears of returning home. She talked about her experience at the clinic and how she had come to realize how important it was for her to stop feeling she must meet everyone's needs but her own. She was still grieving for her husband, she was worried about her children, she was concerned for her grandchildren, she let her mother have too much influence on just about every decision she made about her treatment from the moment she got sick and she was beginning to wonder if cancer had been the only way she could find to finally take the steps to assert herself. She had started by coming to this program against her mother's wishes. She needed to say the words out loud.

"I am the only one who counts in this life of mine, my life is all I have left." She pointed at the empty chair in which her mother symbolically sat and said ... "I don't care if you agree with what I've decided to do. If you don't like it you can screw it."

We were elated at the tone in her voice and the body language which telegraphed her resolve. She was also a little taken aback by her choice of words which made us laugh and cheer even harder. She turned to Tom and said ...

"I need to be more like you, Tom. You're so in charge of your life. I'm glad you were here with me. I think I can say 'no' now without feeling I've hurt someone's feelings. My feelings matter, too."

At that point Tom stood ...

"That's right, you just tell them all to go screw it, and if you need any help doing that you just call me up and I'll fly out here and tell them for you."

Everyone laughed and Tom and Susan hugged. Our therapist who was laughing with the rest of us wondered if perhaps Tom had come up with a new therapy mode. He called it the 'Tom Murphy Screw It School Of Counseling'. We were all in stitches from laughing so hard.

We learned a few months later that Susan not only went into remission but there seems to be no evidence of cancer. Her oncologist has no explanation. I had occasion to see her some six months after the program and she looked great. Her face was in a constant smile, her eyes bright, her body language the language of success. She was organizing a support group for spontaneous recovery patients who were having a hard time dealing with doctors, friends and family who couldn't accept her sudden wellness. To make matters even more wonderful, her arthritis is also gone. She remarried in 1989.

To say there was an element of sadness mixed with unspoken feelings of dread as everyone said goodbye the next morning would be an understatement. We had become a very close knit group during those seventeen days.

Tom had done so well and we had been so encouraged by his progress that we decided to stay for an additional six weeks of treatment. His improvement continued during that period. I knew he had it all in hand when he made an appointment to see Dr. McGarey to 'discuss an important issue'. He asked Dr. McGarey what his plans were for the clinic. Did he wish to make it larger or was he content with it as it was? Dr. M. asked him why? Tom responded ...

"There are lots of people out there like myself who have been turned off to their doctors and their treatment, who are offered no hope, and who have nowhere else to turn. This place is a place for them to go, but how do they find out about it? If it hadn't been for my sister-in-law I wouldn't have known about it myself. What your clinic needs is a good marketing person. Would you be interested in hiring me?"

Dr. McGarey asked Tom if he really felt ready for that kind of assignment just yet. Tom admitted that no, perhaps he wasn't ready just yet, but that didn't negate the fact that the clinic needed someone if it was to reach its population. Six months later we received a letter from the clinic introducing their new Marketing person. Tom felt very gratified that he might have had a part in that decision.

When we finally left Phoenix it would be with plans of returning once a year until Tom was completely well.

THOMAS MURPHY   **Division of Neurology**
DATE OF EXAMINATION September 2, 1988   **L.P.B., M.D.**

This is a return visit for Mr. Murphy, who suffered a most unusual progressive dementing illness. Since I last saw him, he participated in an intensive neuro-rehabilitation program. The results have been remarkable. His speech and memory seem clearly improved. He is still very aphasic and does not know the day, but his social responses are far better than they were before and his conversation more fluent ...

IMPRESSIONS: Perhaps he had suffered an encephalitis and was never fully rehabilitated. We will need to observe him and see if he progresses. That is really the acid test of all this. I think we can still not make a firm diagnosis. I know that I thought perhaps he had Pick's Disease, but I cannot believe that improvement and stabilization are consistent with that diagnosis. We will see him again in 6 months.

On the side Dr. B. offered ...

"Beverly, tell me what you think, do you see a difference in Tom?"

I felt threatened by the question and for a moment I expected ridicule. I launched into my list of what I saw as improvement in Tom, taking on the anticipated argument. About mid way through my tirade Dr. B.'s hand went up in the air as if to signal 'stop'. I stopped talking and took a breath.

"Why are you asking me that question?"

"Because ... I don't know what happened at that clinic Beverly, but I will say this ... whatever you did there, keep on doing it. This sort of improvement just does not happen."

MORE THAN YOU KNOW

More than you know, more than you know
Man O' my heart, I love you so ...
Lately I find, You're on my mind
 More than you know ...

Whether you're right, whether you're wrong
Man O' my heart I'll string along
You need me so
 More than you'll ever know ...

Loving you the way that I do
There's nothing I can do about it.
Loving may be all you can give
 but, honey, I can't live without it ...

Oh how I'd cry, oh how I'd cry
If you got tired and said "goodbye"
More than I'd show
 More than you'll ever know ...

words by: Billy Rose & Ed Eliscu *music by: Vincent Youmans*

CHAPTER TEN

In spite of the improvements Tom made at the clinic, his inability to function in the presence of stress was an ever present fact of life. It took relatively little to send him into a tailspin which always resulted in total shut down. The flight home from Phoenix would provide all the elements of stress so detrimental to people dealing with brain damage, stroke, and dementia and Tom responded accordingly.

The cramped space of the airplane, the noise, problems with moving him over and around people both on the plane and off conspired to rob him of any control. He was terribly disoriented through the whole trip. I told the steward to just bring one tray at a time when food was served knowing Tom was not going to be able to juggle the utensils without help. When Tom's tray was taken away, the mess cleared and mine set down, Tom then announced he had to go to the bathroom. The following sequence of movements necessary to get him into the cubicle they called a rest room on the plane ruined what was left of my appetite and I settled for a can of soda instead. By the time we landed in Houston he was beyond reason.

The airport itself offered nothing but confusion for him. Between the hard surfaces which made sound bounce all over the place, his visual problems, the crowd noise and movement, and his fear of being lost, getting him from the plane, to the luggage, to the taxi was a nightmare. The ordeal would involve my trying to juggle three suitcases, my purse, a carry-on tote, and Tom. He couldn't distinguish my voice from other sounds nor could he follow the simplest of directions such as 'wait here' and 'don't move.' I had to make sure I was physically touching him at all times and that the sound of my voice was constantly in his ear in order for him to keep his orientation.

If both senses weren't constantly reinforced he went into a panic. That panic consisted of immediate movement as he began his search to find me again, a search profoundly affected by his hearing and visual deficits. If I let go of him to pick up a suitcase he was gone by the time I turned around. I couldn't leave him alone long enough to go to the ladies room unless I was ready to launch a full scale search of the airport for him. It never occurred to me to ask for airport assistance for the handicapped. For some reason I still didn't think of Tom as handicapped. How could I not know his special needs qualified for handicapped assistance? I'd had 25 years working with handicapped people. There was no real reason for my having been so blind as to not know assistance was available, but then I was also exhausted.

The scene had to have been noticeable to everyone, in fact I know it was obvious that we were having problems because the crowds parted like the Red Sea as we moved through the airport. One man made some crack about us drinking too much. No one offered to help. Just picking up the luggage was an ordeal. When the air cap told me I couldn't leave the luggage carousel without showing her our ticket stubs, which were buried in the bottom of my purse, I just started to cry, all the while holding on to Tom with my one free hand while trying to find a kleenex with my other. After looking at Tom and seeing what I was dealing with she waved us on. He never stopped moving until I got him into the taxi for the ride home.

I was frankly depressed at the thought of having to return to Houston. After all those weeks of interaction and attention, Houston held all the intrinsic appeal of prison. We were already lonely and we hadn't even unpacked yet. Our next door neighbors, waiters in restaurants and an occasional chat with the clergy on our way out of Mass, were the sum total of our social life. Other than those moments our life was pretty much just the two of us. I feared it would take us a while to get back into the swing of things. We ordered a pizza when we got home, put on a meditation tape after eating, wrapped our arms around each other after climbing into bed and slept the entire night in that position.

Tom was up before me and raring to go. He decided to do his exercise program twice a day instead of once, reasoning that he'd get better twice as fast. I'm not sure I was overjoyed at this declaration, but we had nothing else to do with our time and Tom was so enthusiastic I thought, why not join in his enthusiasm.

For the next few months we began each morning with Tom's program which took about an hour, and then we'd repeat it again late in the afternoon. The morning sessions were always better than the afternoon ones. We started with his eye exercises which involved following the movement of a brightly colored object with one eye and then the other. Then we'd repeat the exercise with both eyes. There were other tasks he had to complete while sitting in his chair and then we'd move to the floor routines.

He'd lay on a rug. I'd put on soft music and we'd start with a meditation. Then I'd lift Tom's right hand, stroke it and ask him to identify it. I'd wait for him to identify his right hand and then focus on his finger, his wrist, the palm of his hand etc. Then I'd move my touch up his arm to his elbow, and then the shoulder. If he missed the body part I was holding, I provided further clues as to function and position such as ...

"This part lets you bend your arm, it is called ..."

And sometimes the clue would trigger the proper word 'elbow'. Sometimes it wouldn't. If he was still unable to find the proper word I'd give it to him and have him repeat it after me before moving on. This process was done on both right limbs, then repeated on the left limbs. The point of the exercise was to reacquaint his brain with his body and help it relearn to distinguish left from right. I hoped to therefore improve his ability to coordinate his movements in simple things like dressing and handling eating utensils, etc. For some reason he always had difficulty connecting with elbows and knees when other parts of his body were recognized immediately. He finished the program with his jumping jack exercise which also helped him coordinate movement and then we'd shower, dress and go out to breakfast.

He was always concerned about how he had done and if I'd seen improvement. It was minimal, but it often seemed like it was improvement. His speed and accuracy gradually improved and he was always so delighted when I noted it to him. He'd ask the same questions over throughout the day ...

"How'd I do, Beverly?"

"You did fine, Tom."

"Was it better than the last time?"

"I think it was."

"Do you think we should do it more often? Maybe I'll get better faster."

"I think more wouldn't help. Let's keep it the way the clinic told us to do it."

"Should we call Black and ask?"

"No, Tom."

And on and on it would go. Always the same, sometimes for 15 or 20 minutes, while I tried to keep my enthusiasm level intact. It was as if he had concocted some sort of test for me to pass. I'm not sure if it was designed to drive me crazy or whether he just needed that much reassurance. Probably a little bit of both. Then again, maybe the truth seeped through no matter how I tried to disguise it, and maybe he knew we were both making believe it was more so than it was.

[No one ever stops to consider the complexities involved in movement. Something as uninspiring as rolling over from your back to your stomach involves many independent movements all of which are choreographed by the brain. Masses of muscles and sinews and nerves all taking direction from one main source of power. Which way does the arm move, what direction do you shift your hip and is it the left or right hip, or is it both hips moving in concert with each other? What muscles connect to what? When the connectors that compute those moves are severed there is little that is ever simple in your life again. It's not that someone with Alzheimer's actually forgets how to do those things, it's more that the mind can't find the information floating around in their brain to enable them to do those things. Often, until the very last stage of this illness, skills return intermittently. A woman I know told me her husband started walking again after being completely wheel chair bound for over two years. Which, given the expectation that muscles and sinews would atrophy, leads me to wonder how that could happen, but it did. Tom would suddenly click into gear and accomplish tasks he hadn't been able to do unassisted for months. The little spurt of skill never lasted for any length of time but it led me to believe that this illness was much more complicated than I first thought and the words *'they forget how to'*, maybe should be rethought or expressed differently. It's the *forgot* part of it that bothers me. *Misplaced* seems to be a better choice. If the former holds, then Tom *forgot* more than many people ever learn.]

The fact that Tom was unable to follow a direction as simple as 'roll over from your stomach to your back', before we went to Phoenix, and he could do it now with relative ease was phenomenal. To not have had the imagination or the sensitivity to recognize his achievement would have been to deflate any enthusiasm he had left. I could easily have fallen into the trap of measuring the distance of how far Tom had fallen and given up before he even tried to recover some of that distance. I decided that as long as he was willing to try, I was willing to help him try and I cheered him on. Boy, did I cheer him on! As long as he believed he was doing better, he actually seemed to be better. He was speaking clearer and his eyes were more focused. That was proof enough that something was working if it was only the result of undivided attention from me.

I never did take the steps to hire anyone to help Tom with his program. However, I did take steps to find a lawyer so that we could find out just how vulnerable we were going to be financially if Tom started to slide again. Something else the clinic people in Phoenix had urged us to do -- I called the Alzheimer's Association and asked for a referral to a lawyer well versed in estate problems associated with dementing illness. They gave me three names. We chose the one nearest our address.

We were told that with the new laws, the spousal home would be safe. If it was listed in my name only the house would not be touched by Medicaid or Tom's 'debt' at all. If it was listed jointly under Tom's and my name the worst scenario is that Tom's half might face a lien, but Medicaid would still not force me to sell the house or move. We had been misinformed on that point. We were also told that as long as all our accounts were jointly held whatever money left in them at the time of Tom's death would automatically go to me. A will wasn't necessary and probate would not be involved. The lawyer told us that Tom was correct in that assumption and it was the wisest thing he could have done under the circumstances. He neglected to tell us to get a power of attorney signed. I think he may have assumed we had done it already.

He told us it was in our best interest to close Tom's retirement funds now because Tom was over 60, he was no longer working, our income was low enough to absorb the additional income on our upcoming tax return, and we could avoid the need to establish a guardianship at that time. Considering that Tom might not improve, waiting would only complicate that task. He also felt that Tom understood the reasons why that act was necessary since Tom was able to participate in the discussion.

We were cautioned against keeping investments in long term programs because we wouldn't want to tie up funds that might be needed for Tom's care. He encouraged us to separate our joint funds into individual accounts so that a precedent might be established in the event that laws changed and funds could be secured in my name for my future and not subjected to Medicaid reimbursement. He also emphasized the need to avoid total impoverishment prior to Tom's going into a nursing home, because the welfare homes that took Medicaid exclusively were notoriously awful. As it stood at that time, if there were enough funds to cover three years of private care, and that facility also took Medicaid funding, then at the end of those three years, if the patient now met impoverishment levels, that facility would continue to care for that person under Medicaid sponsorship.

Keeping the above scenario in mind, it is ironic that children of long term care patients are able to take control of an estate and protect the funds in that estate for their own eventual use, but spouses are not. Children are not held accountable for the continuing care of a disabled parent. The spouse of the disabled person on the other hand, is responsible for that person's care until death or impoverishment as long as funds exist in their names or the well spouse's name.

The current laws that allow tax free transfers of money to children under these circumstances only serve to cheat the tax paying public and provides a bottomless pit of potential abuses amongst family members. With several children in a family and tax free transfers of $10,000 to each a year, $20,000 if both parents contribute, over a three year period that amounts to a considerable cache out of reach of nursing home fees or the well spouse. For families with some resources but not enough to satisfy all the needs of parental care, and inheritance assumptions, made at a time when life was different, one can easily imagine the problems that can arise.

I had no expectations of living high on the hog from the estate after Tom died. If all the assets remained in our possession through our marriage I doubted there would be much left after he died. But I did feel it was fair to expect the house would be mine, which is what Tom promised me, and that the rest of what was left, shared between his children and me.

The problems with the estate were beginning to escalate and I felt particularly vulnerable. I was waking up each morning in a panic over what my future would be like if Tom really did have Alzheimer's Disease. It was a lousy way to feel in the midst of the kind of care and attention he already needed. The dichotomy of this scenario is that thoughts about having all the funds in the estate used to meet his care needs didn't seem to raise the same fears in me. It was the thought of not being able to provide the care I wanted him to have that left me in a panic. The thought of being forced to place him in a nursing home was not a choice I wanted to make. I kept passing the milestones in his care as his needs changed and was beginning to feel I just might be able to do it all, as long as I could afford help. I wanted him to be able to die in his own bed amongst the things he loved and I wanted to be there with him, not called in the middle of the night and informed of his passing.

I also know that Tom didn't want any part of a nursing home. He asked me more than once if I was going to "put him away". As time passed and Tom's ability to express himself in words diminished, he demonstrated his vehement feelings about being moved away from me in other ways. After we relocated to Boulder and after two short hospitalizations for psychiatric overload, he would bounce around in the car seat yelling every time I drove by a hospital or the medical center where his doctors practiced, glaring at me and gesticulating dramatically. He didn't have a clue as to what our new address was in Boulder, but if I took a different route to the diner where we had our morning breakfast, he was furious until we pulled into the parking lot. It took me weeks to figure out what was triggering his tantrums, tantrums that started the moment I went in a direction different from the one we normally took. A look of panic would take over his face, he would start twitching in his seat, banging the dashboard with his hand while shouting *NO!*, over and over.

During the last office visit we had with his neurologist in Boulder, (she started making house calls after that,) it took three male aides to get him to submit to his examination and to draw the blood we needed to check on his B12 levels which were being periodically monitored after he showed a profound B12 deficiency. I had used an ambulance carrier van to transport him from our home to the doctor's office because it was impossible to get him in the car during that period, and I had all I could do to keep him contained after his tests while we waited for the van to arrive. He was combative, anxious, and intensely into his moving mode. Finally I figured out what might be happening and I assured him we were going home.

"My home?"

"Yes, your home."

"Okay."

His entire demeanor changed. He started doing the cute little things he normally did, flirting with me and being generally darling to whomever passed by. He walked up the ramp to the van unassisted when it arrived with no further incident and even waved to the male aide who had accompanied us to the door to help me contain him. He was well into the last stages of Alzheimer's Disease by then and he wasn't supposed to have any such awareness of his surroundings.

I recall an early time in our life together. We were running up 5th Avenue in New York. We had been talking about marriage and it was before the onslaught of doctors entered our lives. I knew Tom had some little quirks but neither of us had an idea that he was facing the life we'd both be facing in just a few months. An elderly woman shuffled from the apartment entrance we were approaching to a waiting cab. Tom stopped to ask if she needed help. The companion who was with her, also elderly, thanked Tom for offering. When we continued on our way, Tom turned to me and said ...

"If ever get like that I want you to put me in a home and forget about me. Better yet ... shoot me."

The reality of that remark is that when the time came, when nursing home placement was a consideration, Tom clung tenaciously to what was home to him. He wanted no part of being torn away from what was left of his life.

I have heard other caregivers share similar incidents with me during my support group meetings. One woman was in tears of relief when she told us her husband had given her permission to put him in a home "when the time comes". Most of us looked on sympathetically. One man remarked ...

"Well, yes they say that. But I don't think they really mean that. I've said that myself, but the truth is I *would* rather die first."

We launched into a discussion trying to figure out what our loved ones really mean when those words are spoken. Who do we believe, our loved ones or our hearts? We came to the conclusion that regardless of what our people state, it is really up to the caregiver to make the decision. It really rests on what he or she can handle and what they can live with that matters.

A Rabbi I met after a talk I gave about caregiving at a local Senior Center, told me that when she hears her elder congregation members talking about not wanting to be a burden to their children, what she really hears is their fear of dying alone and unloved.

I agreed that the *"being a burden"* phrase is really over rated as a statement to be taken literally. People make those comments before they are faced with the horror that something devastating might actually happen to them someday. It's not a demand for action, it's a subliminal plea to the cosmos to not have to face that particular trial in their lives and a basic fear that the people they will have to depend upon will abandon them. Too many people are using those words to justify what really feels like abandonment to their loved ones. And too many who act on those words are finding that they feel as if they *have* abandoned them. This Rabbi offered that she spends more time dealing with the guilt that envelops the nursing home decision than she does counseling families about facing the loss and the grief they also feel.

[There is a moment in the movie *"Fire in the Dark"*, when Olympia Dukakis, who plays a widowed, frail woman reflecting on her own mortality, says to her adult daughter, played by Lindsay Wagner ... "I'm not afraid of dying, what I'm afraid of is what happens to me before I die."]

I doubt that Tom in his wildest dreams could have imagined outliving his brain when he spoke those words. He had no idea of what was yet ahead of him. He thought, or at least hoped, he'd leave his life working full speed in some corner of the world, making piles of money and grand decisions at the age of ninety, having suffered a massive cerebral hemorrhage, in his sleep, preferably after great sex. How could he possibly envision the ignominy of the death he was facing?

As for the reality of placing Tom in any nursing home, the crude fact is there wasn't a nursing home within range of our home that would have taken him when his nightly wanderings and combativeness set it unless he was drugged into submissiveness. There wasn't one Alzheimer's unit in the area. By the time he became docile enough to be acceptable to a facility, I'd already been through the worst of his illness. As for justifying his placement after he no longer knew who I was, or because he needed to be diapered, well, those were landmarks in his care that somehow turned out to be not such a big deal to me. I find those aren't the reasons most people make nursing home placements anyway. They place their people because they just can't do it any longer alone. They just are too worn out from the stress. There aren't a lot of options being offered to people.

[Making the nursing home choice is not simple. The support groups are filled with people wrestling with having had to make that decision. The feelings of abandonment and grief that face spouses and children being forced to renege on what might be characterized as spiritual commitments to love and cherish a spouse, or to honor and give back what has been received from a parent, often leave caregivers with a sense of failure no matter how irrational those feelings are in the face of what continuing to care for them at home alone means.

Circumstances do not always allow for loved ones to be kept at home. Having observed the angst that goes into making that decision leads me to wonder if the *Golden Rule* isn't more deeply ingrained in our cellular structure than many of us would like to believe. Maybe there needs to be heightened awareness of this phenomena. Maybe people need assurance on a deeper level than the surface reasons of the care being too hard, too involved, and too draining. To say to Mom that Dad wouldn't want her to do this for him is a meaningless statement to make. The word sacrifice is thrown at the caregiver as if it's a dirty word. It is time to recognize that *sacrifice* and *sacrament* both come from the same root word and both are ultimately about giving the gift of a selfless act.

The selfless act of caring for and loving someone in spite of the needs a disease like Alzheimer's imposes is a deep expression of commitment and honor for most of us.

One cannot underestimate the bond that develops between the caregiver and the loved one. And there are very basic feelings going on that must be recognized by those who live just outside the parameters of this relationship. When love is not expressed or demonstrated by other family members to the parent with Alzheimer's Disease, or any other illness for that matter, that lack of love deeply isolates the caregiver as well, and it sends a message to them that their commitment is of no more worth than that of the loved one who is actually facing the illness. What affects one has to be absorbed personally by the other because when you truly love someone, you want and need for them to be loved by others.

So when those cards and letters and gifts stop coming because Mom or Dad can't read any more or can't give the required expected response anymore, more is involved than just saving the price of a card or a gift or a stamp. What is involved is rejection, rejection of an ill parent and rejection of a well caregiver. To then force Mom to place Dad in a home before other options are explored and before she is ready to accept that choice, is to force her to sever her bond and it also sends a message loud and clear that this is exactly what is going to happen to her when her time comes to be taken care of. If she gets depressed it may be that she's not only mourning the loss of her spouse, she is also mourning what she perceives as her own end.

Of course, it's too much for Mom to do alone. But what Mom needs is help. She needs her children pitching in, and yes, sacrificing their time and effort, and she needs it done happily. And if the option of home care is impossible, then she needs assurance that she's done the best she could do and that Dad on some level has to know that. And she needs touch and assurance herself that she is loved. And she needs to be supported in her needs to be there with Dad in his new home, everyday, if that is what she desires.

There was an elder gentleman in one of the support group meetings I attended who was in tears relating that his doctor had yelled at him for spending too much time in the nursing home with his wife, a late stage Alzheimer's person.

"What are you doing here? She doesn't even know who you are. Why are you driving 60 miles a day to be here with her? This is totally unnecessary. I don't want to see you here so much any more. It's time for you to move on and start your life over. She doesn't need you anymore."

There was an outcry of ... **Get another doctor!** ... from the other members of this support group. This man was honoring his commitment to be with his wife in the only way he had left. He didn't see the long trip as a sacrifice at all, he was going to spend time with the woman who had been a part of his life for over 60 years, a commitment that gave him a sense of peace and purpose and resolution about his loss of her.

On the other side of the coin are those who can't do it. For family members who never did make the connection with each other and who see no need to start just because a parent or brother or aunt is losing their memory, perhaps placement in a facility where others can at least provide an aura of care and nurturing is the only choice. And perhaps they need to own up to the fact that they can't or don't want to do it. What they must do is stop throwing the clichés around about the work being too hard for Mom/Dad as justification for shifting what is really their guilt on to someone else. If they can't contribute happily they aren't going to be of help anyway. But don't belittle the efforts being made by others.]

In Tom's case, had he been placed in a home, I believe that he'd have lived with his disappointment and his fear without liking it much, made friends with the aides and staff and existed until all ability to express himself faded. However, I was there, and facing the reality of Tom's future in such a place was unthinkable to me as long as I was able to do it.

[Do people really think about what putting someone in a nursing home does to them? Over and over as I've involved myself in various advocacy groups on behalf of the frail elderly in this country, what I hear is that most people want to remain in their own homes and most caregivers want to keep them there. The cry is for help and respite care and planning services. There isn't a person I've met in a support group who isn't dealing with guilt and grief over having made the nursing home decision, a decision often imposed on them by an inability to afford home health care.

Our government has set a system in place that forces many to renege on life long commitments because funds can't be made available to allow the poor and the middle class to stay in their homes. Economic factors and a general malaise in attitude towards the frail elderly in this country have set a standard of treatment of these once productive people that is to be abhorred.

Do any of the government officials who take such a cavalier approach to the care and maintenance of our elderly citizens think about what people and families go through when care needs get critical and people don't have the resources to provide the quality care their loved ones need? Do these officials have a clue as to what it is like to spend the remainder of their lives in a welfare nursing home? Do they have any idea what it means to be drugged and restrained because their behaviors are a hardship on an over-worked, usually understaffed nursing home? Do they even care to consider the loneliness and despair and mourning people feel, even in the best of those homes? If they did, they would make efforts to provide the means by which more people could keep their loved ones home longer.]

---

*   There is never carpeting in the hallways and bedrooms of chronic or Alzheimer patient units because of sanitary and safety considerations. Aside from the obvious cleaning needs, wheelchairs and beds move easier on hard floors. Falls on hard floors account for most of the injuries patients have in nursing homes. To avoid falls, they are 'encouraged' to sit in wheelchairs and if not cooperative they are put in geriatric chairs, a device that more or less controls the more active patient. If that fails, then the 'team' meets and discusses the use of drugs to 'control the behavior problem'.

The hard surfaces also make sound bounce. The sad reality is that most elderly patients suffer from some form of hearing disorder and the noise level in the best of these homes is very high. The sound distortions, especially to an Alzheimer's patient can actually be painful, if not frightening.

Spanky clean corridors and reproductions of antiques in the waiting room may look impressive but they aren't the real measure of what it means to spend the rest of your days there. It all boils down to the staff, and by staff I mean the people who actually do the caretaking. Their awareness, sensitivity, intelligence and imagination are difficult to assess until someone you care about is placed in that facility and no matter what the skill level of these people, time is spread amongst several other needy, sometimes cranky, and often demanding patients. If one convinces themselves that any nursing home is really a home away from home then they are deluding themselves. It is a place where a loved one can be taken care of when you can't, sometimes well, sometimes not so well. But, it is not home! *

We visited the wife of a deceased colleague of Tom's at least once a week while we lived in Houston. Her nursing home was a very expensive home as those places went and from my observations, well staffed and well supplied. We'd find her either in bed or in a wheel chair in the hall with other patients waiting for scheduled activities such as beauty parlor appointments, or therapy, or diaper changing time. We never knew how long she'd been in that spot but I observed that other patients near her were usually still in the same spot when we left, sometimes an hour or more later. Sometimes we found her in the television room where she was subjected to watching whatever happened to be on. She was unable to move her chair herself and couldn't have changed the channel had she tried. It can be torture for someone left in a room with a football game when they hate football. It would have been torture for Tom.

She had suffered a series of strokes but she was still quite lucid. I might even characterize her as one of the more interesting people I met in Houston. She was quick and she was funny. She was still sharp enough to note the changes in Tom and to ask me how he was when he was out of ear shot. She was visibly saddened by those changes. He and she had enjoyed a close friendship in earlier days, their families often vacationing together, and if their conversations were sometimes a little disjointed they still managed to make each other smile. And of course, Tom was very attentive to her, stroking her hair, and kissing her hand and cheek. She seemed to twinkle with the attention.

It bothered her that she often found herself in other people's clothing and that none of her possessions, except for the pictures of her family which were prominently displayed on her end table, were with her. She found herself instead in an overtly sterile plastic covered environment with nothing to indicate anything about her past or her identity except for those photographs. I know her family visited infrequently because she complained about it bitterly and the nursing staff thought I was her daughter, often asking me about her care needs when I arrived. But then knowing what staff problems exist in any nursing home, I don't doubt the constant shifting of personnel left gaps in who knew what about which patients, another problem that only aids in the impersonalization of the patient. She was a very lonely person who related as best she could to those around her. The ward she was on was peopled with chronically ill patients and it was a very depressing place in spite of the prints on the walls and the outwardly cheery atmosphere the nurses and staff tried to provide.

[Once upon a time, some administrator or social worker in a nursing home hit upon the idea of putting photographs of family members in patient rooms and, in the case where end tables weren't allowed, on the doors. I suppose it was an attempt to bring some sense of homeyness into an otherwise sterile environment and help people at least recognize which bed was theirs. They also reasoned that contemplating those photographs might help the patient adjust faster to their new 'placement', after having been uprooted from their homes, wrenched from their loved ones, and their belongings dispersed amongst the yet living or sold out from under them to pay the costs of the nursing placement. Well, of course, that's not the image any of us want to hold as we are forced to make the nursing home decision for an elder frail individual, but I suspect, that is closer to how the patient sees it and feels it. It is the ultimate in terms of fear of the unknown and mourning, deep deep mourning on levels we can't imagine.

And so photographs became **de rigueur**. There is hardly a nursing home on the planet that doesn't have a place to put those photographs. Photographs of people, who for the most part don't or can't visit regularly and when they do are at a loss as to how to relate to their person anymore. I imagine there's even a little competition at times between family members to make sure theirs are the most prominently displayed and the most up to date. For the patient who still has their thinking process, those photographs often come to symbolize everything in their life that no longer exists, but for the demented patient those photographs are particularly meaningless. Their memories are of people the way they looked twenty years ago and most can't focus on something as abstract as a photograph anymore anyway. They can barely focus on the person standing in front of them.

As for the living embodiment of those photographs when they do come to visit, conversation is limited to the weather and talking between themselves because there is often little response from the patient. They watch television while seconds are counted until the grand escape can be humanly made or attempt sociability at lunch amidst the sounds and sights and smells of a roomful of old, dying people. At best it's like visiting a stranger in someone else's house, a stranger who doesn't have enough time to make the connection between the flash of the person standing in front of them, and the real memory of who that person was in their life. By the time the connection is made the visitor is long gone. The moments when personality and recognition surface in the patient are shared with attendants, and cleaning personnel and nurses instead, because they are the ones most in their lives.

People approach the prospect of being placed in nursing homes in one of three ways:

- They decide to embrace it as the only choice left to them and actually find a level of joy in their existence.

- They accept it with benign resignation while nurturing resentment, disappointment and fear, making sure anyone who visits them leaves with either a sense of guilt or despair.

- They go kicking and screaming all the way, some of them dying sooner than they might.

If adjustments to nursing home care are made by patients, and I include the Alzheimer's patient who isn't supposed to know they've been placed in a nursing home, but seems to anyway, it is because the human condition, even in the most debilitating of circumstances still has the ability to accept change and adapt and find comfort.]

We continued to visit Tom's elegant lady friend until an incident happened that made it impossible for him to return. We were waiting to hear of her condition knowing she had suffered another stroke, when an elderly gent was wheeled into the television room where we were and left at an angle that didn't permit him full vision of the television or the room at large. With his back to the door, no one could hear his attempts to call the attendants for help. The attempts he made to be heard were garbled noises that only resembled speech. His face was frozen into a mask, his jaw locked open, his eyes frantic. He was drooling. His hands jerked uncontrollably and he had been strapped into his chair for safety reasons. He had a urine bag slung between his legs under his seat which was half full. An attempt to hide it with a towel had been made but the towel had slipped during transport into the room. I went to find an attendant because I felt helpless to come to his aide. When I returned I found Tom weeping. He asked me to take him home. When we got into the car he told me he didn't want to go back again, ever. He once more asked me to kill him if he ever got like that old man, but this time he started to cry. The 'old man' was only three years older than Tom. We never visited again. Mary had often expressed the desire to die and get it over with to Tom. Less than six months later she got her wish.

I promised Tom that day, that as long as it was within my power he would remain at home with me amongst his things and I would do everything I could to keep his life as normal as possible. I had no idea what that vow would mean in terms of energy and resolve. The hard truth is that this illness made both of us prisoners and each of us was the other's jailer. There were days when I wondered which of us had the keys. What kept me going was the knowledge that it wasn't much easier for those who had placed their loved ones in homes. There is nothing easy about any of this.

═══════════════

Back in Texas Land I was facing the enormity of the isolation that had taken over our lives and hiring anyone to come and spend time with Tom so that I could get away for an hour or so was not an easy thing to do. My first and last foray into home health care for a while happened when my doctor decided I needed some minor surgery to correct the problem detected while I was in Phoenix. I needed to be in the hospital for four hours and I needed someone to stay with Tom while I was away. Tom's family wasn't available so I called a number of home health agencies but most would not service the suburb in which we lived. I finally found one that would do an assessment and provide someone to stay with Tom.

The meeting in our house went smoothly enough although Tom was not on good behavior. His pacing had picked up and he was very agitated through the interview. Tom was not someone who was going to be easy. As his illness progressed he got more and more erratic. I thought we had the date and time set with the agency, but when the day arrived, no one appeared. There had been a mix up on the date and the agency was trying to find someone to fill in as fast as they could. It didn't happen.

My doctor not wanting to put off dealing with what she now referred to as a *pre-cancerous condition,* tried to convince me a shorter procedure done in her office would be just as advisable, and I should bring Tom.

[Sure! Shorter! Why not! Bring Tom! Right!]

She had no idea what she was in for. He was already upset and anxious by the time we arrived at the office. I tried to explain to Tom that I'd be in the doctor's office for at least half an hour and he'd have to sit quietly by himself during that time. While Tom understood the need for the procedure, he had lost his sense of time. Half an hour, half a minute, held little difference to him. I told him several times not to worry while I was out of the room and that as soon as it was over we'd go home together. I might has well have explained it in Hungarian.

[Talk about going into treatment with a positive mind set. Talk about having a moment of quiet so that I could receive the treatment in as positive and serene a manner as possible. Talk about dreaming.]

I was barely on the examining table when Tom started. He was belligerent and convinced I was dying and they were lying to him. While I laid there counting the minutes I could hear him pacing up and down the hallway with assistants and secretarial staff trying to placate him. At one point he let go of a barrage of four letter words, something that was totally out of character for him. He simply never resorted to such language. He was absolutely furious. I could tell the staff was afraid of him and there were several times when my doctor shouted to the nurse to keep him out of the room. You must keep in mind that all this is going on with my feet in stirrups.

[Candid Camera, where were you?]

Tom was convinced he'd never see me again and I was convinced I had terminal cancer. On top of everything else why not? Hell, it wasn't unheard of for the well spouse to die before the sick one. Why should I be exempt? On some bizarre level I almost welcomed the thought. There was no valid reason for me to have to go through this nightmare. The whole freaking world could drown in a ten ton vat of camel spit for all I cared. I had never felt so abandoned, so alone, so unloved, and so betrayed in my entire life, and I still had to go home with Tom, the love of my life.

Camel spit?
Well, it did have a certain ring to it, Lord.
It did get My attention, Beverly.
Well then, there You are. It worked.
Do you feel better now?
Oh, I'm all right. I'm too darn mad to give up and besides I'm all Tom's got. I can't give up. He needs me and I guess I still need him.

However, it was time to rethink the problem of getting a break once in a while. My reality was very confining for a lot of reasons not the least of which were Tom's needs. It was also apparent to me that except for situations such as doctor's appointments, I had no where to go without Tom. I didn't have a life anymore. I didn't even have peace and quiet to myself anymore. I was aware enough to know I should be building something of a life away from Tom but I didn't know anyone in Houston apart from Tom who was accessible to me. Tom on the other hand might also have benefited from interaction with someone other than me but he would have none of it. Bring someone else in to watch him? If he was adamant about that situation before the move to Houston he was even more so now. He was determined that I was going to be the only person in his life by now. I was the only one he was able to count on. He was safe and secure with me and he was not about to establish any type of a new relationship with strangers. Bringing in an attendant at that point in his life would have been further proof that the ship was sinking. And, I was a coward. I didn't have the energy to take the bull by the proverbial horns and hire someone to stay with him. It might have been emotionally healthier for me to have forced the issue, but it seemed easier to just plod along.

I did call the Alzheimer's Association for information on adult day care programs for people like Tom. Programs usually run by Senior Centers, often on a drop off basis, where planned social activities for Alzheimer's people were designed to keep them motivated and active. Programs much like the one I visited while I was still in New York. I reasoned that if Tom could envision such activity as training, or helping others, I'd at least get a few hours a week to myself. While there were adult day care programs in the Houston Metro area, we were located outside of the parameters of those programs and the logistics of travel and pick up would have held me prisoner anyway. They recommended that I start attending a support group and gave me the address of one in our area. The one time I attended turned into another disaster.

It was the same old story, who would stay with Tom. He kept telling me to go to *my meeting* thinking it had something to do with my old job. I let him think that, it seemed easier than mentioning the dreaded "A" word in his presence. I decided to take the plunge and leave him alone. I would only be away a couple of hours and with him insisting he wasn't a baby, I agreed to go. On the side, I asked a neighbor to look in on him while I was away just to make sure he was all right and so that someone would know he was in the house. He told me he'd tell Tom he was just passing by and maybe invite him over for a beer. It seemed like a good plan. However, it didn't work that way!

Tom had lost track of time by then completely. He'd panicked shortly after I left and in his wanderings around the house looking for me had inadvertently shut off all the lights. Now in the dark, he was unable to find the switches to turn them on again. The neighbor seeing a darkened house figured I had taken Tom with me, although he did try the door bell with no answer from Tom. He had no way of knowing that Tom yelled hello to both the door bell and the telephone in those days and was unable to figure out which was which anymore, and so, depending on where he was in the house when either rang, determined whether or not his calls of *hello* would be heard.

Tom later told me that someone tried to get in the house and he was very afraid. When I arrived home he was a total wreck. He had been standing in the middle of the living room in the dark for I don't know how long, afraid to move for fear of falling and hurting himself, and had been so frightened he had wet himself. The night had been a trauma all around. I wasn't ready to admit that Tom had Alzheimer's Disease and I certainly wasn't able to talk about it. I cried most of the time I was at the meeting as one by one other members of the group talked about what was going on in their lives. When it came my turn to talk, I couldn't. I muttered something, grabbed my purse and fled. Maybe later, maybe after all the hysteria was over and I had time to pull my emotions together. On the way home I reconnoitered and decided on a different plan of action. Then I opened the door and found Tom as he was. That sealed it, he was not to be left alone again, ever.

The next morning I asked our doctor to recommend Tom for speech therapy. He agreed, based on the progress Tom had made at the clinic in Phoenix. I set up the program in a local medical center and Tom started his sessions which allowed me to drop him off for two hours while I shopped. He saw the sessions as training and went into it enthusiastically. We also started going to an acupuncturist three times a week for two hour sessions. More time for me to read or work on my needlework without interruption. There was a marked improvement in his speech after each session, improvement that slowly disintegrated over the next two days. With the acupuncture boosts and the speech therapy sessions our ability to communicate with each other improved and we were once again able to enjoy a movie together and life in general. We had laughter back.

However, once the stress that was constantly bombarding us from the courts took over, he was no longer able to concentrate on the speech therapy, nor could he lie still long enough for the acupuncture treatment. We quit both programs and the two of us gave up trying to get well, the chores of surviving had become too demanding.

We had also been spending upwards of three hours a day on his therapy program by then and although the speed and quality of his response to those exercises seemed to improve, his ability to function on a daily basis did not. He now needed more help getting his clothes on. He could no longer balance on one foot while he put on his trousers and was resisting sitting down while I helped him. It was as if he saw sitting down as another way of giving in. So we'd hop around the bedroom every morning while I found places for him to lean against, mostly me, while he stuffed his feet into his clothes. We stopped the therapy program at that time as well. There didn't seem much point in doing it any more.

The wandering that had manifested itself in the airport was now apparent in any public place. Grocery shopping had become the bane of my life. I had to keep one hand on Tom at all times or he wandered down the aisles and out of the store following anyone who remotely looked like me. It didn't take regulars in the store long to notice us. It was difficult not to notice, with my calling Tom's name out loud, listening for his response which generally had a tinge of panic in it, while I tracked him down. I'd go through the checkout line with him wedged between me and the customer's cart behind us, while I emptied the groceries. He'd help by taking things out of the customer's cart. Most strangers caught on very quickly to our odd behaviors. Sometimes they helped, sometimes they smiled, sometimes they moved their carts into another line while avoiding eye contact with either of us.

Getting him and the cart to the car presented the next obstacle. I tried to instill the response to stop moving when he missed me. It didn't work. Out of sight meant he was lost and he had to find me and he was very fast. In a moment he could be half a block away and all I'd done was throw my purse in the car and open the trunk. Sometimes a stranger would come to my rescue, sometimes I chased him a block or two before catching up to him. Calling to him only confused him more because he could no longer determine from which direction my voice was coming. By the time I'd turned him around he'd be in a complete state of anger and confusion, and we still had to get the bags into the car. That translated into broken bags, broken bottles that hit the pavement instead of the trunk, apples rolling across the lot, the loaf of bread that got stepped on. He refused to just sit in the car while I took care of it. He needed to help. It was hateful, and there was still the ordeal of getting it all from the car to the house.

I remember reading about the phenomena of wandering in a book on Alzheimer's Disease. I wish to tell you that nothing you can imagine covers the experience of living through that phenomena. It is activity that never stops. In our case, it began with little compulsions to move, sudden exits from chairs, a quick walk through the house and progressed to an uncontrollable mania that often became frenetic and furtive in character that, in our case, lasted until he was bedridden. It was as if the only recourse left to Tom was that of trying to outrun the destruction of his brain. It was endless and there was virtually nothing I could do to stop it or change it. The only recourse I had was to try to contain him.

He could still handle door knobs but locks were out of his range. I had dead bolt locks without knobs installed on the front and back doors so I could keep him from leaving the house while I was cooking or cleaning. The key was on a chain around my neck which never was taken off. Locking the doors however, created other problems. He was furious with me for locking him in like a child. I couldn't win.

God, if there is anyone who actually believes I have married Tom for his money, then send them here for a few days and they can find out for themselves what a free easy ride this is. I am so tired of the lawyers and the court officials and the horse opera going on over Tom's remains that I could scream. Can't they see how stressful it is to Tom, to me? Can't they see how much I care about him? No one in their right mind would do this just for the money. Surely they don't think I married Tom for his money. There isn't enough money to pay anyone to do this. Why do they have to be so unfeeling? Why do they have to be so mean spirited about everything? Why do I feel that they are setting me up? What if what has happened to Tom happens to me? What will I do, who will take care of me?

226

I can't answer those questions for you, Beverly, but at least you're not blaming Me for all the troubles. I'd say that's a step in the right direction and let us not forget you're talking about the court system. Have you ever heard the joke about the first lawyer to make it to Heaven?

Yes I have, and no it's not funny. I need to know what to do next. What is my next step?

Grow up, Beverly! If everyone lived by the Golden Rule there wouldn't be any need to call on Me for help now would there?

That's it? That's your answer?

What do you want from me, Beverly, poetry?

A crash of thunder might help.

One thing I didn't have to wonder about as our involvement with the legal establishment increased, was the effect it had on Tom. He was devastated and increasingly obsessed about his estate to the point where I couldn't placate him. His rumblings about it went on incessantly. He insisted that I transfer our accounts to a national bank instead of the local one we were now using. Like everything else that clicked in his mind, the money issue took precedence over all other thought function and there was no deterring him from his resolve to protect it from court control. I tried to explain that changing our funds around was pointless because I had to give our lawyer a complete accounting of our assets anyway. What he wanted was irrational but I was caught in the middle of being a dutiful wife and taking charge knowing that no matter what I did would only be cause for more scrutiny of my motives.

God! How am I going to straighten this mess out?

Just hang in there, Beverly.

Hang in there? Haven't I done enough hanging in this lifetime? Isn't it time for me to move on to something else?

Such as?

How about peace of mind, Lord. It would be really nice to have peace of mind instead of this quagmire of a life we've got now.

Think about this, Beverly, you have an opportunity in front of you. It's up to you to use it.

Opportunity? Are You trying to tell me that everything happens for the good, Lord? Because if You are, I'm not able to see it, not with what's going on.

Yes I am, Beverly, and yes you can.

Gee thanks! That was a big help!

Actually, it was. It was about that time that I realized there is no such thing as the bottom of the barrel. No matter how bad things get, it is important to know that things can always get worse and you had better find something good in what you still have to hang on to or be lost. My definition of the word normal had always been flexible, how flexible was yet to be tested but unbeknownst to me, I was already on the road to experiencing the range of that definition. They say that strength of character is formed through adversity. I thought dealing with Tom's gradual demise would be more than enough adversity for me in this lifetime. I didn't need the problems Tom's estate were imposing in our lives. Our life was hard enough without feeling I was under the microscope for every nit picking decision I made about our life and Tom's care from the moment we met. Talk about living in the past. I was residing in a crate full of receipts trying to justify my existence. It was more than hateful, it was obscene. I felt my character was being assaulted and more than that, my commitment to Tom demeaned. How could any part of this have a positive side? The answer is that this experience allowed me to find my strength. I found out what I was made of. And I discovered how much I hate to be underestimated.

228

THEY CAN'T TAKE THAT AWAY FROM ME

The way you wear your hat
The way you sip your tea
The memories of all that
Oh no they can't take that away from me

The way your smile just beams
The way you sing off key
The way you haunt my dreams
No, No they can't take that away from me

We may never ever meet again
On the bumpy road to love
But I'll always always keep the memory
of ...

The way you hold your knife
The way we danced till three
The way you changed my life
No ... they can't take that away from me
No ...
They can't take that away from me.

words by: Ira Gershwin   *music by: George Gershwin*

CHAPTER ELEVEN

July 1991

Dear Beverly,

You asked if I would share some of my memories of Tom with you.

We had two names for Tom. He was most often referred to as 'The Silver Fox' because of his white hair and his extraordinary skills at bringing in business, but there were also times when we referred to him as 'The Tsar'. Tom exuded authority. It wasn't so much that he demanded to be treated as an authority figure it was more that Tom was the authority. He could be hell on wheels and you certainly could disagree with his management style but then he was also under a hell of a lot of pressure.

He had a plaque on his desk that read:

*Climate is the impact of my behavior on the
attitude and the performance of my subordinates.*

In terms of his use of the word subordinates, Tom considered his subordinates sacrosanct. He hand picked the people who worked for him and we were his people. This implied a level of ownership but it also carried a great deal of security for those of us in his group. If there ever was a foul up, he took the heat. There were times when he should have placed the blame where it was deserved but he never passed blame down the line. However, he was not someone you wanted to disappoint or anger. You learned very quickly that if you were the one to foul up, it was in your best interest to tell him the truth of the situation. If he caught you in a lie, or in a cover up you were history. It was as simple as that.

The up side was that we made very good money. We got the highest percentage pay increases in the Tiger System. Tom saw to it, and we knew that as long as Tom prevailed, we had work. No one ever got very far messing with his people. No one ever got very far messing with him.

I will never forget a run in he had with Bobby Kennedy in 1972. Tom was president of Bell Equipment at the time and a piece of equipment needed repairs at one of the missile sites. Tom immediately dispatched one of his men to take care of the problem. The man was a union member but not the union currently in favor with the Justice Department, of which Bobby Kennedy was head. The upshot is that the union members threatened to strike if Tom's man wasn't removed and their own man put in his place. When Tom's man refused to leave, Kennedy had him physically removed from the site. Tom hit the roof when he got wind of what had happened. He immediately phoned 'Bobby', the ensuing shouting match ending with Tom's comment; "You might run the Justice Department, Mr. Kennedy, but I run Bell Equipment, and no one touches my equipment without my authorization"

Although Kennedy was not someone to back down easily, Tom's reputation was just as formidable. Kennedy was no threat to his career and both Tom and he knew it. The end result of the confrontation was that Tom's man was allowed to make the repairs, and Kennedy removed himself from further contact with him.

Tom had no use for playing the corporate game which is why he preferred operating on a consulting basis, and less use for anyone using him to oil their way up the corporate ladder. He dealt with only the top personnel, running his operation from their offices and answering to almost no one. In order to insure his autonomy he always brought his own staff with him. That staff included his office personnel as well as those of us who worked with him on projects. I, as did most of us, kept a bag of clothing in the office at all times as there were occasions when I didn't even have time to go home before I found myself half way across the globe. We answered to no one but Tom unless otherwise specified by him. It saved us a great deal of grief from corporate politics and also afforded him protection. Tom was someone who generated controversy. There were people who hated his guts. I remember one little man in particular.

Animosity between Tom and this person had been building for months. Tom was in the Middle East on a major project and it was thought out of reach when this person made his move. He fired one of our group for insubordination and warned us not to contact Tom because he was on his way out and our jobs were in jeopardy as well if we didn't play ball. We, of course, contacted Tom immediately and he was on the next flight back. Imagine the surprise of this person when Tom quite unexpectedly walked into his office the next day.

The air was electric as Tom arrived. We were almost giddy waiting for the explosion. Needless to say, all of us who were within reach managed to be in the office that day. We'd all seen Tom in action before. It was going to be too good of a show to miss. Instead of the fireworks we expected however, Tom walked into this unfortunate person's office, handed him a sheet of paper and walked out without saying one word to him. We were stunned. I asked him what happened ...

"No one fires my personnel. I just handed the little shit my resignation."

"You can't do that. He doesn't have jurisdiction to even accept it."

"That's true, that's true ... and, he's going to have one hell of a time explaining it. By the way, all of you are resigning as well and be sure and take your records with you when you leave."

One by one we returned to our desks, wrote out our resignations and put them on the desk of a, by now, very unhappy camper. Without a word and without exception, each of us, Tom's entire staff, office personnel included, packed our files and followed him out of the building.

About two hours later, the company CEO found us in a restaurant a few blocks away where we had gathered to discuss our options. Tom retired to a corner with him and a few minutes later returned to inform us we were to report back to work the following morning. We were all of us, including the man who had been fired, getting new contracts. We ended up with salary increases while Tom clarified his autonomy. Incidentally, there was one glaring absence in the office when we did return.

From my observation, Tom was literally unbeatable in a corporate fight. I don't think he ever underestimated anyone and perhaps that was his secret of success. He always seemed to be three steps ahead of everyone.

As for working with the man, there were a number of people who learned a hell of a lot from Tom Murphy. There are those of us who recognized this and will always be grateful. There are others who fell in love with themselves and forgot where their opportunity originated. They got wrapped up in themselves and lost perspective. Tom was more than just competent. He was good natured, he was imaginative, he was generous, and he was a man of honor. Mainly, working for him was exciting. There weren't many like him.

Good luck, Jim O'Leary

April 1989 rolled in on a storm. Conversation between family members and us had ground to a complete halt. Lawyers had now entered the scene and our lawyers were talking to their lawyers with little movement happening regarding what was being characterized as estate issues. Anticipating that Tom's competence would be called into challenge I started the process to have him re-evaluated. Our new doctor recommended a neuropsychologist and rushed copies of Tom's medicals to him with a letter stressing the importance of getting Tom a timely appointment. The testing sessions were barely finished and we had yet to get the results when we got the news that members of Tom's family had gone into court without notifying us and had gained a temporary guardianship of our finances and his body. Our accounts were frozen with the exception of those funds I had changed to Citibank and a CD Tom had insisted I put in my name temporarily. Citibank decided that until a permanent guardian was appointed, no information about our accounts would be released without a court order. We had no idea what a guardianship would mean in terms of our daily lives.

For one thing we weren't even notified our funds had been frozen until we tried to cash a check the Court had ordered released for Tom's daily care and the local bank we had been directed to use refused to honor it. It took another day in court to ferret out which account we could still use. Our life had already moved out of our control and into the control of the court system.

Our first chore was to overturn the temporary guardianship, and challenge the claims of Tom's incompetence. Armed with the report from the neuropsychiatric exam which recommended that Tom have his say, I thought we still could make the mess all go away. The report addressed two questions in relation to Tom's competency.

1. Is Mr. Murphy competent to make legal decisions?
2. Can Mr. Murphy help to choose who will manage his affairs?

In response to the first question, Mr. Murphy evidenced severe linguistic and perceptual deficits. In addition, his memory skills, for novel verbal and nonverbal stimuli, were significantly impaired. Although Mr. Murphy evidenced some ability to solve verbal problems, this was an inconsistent skill at best. Because of these severe cognitive deficits, he was unable to read with adequate comprehension or to solve mathematical problems. In total, it is my opinion that Mr. Murphy is not competent to read legal documents with comprehension or to manage his fiscal affairs. In addition, a complex legal document could not be read to Mr. Murphy with the expectation that he would comprehend the aurally presented material.

Secondly, Mr. Murphy's cognitive strength is his previously stored memory. In addition, as mentioned above, he is able to inconsistently answer some relatively complex verbal questions (e.g., Name one advantage and one disadvantage of labor unions), even with his expressive language deficit. Throughout the evaluation process, Mr. Murphy was able to get his desires across and he stated some strong opinions about aspects of the testing sessions. Finally, when discussing the results of the evaluation, these two questions were brought up by Mrs. Murphy in a general sense. As I began to address the questions, Mr. Murphy expressed strong emotions about his feelings and began to cry. Overall, it is my opinion that Mr. Murphy can assist in the selection of his caregiver and the individual that he would like to manage his fiscal affairs. This determination, however, should be undertaken in an extended interview session and conducted by a neuropsychologist who is experienced with interviewing individuals with linguistic deficits. This individual would need to be aware of the pertinent issues in this legal case so that the appropriate questions can be asked in a number of different ways.

In response to your suggestion of my being appointed to be the person who interviews Mr. Murphy, I would be willing to undertake this interview if the court would ask me to do so. I am also able to provide you with the names of some individuals who could also undertake this process.

Dr. R. Ph.D.

This report was ultimately ignored. The new lawyer we had just hired told us that if Tom responded in my favor as he expected, the other lawyers would claim he had been *brainwashed*. The launch of a medical battle of experts would put Tom under extreme stress and it would cost a fortune. While I had no doubt that Tom would name me as his guardian, I was told there would be a counter action if for no other reason than to maintain neutrality in determining Tom's care. I was finally convinced that the only one to suffer if we pursued the interview would be Tom. I have always regretted that decision but I just couldn't see putting him through any more stress than was already happening. The report was never presented to the Court, but I knew that Tom placed his trust in me over everyone else in his life and its not because I brainwashed him or did anything more sinister than be there for him. I would like to clarify this brainwashing thing however.

[It is impossible to brainwash a person who has Alzheimer's Disease or dementia and I have serious doubts that those suffering from brain damage resulting from a closed head injury are any more susceptible either. Brainwashing involves the programming of recent memory to influence behavior differently than it might be manifested under normal circumstances. Since recent memory and the ability to organize information are the first things assaulted by dementing illnesses, and closed head trauma, brainwashing is really quite impossible. One has to be able to remember the new programming for it to be effective and more important, one has to be able to locate it in the brain once it's been imprinted, if it can be imprinted at all.]

By the time Tom was facing this particular chapter in his life, it was impossible to imprint anything new for more than a few seconds. He was well into the mid stages of Alzheimer's Disease by then. If anything, his old memory, memory older than my entering his life had taken over, memory that was more deeply seated in his essence as a person than in actual data input. The idea of *brainwashing* someone like Tom might have been an interesting notion to someone on the outside looking into the behavior of an Alzheimer's person, but one that was simply preposterous. And it's not a notion limited to a few. It is a notion that not only persists but seems to be a favorite misconception family members all over the country assert when life with an Alzheimer's person becomes strained. I guess it's a logical conclusion to draw when Alzheimer's people draw away from certain family members especially when other family members are doing the day-to-day care. The only problem is that the logic doesn't apply in these cases. There is no definable logic as to how an Alzheimer's person perceives anything. Once they enter the mid stages of Alzheimer's Disease their logic is unique to themselves and has little to do with the real world around them although there is often a seed pearl of reality at the base of their response. The problem isn't in the input of information, the problem is in how the information is processed. Figuring out behavior becomes a full time occupation for the primary caregiver and one that has little reward because figuring it out doesn't mean you can do anything to change it.

I am reminded of Martha, a member who attending the support group I led for late stage caregivers. She arrived late one meeting and in great distress. Her sister, who was living out of state, who never wrote, never called, never sent their mother a card or a gift, was accusing Martha of brainwashing their mother against her. She had finally come to visit and the mother refused to acknowledge her. The mother wouldn't even look at her, sitting in her chair rigid and unmoving all the while giving sweet attention to Martha. Martha said this was highly unusual behavior for her mother. Their relationship was sound but it certainly was not one in which the mother finished every comment with the words ... "God bless you, Martha", which is what she did all the time her sister was present. It was as if she was doing it on purpose just to annoy her sister.

I had to ask the following questions of the group. Was this brainwashing or was it merely a mother's way of displaying her hurt and dissatisfaction towards a daughter whom she now perceived as uncaring about her? Then again are Alzheimer's people capable of perceiving actions that aren't overtly nurturing from others and if so are they even capable of making their feelings known when severe language deficits interfere? We all thought so. From our close experience with our loved ones we knew it was so.

During the first year of our marriage I took the time to scout out possible programs for Tom in the event that Tom actually was facing Alzheimer's Disease. I needed to know the cost and availability of care for him so that I could continue to work if we were to even consider staying in New York. This agency was reported to have one of the best adult day care programs for Dementia patients in the city. I had time to observe the activities room before beginning my tour and noticed the interactions of many of the patients and staff while I waited. One of the staff seemed singled out by the patients. When she approached the patients, some of whom were in wheel chairs, each one either turned their head or moved away from her. They ostensibly ignored that she had entered the room. One patient pulled a face at her when she walked by. I started to laugh and the social worker directing this program, whom I knew through my years in the field, let a little chuckle out as well.

"They don't seem to like that person very much."

"Well, she's a little rigid and not very friendly. As you can see, even these patients have figured her out. I am amazed at the feelings these people are able to express when the impression, given the stage they're at, is that they are incapable of knowing what is going on. Most of them have severe language deficits. Why are you here for the tour?"

"My husband may have Alzheimer's Disease, and I'm trying to get a grasp on what to expect if that's what we're dealing with."

"God, for your sake and his, I hope not."

"Yeah, me too."

As my support group members listened to Martha's story, we wondered if those who never involve themselves in the day to day care of an Alzheimer's person will ever understand the scope of what that care involves. And yes, bonds do develop as that care is administered. Does even that bond have to be scrutinized? Apparently, Martha was not only responsible for seeing to every waking need of a mother who was now facing incontinence but she was also somehow responsible for the feelings of a person living out of state who showed little apparent interest in any part of her mother's care except to criticize. Somehow it was Martha's fault the relationship between her sister and her mother wasn't wonderful. Martha commented that being accused of brainwashing her mother was almost as stupid as the other charge that had been levied against her. Apparently her sister had also uttered those words every caregiver hears at least once in their career as well.

"If you didn't do everything for Mom she might still be able to do something for herself."

As if it is every caregiver's mission in life to make our people forget how to dress and toilet themselves. No wonder Martha was mad.

One man in our group asked, rather sarcastically, if brain-washing could possibly help him get his wife to use the bathroom by herself again. Another man started to laugh and offered that perhaps brainwashing could help his brother dress himself again. Someone else mentioned her husband being brainwashed into remembering she was still his wife. However, while all of us in that group had had similar experiences at one time or another, the beauty of the group was that invariably the opposite side got a chance to air. A young woman brought up another aspect of this situation.

She offered that perhaps Martha's sister isn't really so terrible. Maybe she's just frustrated at having family needs that keep her away, and maybe her calls to her mother and to Martha have been unrewarding and so she finds it's harder and harder to call at all. And maybe she misses the holiday events because she's so out of the loop they're on her before she realizes it. And maybe she's suspicious about how the estate is being spent because she is getting no information and she doesn't know what the scope of the care entails. The woman speaking, was an adult child facing the same situation Martha's sister had to deal with. She was also a long distance caregiver and she also knew how difficult it is to feel a part of a parent's life when that parent becomes such a stranger so quickly. Her own family needs just didn't permit the contact her brothers and sisters had with her father, who is in the late stages of Alzheimer's and her feelings about not being there were expressed in terms of guilt, and jealousy, and being isolated from her family.

Martha decided that perhaps it was time to sit down with her sister and talk about what their mother needed from the family instead of what the family needed from her. One thing we all agreed on, however, was that when it came to family dynamics nothing was ever simple again once Alzheimer's entered the picture.

―――――――――――――――――

[Oliver Sacks in his book, **The Man Who Mistook His Wife For a Hat,** contends that aphasic patients, that is patients who were rendered incapable of understanding words, none the less understood most of what was said to them, in his studies with this group. His work with extreme neurological problems has set him apart as one of the great observers of the unique nature of the human brain. Although his research is not about Alzheimer's patients specifically, much of what happens to an Alzheimer's brain is not that dissimilar to what happened to some of the brains Dr. Sacks encountered. Alzheimer's patients exhibit marked aphasia as the disease destroys their brain tissue as assuredly as a tumor, or a stroke destroys tissue and I had to wonder as I read Dr. Sack's books, if it makes a whole lot of difference how the brain damage occurs. It seemed to me that aphasia is aphasia. The only real difference is that with Alzheimer's Disease the damage that occurs is progressive and constantly affecting different functions because the attack is almost random in nature and the damage becomes more and more profound. However, if Dr. Sacks' observations and the observations of those of us who live with an aphasic patient are correct, then our actions do speak louder than our words. The following event demonstrates how Tom managed to function when he was already dealing with severe brain damage. Damage that testing said made it impossible for him to follow complex material at all.]

The day Tom was made a Ward of the Court, I was ordered to take part in a deposition in order to determine how estate funds had been spent by me. Both Tom and I appeared for this meeting which did not make the lawyers happy. After some discussion Tom was told questions would not be directed to him and he was not to speak at all or he'd be asked to leave. As for threatening to remove him, I was the one involved in the deposition and my testimony was essential to satisfy the judge that I was not misusing funds. I was also the only one who was going to take Tom to the bathroom and control him. There was no way Tom could be trusted to stay outside of the deposition room on his own, and so the threat to have him removed if he spoke out of turn was a hollow one. There would be no deposition without Tom present. He knew it and so did I. I also knew it would not be possible for Tom to not make his presence felt as he saw fit. He never had before. Why would he start now?

He injected his feelings and his comments into the proceedings throughout a very long and tiring day. His remarks were relevant to the subject matter being presented, and each one was duly written into the record by the court stenographer. He was following a long complicated relating of money expenditures that covered the three years of our marriage in spite of his having been legally declared to be unable to do so. One of his comments was so cuttingly on target and so sarcastic that a number of us burst out in laughter.

[So much for The Ward's inability to follow what was going on!]

It was amazing that a room full of lawyers could hear how relevant his comments were and ignore them. But then, of course, I must have brainwashed him. And, of course, they were doing their job.

Excuse me! ... I thought "The Ward", was supposed to be the one incapable of understanding what is going on. God! Tell me, am I crazy?

What do you think, Beverly?

I think this whole thing is unbelievable! That's what I think. Incidentally, are You taking all this down?

There's a time and place for everything, Beverly.

Please don't get too obscure on me ... I'm having trouble dressing myself these days.

Beverly ...

What?

Don't let your anger run away with you.

Anger? You tell me, how am I to deal with all of this? The Love of my life is dying on me, I can do nothing to change that and we have to face this particular heap of guano on top of everything. Who are these people? What manner of people are they? I can't tell who is on our side and who is the enemy anymore. They stand there mouthing the words that this is all on Tom's behalf. Tom's behalf my foot. They all walk in laughing with each other, discussing golf scores and who's played tennis with who lately. What are they, all members of the same country club? Isn't there any decorum anymore? Isn't there a hint of how devastating this is to our lives, in any of them? I can't stand it. They act as if Tom is stupid. They act as if I'm stupid. It's as if neither of us exist. How can Tom fight this illness in the midst of all of this? How can he even want to live after all this?

You can't assume Tom's fears or his sadness for him, Beverly. In fact, you're the one he's worried about.

Then what about my fears? What about my sadness? I take care of this man 24 hours a day. I put up with his petulance, his confusion, his demands, his needs. I love him. Isn't it obvious how much I love him? I run around like a cat in a giant litter box trying to find ways to keep him functioning. What about me?

What do you need, Beverly?

Thank you ... would be nice.

And if you don't get a proper Thank You, what do you do, drop him and run?

Of course not.

Then do what you do for Tom for the right reasons or don't do it at all. I don't know what else to tell you, Beverly, it's the only offer I've got right now and it's the only choice you have that matters. You'll get through this, but only if you decide to.

By the time the deposition had ended, Tom's resolve to prevail was completely crumbled. The enormity of the situation hit him hard. He started to deteriorate and over the next few months lost all he had gained at the clinic. As for our participation in the continuing, often postponed court proceedings, I have never felt so ignored in my life. Tom and I weren't ever given the opportunity to express ourselves in words. We never had our say. It was all done *in sotto voce comments*, at the bench, and in meetings behind closed doors where our fate was sealed without us being present. When you're the Ward of the Court you might as well be dead.

The appointment of a Guardian Ad Litem was greeted by both of us with all the enthusiasm of being condemned to bureaucratic hell. I was under the mistaken impression that his job was to represent Tom and sort out Tom's desires from some impartial place. I was wrong. What he turned out to be was another body to pay. What I didn't realize was that he wasn't representing Tom at all, he was representing *Air*, a non entity now called The Ward, who had become a legal definition of those words. His job wasn't to reflect Tom's wishes or concern himself about how Tom was responding to what had happened, because his job was to reflect on the legalities involved when someone is incompetent only. If he was moved by the effect of the court action on Tom it was his duty to get past that. He wasn't there to care, that wasn't his job. He couldn't be swayed by any input I had to offer because I was the potential enemy and his job was to 'protect Tom'. He couldn't listen to Tom's family for the same reasons. Most of all he couldn't listen to Tom, because Tom was Air.

* *Guardian Ad Litem: A court appointed figure head who collects his legal fees for speaking for a disabled incompetent person or minors. Obviously if his appointee is competent his services are no longer needed. He is there to protect funds and the disabled person's legal rights. His fees are paid for by the disabled person's estate if the disabled person has an estate. If he's particularly adept he can manage his task without ever having to look his charge in eyes.* *

I gave copies of Tom's medicals to this person as requested. Who knew what would happen if I refused to cooperate? He wasn't qualified to interpret them and he didn't call in people who were qualified to interpret them. Dr. P's reports and the testing reports with a very depressed performance score on an IQ test, a score profoundly affected by Tom's visual deficits, were included in the package, and that's as far as any of the legal thinking process went. He told us he was going to make the recommendation that Tom be considered a Ward of the Court. Let me make this clear, this particular guardian ad litem wasn't a bad person, he was as cordial and as socially appropriate as anyone else who flitted by our bodies in those days, he was just a person doing his job. Like everyone else. But Tom was dehumanized by the process of that job and I felt maligned and abandoned and ignored in the process.

The prospect of what we were facing in the Texas Courts had me in knots. I couldn't sleep, I was extremely anxious at the thought of what might happen and I was terribly upset over what it was doing to Tom. If I wasn't appointed guardian of Tom's body we were in for the nightmare of our lives. A Court appointed guardian meant that a stranger could order Tom into nursing home care any time and with no funds of my own to launch a legal battle to stop it, there would be little I could do on Tom's behalf. There was a real chance that my influence in his care could be effectively stopped cold. I could not get myself to share that reality with Tom. He would have been thrown into a complete state of panic.

As the first day in court approached Tom almost seemed rejuvenated by the challenge. I now think that it was anger that was propelling him. He was someone who always rose to the occasion and he was not going to be less at this stage of the game. However, I was watching what was fundamentally his essence in operation. The constant questions, the demands to call the lawyer over and over, the level of his frenetic activity told a different story. The bravado soon wore off to be replaced by confusion and hurt. Tom was not going to be able to bulldoze his way through this. The energy might still have been present but the ability wasn't. I spent what time I could find scrambling to organize four years of records into something intelligible. Thank God I had foreseen the need to keep everything, and thank God I routinely cross referenced it all. My paper trail was as clear as a road map.

Tom picked his 'power' wardrobe the day of his competency hearing, a black three piece Savile Row suit. There aren't many men who can carry off black in daytime the way Tom did. With his white hair and his attitude he was without doubt the best looking, best dressed, most impressive man in the entire court building. He was determined to hold it all together. He was going to show the court that he was still in charge. He showed no one. None of his effort mattered. From that point on Tom would not be included in any of the proceedings. Nothing that pertained to his life; past, present or future would be regarded with any significance. He had the unique experience of being totally ignored as a human being. From that point on Tom would always be referred to as 'The

Ward'. He didn't even get to answer his own name when it was called by the bailiff, a lawyer answered for him. Tom Murphy, who had once set the world on fire. To take his last vestige of control away, for what? Why not just blow his brains out and get it over with?

It is impossible to describe the effect it had on him. Helplessness, disappointment, and rage only began to scrape the top of what he was feeling. Helplessness, disappointment, and rage, the three most destructive emotions in human experience. Three things Tom had rarely experienced in his entire life and never in combination together.

If everyone in this drama consoled themselves with the thought that Tom didn't have the comprehension to understand what was transpiring, they were wrong. If they thought Tom was unaffected by all the machinations, they were wrong. Tom's thought process might have been erratic, he might have had difficulty integrating nuances, he might have asked the same stupid questions over and over, but he also understood the same stupid answers over and over, getting as an extra boon the pleasure of realizing the enormity of the situation over and over. If they thought Tom was unable to feel betrayal and disappointment anymore, they were wrong.

We lost it that day. I just started to cry, Tom was simply enraged. When we got home from court he stormed into the house. He went to the wall that held photographs of his life. One by one he tore them off the wall and threw them around the room. There was glass and broken picture frames and pieces of photographs all over the place. He repeated over and over ... "It's all over, it's all over." He was right. It was all over the moment he was made a ward of the court. Everything else that happened after that was out of our control.

He turned to me, his arms outstretched as if pleading with me.

"Get me away from here."

"We can't move, Tom."

"What do you mean we can't move? I want to move ... now!"

"We no longer have control over the money, Tom. We're stuck here until this mess is settled."

"How did that happen?

"Stupidity, I guess."

God! How could I be so stupid?

Beverly.
What?
Get a grip.
Do I have a choice?
Not really.

"Beverly."
"What, Tom?"
"Do you still love me?"
"God, Tom, what do you think? It's going to take a lot more than this to get rid of me."

As Tom's anxiety increased it translated into demands and unbelievable stress on me. He had one track still in operation in his brain and that focused solely on our lawyer. Unfortunately, our lawyer was now considered my lawyer and largely ignored. Regardless of the army of legal and financial people now accompanying us into court, which appeared as soon as the determination was made to put the whole disposition of the estate into the hands of strangers, in Tom's mind the only lawyer he trusted was the only lawyer who was still listening to us and that was the lawyer we had hired. However, he expected that person to be at his beck and call, day and night. He wasn't. He had office hours like the rest of the civilized world and an answering machine.

God, I have a question for You.
What is it?
Why is it that lawyers always time delivery of their mail to arrive after 5 p.m. on Fridays when it's too late to do anything about the contents of the mail. And is it written somewhere that lawyers can only serve papers, after 5 p.m. on Fridays or at 8 a.m. on Saturdays for the same reason. I mean is there a course they take that touts the importance of driving people crazy during the two day wait between Friday and Monday before issues that take your life away can be dealt with?
Good question, Beverly!

Every notification we received happened on a Friday, after it was too late to contact our lawyer, giving us what seemed like an unending series of weekends to wait before we could even tell him

246

what was happening. Unfortunately Tom was also unable to hold what 'closed for the weekend' meant in his mind.

[I should have tried brainwashing.]

Since Tom had never been formally served notice of an incompetency hearing and to insure yet another weekend of mental anguish, papers arrived 8 p.m., on, you guessed it, a Friday. He had to stand there while a court officer read the summons to him. He was to appear in court to be adjudged a disabled person and have a fiduciary guardian appointed to make decisions for him regarding himself or his property or both. He was advised that he had the right to attend the hearing, and if he was unable to understand the proceedings, someone, would be appointed to 'explain it' to him.

Tom looked at me with tears in his eyes. It was difficult for me to know who's tears were reflecting who's.

"Tom, I am not going to give up, so please, don't you. You have to stay strong for me, Tom. If you lose it, we're both dead."

"Bevaly ..."   (It was the first time he had mispronounced my name.)

"What, Tom."

"I don't even exist anymore."

"First of all, you do exist so I don't even want to hear you say that. Second of all, I love you, Tom, and nothing can change that."

I made two trips to the lawyer's closed office that weekend to prove to Tom that our lawyer wasn't available until Monday. But then, who knew if Tom even knew what Monday meant anymore. Tom never gave up having me phone our lawyer however, even after hearing his answering machine message for the eighth time. I was ready to rip the phone out of the wall. But that wouldn't have stopped him from ordering me to make the calls so why bother.

Needless to say, we were at the office the moment it opened. Our lawyer was in court all day and had been appraised of the situation. We were told to go home and he would call us later in the day. Tom refused to leave until he could speak personally with him. I managed to get him to leave long enough to get lunch but for all intents and purposes we were there the entire day with Tom pacing non stop. He was unable to sit for more than a few minutes at a time and this at great effort on my part. He drank enough coffee to float a battleship and, of course, he then had to go to the bathroom frequently. Our lawyer's staff got first view of what life with Tom could be like. Between the trips to the bathroom with our voices emanating from the confines of that room with my pleading with Tom to stand still while I got him *arranged*, his constant demands on the secretary to reach our lawyer, and my fruitless attempts to contain him, it was 'The Day From Hell'.

Our lawyer was appalled by Tom's condition when he finally returned to the office and he immediately put a call into the Guardian Ad Litem to appraise him of what the stress had done to Tom. We were told it had been noted.

God! Its all so civilized ... The world is crashing down around us and its all so freaking civilized.

As a result of that day in court I was told that nothing Tom told me to do with our finances as matter of course in our marriage was valid because Tom was known to be ill before our marriage. I pointed out that no issue with our marriage had been voiced by anyone in the family at the time and Tom was supposedly considered competent up until the court made him a Ward. Our lawyer just nodded.

[I believe using the words common sense in relation-ship to any Court driven action is what they call an oxymoron.]

Apparently, something exceedingly nefarious had been done when Tom had me include my name on our accounts and holdings. Apparently joint accounts between married individuals was a new and previously unknown innovation in spousal financing in Houston. I wondered if any of the wives' of these legal eagles were on their accounts or deeds.

In February, two months before the cold war turned into 'Wounded Knee', we were in a car accident. It took two tow trucks to separate the vehicles and no, it wasn't a subconscious suicide attempt. Our car was shaped into a right angle when I later saw it at the junk yard. Both of us ended up in the emergency unit and the paramedics were amazed that neither of us had been seriously injured. Tom had been bounced around but sustained no injury. I walked away with scrapes and some major bruises. Tom refused to get into another medium sized car after the accident.

Aside from anything else, getting him in and out of bucket seats was becoming a problem. The entry space was too confining and I could see that this seemingly simple act was no longer automatic. I'd have to pull the car seat all the way back while keeping one hand on Tom or he walked away. I'd then have to move him towards the open door of the car and tell him to get in. Most often, simple clues were enough for his body to 'click in'. If not, it took a couple of tries to get him in. I found it was easier to just turn him around and start over if he didn't succeed on the first try. It was similar to the process that impeded his finishing sentences. He either got it on the first try or he had to completely reconstruct it from the beginning. It was impossible for him to pick up anything where he had left off. If he didn't 'click in', we then had to contend with his ensuing panic which only impacted the situation more. Nothing would ever be simple again. His ability to make his body respond to old movement patterns was eroding. It impacted every situation in our lives, booths in restaurants, and seating him at the dinner table, and getting him through a revolving door, just to name a few.

Two years later there would be times when it took up to twenty minutes to get him into a car. There would be times when his body stiffened in mid motion and he'd freeze in that position unable to retrace the movement or finish it. There'd be times when it took the combined effort of my two sons and me to literally stuff him into his seat with all the accompanying combative behavior flailing about. There'd be the times when we simply turned around and returned to the house. At the time of the initial court action however, all I had was an inkling of what was to come and buying another small car with bucket seats was clearly out of the question.

We had other problems with the car. Tom couldn't figure out how to open the door by himself which became one more thing for me to do for him. However, he managed to accidentally open the door on his own while I was driving 55 mph on a couple of occasions while groping for the window knob.

With various rebates available to me because my father had been an employee of Chrysler, and the insurance money from the accident, the New Yorker we bought cost half the list price. It had a bench front seat the height and position of which could be controlled from a panel on the door of the car. The panel also allowed me to operate Tom's windows from the driver's side and I could reach the seat belts without becoming a contortionist. The car would also accommodate a wheel chair at some future date and the door opening was wide enough to give Tom the range of movement he needed to maneuver. Most of all, he felt safe in it.

How to keep my head while I watched him deteriorate? How to remain as impassive as possible so that he wouldn't know the grief I was feeling inside while I helped him handle his? All of these thoughts were racing through my brain while I was being questioned about the expenditures of funds on what was characterized as a luxury car and why it was registered in my name.

[Has anybody noticed yet that Tom can't drive?]

I explained all of the above which satisfied the interest in that purchase. The final comment was ...

"So you purchased the car for Tom's needs."

"Right".

Then I explained why my name was put on our joint checking accounts, and why we closed out Tom's retirement accounts which "were there for the purpose of being used for his retirement."

[Hello! Is anyone out there? Has anyone noticed that Tom is retired yet? Does anyone understand that he is getting disability because he can't work any longer? Is there something terribly profound about this?]

I explained why the house needed renovations and why the existing layout of the house was a problem for him given the progressive nature of his illness. I had the documentation to prove my clothes were bought in Target and Marshalls instead of Bonwit's and Sacks, and, oh yes, there were no hidden bank accounts. I guess it would be an understatement to say I was fast realizing the level of scrutiny I was under. However, I had the documentation I needed to support my defense that no money had been squirreled away for my own use, everything was accounted for, the house renovations were necessary, the trip to Phoenix was successful as proven by Dr. B's report and yes I didn't care if all of the estate assets were spent for Tom's long term care.

One of the lawyers asked me if I'd ever heard that Tom only had six months to live prior to our marriage. This would be the same man who stopped me after court some days later to tell me how much he admired the way I looked after Tom.

> [... and they tell me that lawyers are a breed apart. I wished I could separate my emotions from the rest of my life that way!]

Our lawyer refused to allow me to answer that question. I was sorry because it was the one question I expected and the one question I was ready for. We'd been married for three years at that point, so the significance of the 6 month death sentence was long past due and I was still giving Tom the most attention he had had in his entire life. And if asked what I expected to get out of marrying Tom, I was going to tell them all about the great sex we were having.

I had one goal at that time and that was to move us from Houston as fast as I could. I also needed to get us temporarily away from the constant stress surrounding us. I called Eileen Black at the A.R.E. Clinic in Phoenix and told her what was going on. I wanted to know if I could bring Tom back for another two weeks of treatment. He had refused to continue with his speech therapy and he was becoming more and more agitated and demanding as the days passed. His experience had been so good there I hoped we could regain a grasp on the whole situation. I emphasized that I wanted Tom in daily therapy sessions with their psychologist and ventured that I could use some supportive therapy myself since I was beginning to experience anxiety and sleeplessness. We set some tentative dates and rung off. I was then faced with getting approval from the court for the funds and permission to return there.

Tom's neurologist agreed that removing Tom from the stress was essential. He was deeply upset at the turn of events and wasn't surprised that Tom had started to deteriorate. Who wouldn't under the circumstances? He couldn't imagine a worse scenario for him. He also tried to support me in my efforts to care for Tom. He hoped I realized what was happening had nothing much to do with me personally and probably more to do with being Tom's second wife than anything else. That was not new news. It was the comment all the lawyers made in my direction.

"The courts are full of this stuff", they'd say.

"And you're all getting rich on it", I'd think.

I explained to our doctor that we also intended to relocate to Boulder as soon as I could get the court approval. My sister and her family were there, my sons were relocating there and both of us would have a real support system in place. I had one goal at that time and that was to get Tom into a loving and caring environment, one we could both count on. Dr. B. agreed a permanent move out of the area was in order as much for my peace of mind as for Tom's and offered to support both the return to Phoenix for treatment and the move to Boulder in writing.

May 1989, The Guardian Ad Litem petitioned the court to appoint a corporate fiduciary to be named guardian of the estate of Thomas Murphy. I was told that if I were to be appointed as Tom's fiduciary guardian, I would probably face one court appearance after another in order to justify every expenditure I authorized on Tom's behalf. It was also going to be up to the discretion of the Court to authorize our move out of Houston. Tom's body was in Houston and the money was in Houston. Even if I decided I wanted to live elsewhere, getting permission to relocate was going to be a miracle. The only straw that was held out for me was that I was to be named guardian of Tom's body mostly because I was willing to do it, and I would do it for free. That meant I was now responsible for Tom's well being, his care and his sense of himself, without any authority to order the expenditures to make any of that possible.

In recommending acceptance of this proposal I somehow missed the information that by agreeing to the removal of my name from all of our accounts and holdings I would no longer have any credit of my own since I no longer had access to any funds for myself, nor would I be able to afford legal help to defend my interests in the estate since the trust would now cite paying my legal fees as a conflict of interest. I was told that since there was no will, the estate would now be subject to probate and both Tom's progeny and I would share in whatever the laws of the state in the jurisdiction of the Trust ordained when Tom died. In addition, we would now be paying three lawyers, bankers, an investment broker, and various 'court appointees out of what was left. Any profit the

"Trust" might generate above what I had been getting on investments would now be offset by fees and there would be lots of fees. I would now be subject to question on everything I needed to run the house and Tom's care. My care, my sanity and my needs were now at the bottom of everyone's list. I was now officially unpaid help.

This would be most graphically demonstrated a little further down the pike when I was questioned about my rental of videos and asked if those videos were rented solely for Tom's amusement. It was my duty as Tom's wife to take care of him but it wasn't all right for me to receive money for those services, services for which they'd gladly pay others. If I chose to work while someone else watched Tom, my share of the budget would be downgraded according to my earnings in order to offset the cost of Tom's care in my absence and of course there were still the legal issues of my obligations if and when the money ran out. I was the only one accountable.

The fiduciary guardian was responsible for conserving the estate for all the heirs, however they could recommend payment of any of their fees as they saw fit. When all was said and done in Texas, nearly $80,000 had been spent on legal and court fees and the cash register is still clicking.

I was ordered to sign over accounts that were jointly held by both of us and I voluntarily signed over the one CD Tom ordered me to put in my name when the whirlwind started. I was questioned about whether the $2,000 IRA that was still in my name was really mine. Can words describe this? It wasn't a total loss, I got a letter from the Trust thanking me for my cooperation.

[And I thought indentured servitude was something that went out with the Pilgrims. Silly me!]

Questions about Tom's medical care, except for ordinary daily care would be taken out of my hands and his. Questions about life support, treatment, continuance of care that was contrary to his wishes would now be in the hands of the court since Tom had also neglected to establish a living will or give me a durable power of attorney on medical issues. I wondered if I'd be allowed to bury him after all was done with, or would the final travesty be the court battle over his remains.

Aside from anything else, the bottom line was that there was still no prognosis for Tom. Tom might just live out his normal life span, then what? Longevity was well established in Tom's family. The court in the meantime was petitioned for funds to be provided for the cost of travel, lodging, and treatment for Tom at the A.R.E. Clinic in Arizona. The court agreed since they were mandated to provide medical treatment for him and I had rallied all his doctors to support the request.

Our lawyer, who was now considered my lawyer, would hereafter be ignored because I didn't exist anymore as a voice in our financial affairs and everyone knew I didn't have the money needed to become one. In fact, he wasn't even permitted to take part in the final negotiations because he kept raising issues no one, including the judge, wanted to deal with. The next step in establishing the 'Trust' would be a formality. Our presence wasn't even required. As I saw it, we had no choice in the matter. The whole thing had been taken out of our hands. We left for Phoenix knowing we were about to be screwed.

Tom and I were victims of theft. However, something much more grand than money was at stake. Something much more precious than that was taken from us, something so precious that it is impossible to even calculate its worth, and it was taken heartlessly without an inkling of a notion of how irreplaceable it was. The ignominy of it all is that no one even recognized it as having value.

Time had been stolen from us.

The last best year of our lives together would be spent fighting for survival and grasping at sanity instead of being allowed to experience what was left of the joy of each other's company and love. I didn't know if I could ever forgive the loss of that.

254

I CONCENTRATE ON YOU

Whenever skies look grey to me
And trouble begins to brew,
Whenever the winter winds become too strong,
I concentrate on you.

When fortune cries "Nay, Nay!" to me
And people declare "You're through,"
Whenever the Blues become my only song,
I concentrate on you.

On your smile so sweet, so tender,
When at first your kiss I decline,
On the light in your eyes, when I surrender,
And once again our arms intertwine.

And so when wise men say to me
That love's young dream never comes true,
To prove that even, wise men can be wrong,
I concentrate on you,
I concentrate
And concentrate
On you.

words and music by: Cole Porter

CHAPTER TWELVE

I'd hoped we could put what was going on in Texas on the back burner as we started our drive to Phoenix. It was a foolish wish. The happenings were impacting our lives in ways far beyond what either of us could have imagined. However, we tried to make the best of the time we had away from the madness.

Phoenix held the promise of offering respite for me. I needed time alone away from Tom and I needed to have normal conversation with someone, somewhere soon or go nuts. I had no outlet in Houston, no family, no friends, no one other than Tom on a day to day basis. The isolation was consuming. No aspect of my life was my own anymore. Everything revolved around Tom and his needs and scrambling to get some semblance of control back into our lives. I couldn't remember when I'd been able to laugh at a simple joke, or talk about a movie, or just sit and find a quiet place. Every minute of the day was more or less spent in readiness for combat. The only thing that kept me going was the total belief in Tom's love for me and mine for him. We still had moments in spite of it all and those moments were still of value.

Tom decided to return to the Catholic Church which he did shortly after our move to Houston. It was a natural progression for him, it was familiar and it gave him comfort. We attended Mass at least once a week. My experience revolved more on helping Tom stand and kneel on cue and steering him down the aisle for communion than furthering my own sense of peace, although I still managed to find moments for myself. Father Jim told me I was going to get my wings this time around. I was still trying to figure out if he was speaking metaphysically or figuratively when we left for Phoenix. I decided I wanted big fluffy ones. I hoped Phoenix would give me time to examine a lot of things on my mind.

Tom's re-evaluation showed improvement in his ability to do his exercises. However, it was also apparent that little of that facility had translated into improved functioning. Those abilities had obviously deteriorated. His speech had remained marginally stabilized and perhaps the exercises had helped in that regard. Considering the stress we'd been under they probably helped a lot more than could be measured. There was also one glaring difference in the Tom Murphy who had been there a year ago and the Tom Murphy who walked in the door this time. His spark was gone. I would find he had a different purpose for being there this time.

That time alone for me never happened. Instead I found myself sitting outside his treatment room invariably called into his session to reassure him I was still there. The moment he missed me he had to see me and there was always an element of panic in his demeanor until I appeared. I guess it was natural for him to wonder if I was going to jump ship. I don't think there was ever a time in his life when he felt so vulnerable. I assured him over and over in every way I could imagine that I wasn't going to leave him. We ended up in what seemed like marathon counseling sessions because that was the only thing Tom wanted to do ... talk. He talked about his fears, his anger, his disappointment, his sense of loss, his death, whether I could live without any money, my death. It was clear that he wasn't there to get physically better, he was there to deal with the awareness that he no longer had a life and he had better tie up the loose ends while he could still think. In some ways he was also there to mourn. He even had a dream for the occasion.

"I'm at Astor Place in New York City. I'm walking towards the subway when I notice a young nun ahead of me. She is headed down the stairs to the subway. She's wearing a beautifully tailored suit ... grey. There's a silver cross over her blouse, it's the only way you can tell they're nuns anymore ... that silver cross ... and she is very beautiful. There is also a large brooch on her lapel. A large silver 'C'. It's very ornate and quite striking. As she moves ahead of me I notice a young hoodlum following her. He is close behind her as they enter the tunnel. I don't know what he's up to, but I have the feeling he isn't up to any good so I hurry to catch up to her. The hoodlum starts to approach her but I step in between them. I tell him to move along ... very few people stay when I ask them to move along, you know ... I stay with her for a few minutes until the train

*arrives and make sure she gets on without further
trouble.*"

Eileen Black, who was once more working with Tom asked him
to focus on the most significant thing in his dream. He immediately
mentioned the brooch. She asked Tom why it was shaped in the
form of a 'C'.

" Does the 'C' symbolize something to you, Tom?"

"C could be church. Church is all encompassing.

"You mean like a sanctuary?"

"Sanctuary! (long pause) You couldn't take a person out of the
church ... with violence. (long pause) I may be the sanctuary."

"Do you need to be protected, Tom?"

"No! I was the one who did the protecting. My mother ... My
family ... I stop ... Most people don't stop if someone falls. I stop.
I feel protective to those more vulnerable. I always felt good
helping people. My brothers said I was going to land in jail helping
someone some day."

He sat quietly for a few seconds as if trying to remember
something and then he started to speak again.

"... a bully! When I was about twelve there was a bigger kid,
and he came over and picked a fight. I told him, I don't want to
fight."

"I'm gonna make you fight! I'm going to beat you up, he said."

There was a long pause as Tom shifted in his chair. His body
stance changed, his back straightened, his eyes narrowed as he
gazed into the camera taping this session. The transformation
occurred in only a second or two. When he finally spoke his voice
hadn't risen in volume or timber but the power behind the words he
said made the hair on my neck stand on end. He had transformed
himself back to the age of twelve and he was looking directly into
the eyes of that bully.

"... and I said to him, I told him ... Now! When you do this!
Your first blow ... You have to kill me. Because, if you don't, I
will do my best ... to kill you!"

Tom then waved his hand in the air as though to dismiss the
image and looking back at us he continued ...

"He walked on. They only pick on underdogs."

As he finished speaking he shifted in his seat again, returning to his former stance. Tears came to his eyes and he started to wipe them away.

"You're very good, Black."

"Good at what, Tom?"

"Getting into me."

The vulnerability he was feeling colored everything he did and said at the clinic during the next two weeks. We both had our work cut out for us. There was one particularly emotional session we shared when Eileen offered him two possible alternatives. He could either get well, or he could die. If death was what he had resigned himself to, then was there anything he needed to resolve first? Tom's response centered around me and his fears that my anger at what was happening to our lives was going to do me in. He was worried about my soul. He feared I was going to ruin my chances to move on after I died if I didn't let go of that anger. He actually used the words ...

"I'm going to a better place and I want to know that *Bevaly* is going to be there with me."

He was fearful about my being able to survive if all the money was gone by the time he died. I tried to reassure him that I'd be all right. I'd have my pension, I could still work, I had two sons and a family I could count on for help. The conversation then moved back to whether or not my soul was going to be able to meet up with him again. He told me over and over that I had to let go of my anger. It was going to do me in. He once told me, in response to a complaint I had about what I characterized as an insidious assault from a colleague, that ...

"Most of the people we think hate us don't even know we're alive."

He said those words again while we were in Phoenix as I sat there still answering the implied charges of misconduct made by people who had no place in our lives.

"You mustn't waste energy on them," he kept saying. "You must be able to blow it all away."

Eileen tried to get him to focus on his own anger. She asked him how he felt about his illness ...

"I've had one hell of a life, Black!"

"Don't you feel cheated, Tom? Don't you wonder ... Why me?"

"Why not me? We're all going to die some day. I don't think how is up to God or me. What happened to me isn't great, but then I might have died in the war and had no life."

"It can't be that simple for you, Tom. What about what's happening in Houston? How do you feel about that?"

"I've been raped." (long pause)

"I'm trying to blow it all away."

He was following the same advice he'd given me a few years earlier, once again when I arrived home complaining about my job. He told me that whether or not I enjoyed my work was totally up to me, it had nothing to do with the people I worked with, not co-workers, not clients, not the bureaucracy.

"Hell, there isn't a job in the world that isn't a bureaucracy. It's entirely up to you whether you like your work or not."

At that moment I thought he was being unnecessarily simplistic when what I thought I needed from him was commiseration about my terrible state of being, but he would have none of that.

"Stop fighting life", he said, and changed the subject. I could have been very resentful of his unasked for advice but something in me heard what he was saying. Something in me remembered words my father used to say when my mother or my sisters or I ranted on about things we couldn't change ...

"You know, life is lot like drowning, it's not so bad once you stop fighting it."

I used to laugh that comment off, thinking what in tarnation does that mean? Suddenly I had an inkling of what both my father and Tom were trying to say to me.

The next day, although still annoyed at having to resubmit my request for approval of a vocational plan for someone with ALS, a someone the agency did not want to work with because of the terminal nature of his illness, I tried a different tact. I went into work with a smile on my face. I decided at that moment that everyone in my office including the person giving me a problem about this client's plan were people to like instead of people to take umbrage with. I had to rewrite my request, but I did it with a desire to make it meet the requirements needed instead of spouting off and getting nothing accomplished. I even managed to get a sense of satisfaction out of it. The plan was approved.

The last two years of my job were the happiest most productive time I had during the 25 years I worked for New York State. I actually enjoyed going to work and it's not because anything changed on the job. I changed. It was a sort of epiphany, a civil service epiphany. Talk about the impossible happening. Could the impossible happen again?

Tom's words to me were loud and clear but there was also another message behind his admonishments to let my anger go. I realized Tom knew our life together was going to be very limited and he was planning for a future for us that wasn't necessarily going to happen in this lifetime. The need to hope that we'd still have that chance together was the only thing I had to keep going. I already knew that hateful thoughts towards anyone would only serve to delay my own spiritual growth. Intellectually I knew nothing was worth that. I'd been wrestling with those feelings as long as I could remember. How does one put all that intensity aside? Tom reminded me that it was a choice I had to make and it could be as simple as that. What had happened in Houston had nothing to do with him or me. It didn't change who he was and he didn't plan to go to his death hating anyone. He didn't plan to go to his death with me hating anyone not if he had anything to say about it.

The problem is that it wasn't anger I was dealing with, it was rage. I couldn't fathom the personal attack I had experienced. But the callous, indifferent way in which Tom was being treated, that was a wound that wouldn't heal. He deserved better than that. I hurt so deeply for him it clouded my mind.

I had a long way to go if I was going to get this particular chapter closed. I also realized that I had taken Tom's burden on as my own and I wasn't helping the situation, but I wasn't ready or able to let go of any of it at that point. I was in the heat of battle to get us out of Houston and the adrenaline surge was the only thing keeping me functioning at that time. The only reassurance I could give Tom was that I loved him, I'd survive with or without the estate and yes I was trying to put the happenings in Houston into some sort of perspective. It was difficult for me to think in terms of forgiveness which is what the people in the clinic and Tom were trying to impress upon me. That was a task that was still in the future as far as I could tell. The tasks at hand were already taking up all of my thought process and energy. The tasks of watching and knowing that Tom's awareness was probably the best it was ever going to be. From here on in it was going to be down hill. I now knew his existence would eventually be reduced to eating and sleeping and being kept dry and clean. I was still wrapped up in feeling responsible for what Tom felt and understood about what was happening in our lives and I just wasn't ready to let my attachment to him go long enough to even think about myself. I felt like a mother who had to defend her child, and the rage I felt was just as deep and complete. Forgiveness! That was a term that was not within my capacity at that time.

[Tom told me that forgiveness doesn't absolve people of the intent behind their deeds it means that you have stopped needing to prove you're right. It means letting them be, as they are, to live their lives and learn their own lessons while you get on with your own.]

Ultimately, I was able to understand what he had tried to tell me. But at the time of our visit to Phoenix I was in a very different place. The best I could do was acknowledge that I had a lot of work to do on my emotional and spiritual state of being. Perhaps I'd have time to think about it later. Perhaps I wouldn't care to hang on to it all so much by then. Perhaps something else would fill that particular void. Perhaps I'd have time to do that when we got our lives back. By then, the only awareness I'd have to consider would be my own. I'd deal with forgiveness then.

That task filed away for future reference, I suddenly realized how angry I was at Tom for giving up. I was very angry that he wasn't there to get well. I suddenly found myself having to shift from making him better to accepting our fate as a couple. I thought he was the strongest, most pervasive person on earth. I thought if anyone could beat this thing it would be Tom Murphy. I thought my love for him would give him the impetus he needed to rise above it all. How dare he cave into this illness. How dare he let me down. How dare he give up and die. I believed in him. If the word 'why' loomed in my mind at all, it was 'why' was he letting me down? Why was he choosing to abandon me? The answer to that, of course, is that he wasn't. It was really up to me to see that and eventually I did come to terms with that.

I had carefully avoided the consideration of what a death due to Alzheimer's Disease, or whatever it was that was destroying Tom's brain, would be like. Tom succumbing to that? No! I couldn't avoid it any longer and I was terribly frightened. I didn't know how I'd manage financially if I was left with nothing at Tom's death. I didn't know what kind of work I could find at my age in an area where my experience was meaningless. My job didn't exist outside of New York. How could my family help me out, they were barely able to help themselves. How would I manage when Tom became incontinent? Where would I find the strength to face his decline? What would I do when he could no longer communicate his needs? I went into mourning for what had already occurred in our lives and in anticipation of what was to come.

> *   *How do you choose the time to say goodbye to someone who continues to live long after the ability to communicate is gone?   Elisabeth Kubler-Ross talks about the stages of dying.   All I can say is that with Alzheimer's you don't go through those stages just once, you go through them over and over and over.   There are no perimeters to this illness, no time frame, no reference points, just the knowledge that it hits everyone differently.   Just when you think you've got it all in hand you suddenly realize there's something else to mourn, there's one more thing he can't do or express and you are plunged into darkness again.   It seems to never end. You can't hide from it, you can't control it, you can't fathom it.* *

I grieved in ways I never thought possible.   I discovered I not only experienced my own loss of Tom, but as his awareness deteriorated I grieved in his place for him.   I'd manage to go for days, weeks, sometimes months just plowing along, actually happy that he'd stabilized and we had a routine we could count on and then the reality would hit again, sometimes triggered but some seemingly insignificant event.

Tom lost his French regimental beret.   It was hours before I missed it.   I spent days crawling over every step we'd made hoping to find it.   I left messages in restaurants, stores in the mall, stores in front of parking spaces we had used, everything just short of an ad in the local newspaper.   I blamed myself for not being more vigilant.   I cried for days.   To this day, every time I think about that hat tears fill my eyes.   On some level it had come to symbolize all of Tom's humor and joy of life to me and it too was gone.

The amount of energy it took to maintain even the basic amenities of life was Herculean. For the moment, (it was always for the moment), Tom and I handled things as best we could. It was a matter of living out the rest of our lives and of treasuring what we had left together. We were told to keep our goals simple and live each day one day at a time. We were given this advice as if we had a choice. With Tom's attention span reduced to less than a thirty second cycle we got a crash course on the reality of what living in the moment is all about. The real challenge was finding joy in any given thirty seconds. The amazing thing is that we did just that. When people ask me how we found that joy I now know it's because we chose to find it.

We made a pact with each other. I promised I'd be there for him until he died. I felt there was a power in me that would give me the ways and means to meet that promise. We'd be all right. I'd be all right. I also told him he had better be there waiting for me when it was my turn to die or he'd find out what anger was really all about. He promised me he'd always take care of me. I believe, even from this vantage point that he has kept that promise. We also made love. It was the only thing in our lives that still lasted for more than a thirty second interval.

As the two weeks in the clinic passed he improved, showing once again what understanding, patience and interest could do for him. Their clinical psychologist felt there was sufficient improvement to warrant the recommendation that Tom be removed from the stressful environment in Texas as soon as possible. He felt forced continuation there could actually endanger his life.

Once again I took a deep breath thinking we had things under control. I was wrong. Several nights after we finally faced our real fears, Tom stopped sleeping. Tom was someone who was asleep the moment he decided to sleep. Friends spoke often of that particular trait of his and for those of us who suffer from residual insomnia it was also a source of envy and occasional annoyance. I had come to the point where I depended on his sleeping. It wasn't easy for me to wind down at night and knowing there'd be no interruptions from him made it easier to finally drop off myself.

It started one night with trips to the bathroom, not just an occasional trip, but trips ... countless trips. Since he couldn't be sure of his aim or whether he had his pajamas arranged properly it meant that I had to make the trip with him. He couldn't find his way around the motel room without help, the darkness increased his disorientation and his hands which he kept in front of him like Frankenstein's monster, cleared off tables, counters, lamps, anything in their path. It was almost as if he was sleep-walking, only he wasn't. He might return to bed and drop off to sleep immediately, or he might not. I on the other hand, after cleaning up whatever it was he left in his wake, often having had to change his pajamas, would be wide awake by the time I got back to bed. I'd just begin to drop off when the whole scenario would repeat itself. It was hell, the pattern repeating itself over and over. He'd rise out of bed, hit the floor with his feet, announce he had to go to the bathroom and then the furtive moving around the room would begin. It was unbelievable.   He'd manage a sufficient number of cat naps to allow him to still function during the day. I felt like the walking dead. The pattern ran a five night cycle from one solid night of sleep to no sleep. It started during the last of our stay in Phoenix, and continued in varying degrees of intensity until he could no longer walk, some four years later.   Once he was bedridden his wakefulness was at least contained in one place and I could then sleep in some semblance of peace.

> * *Nothing is worse than being deprived of sleep, nothing! When you are chronically deprived of sleep you have only one hope of survival. You learn how to prioritize your life and you find the lowest common denominator that still allows you to function, or you die.* *

We drove home by way of Boulder, arriving at my sister's house on Memorial Day. I wanted to look into medical resources for Tom there and get some idea as to property possibilities. We planned to spend the holiday with my family but as soon as we arrived Tom announced he wanted to look at houses. I tried to explain that we didn't have permission to move and there'd be no one to show us around anyway because it was a holiday. Tom dug his heels in and was so obnoxious about it that my brother-in-law Jack called his realtor just to placate Tom.

"We're here, I want to look at houses ... now!"

Carlo was home. Not only that, Carlo had no plans and he'd love to show us around.

"God, I just hate it when he gets his own way. Look at him, he's positively smug."

We needed a one story house, a simple floor plan, a basement and at least one bathroom large enough to accommodate a wheel chair or hydraulic lift. I also hoped for a master bathroom with a shower stall instead of a tub. I could now see that getting Tom into a tub was a lot harder than walking into a shower stall and Tom always preferred showers anyway. The bathroom was becoming a major obstacle in our routine every morning. When they say it's the most dangerous room in the house, trust me, it is. It's more than just slipping on wet surfaces, its keeping the electric razor away from running water, keeping breakables out of reach, finding safe places for cleaning supplies, regulating water temperature so that scalding can be avoided or removing knobs altogether. Its having as little as possible in view so as not to clutter up an already cluttered mind. Tom's movement was so erratic that he was in danger of slipping even with non skid markers. We'd always showered together so my knowing it wasn't safe for Tom to be in the tub alone was hardly noticed by him.

Our bathroom in Houston was so tiny that it was extremely difficult for him to navigate it without help. There was only a cabinet door width between the toilet and the vanity. The vanity gave Tom a very narrow margin of error in movement. I had to position him by that space while I stepped over the toilet and into the tub where I then coaxed him through that space and into the tub. Once he got through his pain response after banging his thigh on the corner of the vanity and stubbing his toes as he misjudged how high to pick up his feet, I'd finally get him in the tub.

I was now washing his hair for him because he didn't always get the soap out completely. He rather enjoyed the attention but one day he became rigid when I tried to move his head under the water. The more I tried the more panicked he became. The result was his flailing about with soap in his eyes and my being knocked out of the tub and over the toilet. Fortunately neither of us were hurt although I did end up with a couple of technicolor bruises. I went out that day and bought a hand held shower. That solved part of the problem. I no longer had to move him towards the water, I could move the water towards him.

Stairs were also a problem. He could go up and down alone but I had to position myself in front of him on the down trip and behind him on the up trip. It was only a matter of time before stairs would become a part of his past. Since the only bath was upstairs we were facing major problems with the house in Houston.

After crawling though the sixth house, that Memorial Day with Carlo, Tom and I were both fairly depressed. Nothing we looked at met our needs and all of the properties were over priced and in need of major renovations. It was then that Carlo told us he had one more house to show us. An hour later we walked into our new home. It was a ranch with a full basement, three bedrooms and a spacious dining-living room. The floor plan was simple and easy for Tom to navigate and it was carpeted, which would cut down on the noise factor. Whole areas could be easily set off for him to wander in peace and safely. It had a large bathroom with a tub and a master bathroom with a shower stall. It was not only in our price range, it was a 'buy'.

As for medical treatment facilities, there were adult day care facilities that worked exclusively with Alzheimer's and other dementia care in the area. There were nursing homes with Alzheimer's units should Tom need to be placed at some point in the future, and I already had referrals for several excellent geron-tology and neurology specialists in the Boulder community. There was a great deal of research going on in Dementia in the Denver Metro area, and the whole area was fast becoming a retirement haven with excellent facilities available in the care of an elder population. And there were Trust firms throughout the Denver Metro area that would accept transfer of the Trust account to Colorado. We couldn't have asked for a better area in terms of meeting Tom's present and future needs.

Our lawyer told me to make an offer when we phoned him. Thanks to Tom's stubbornness, we now had a house in Boulder. We had thirty days to get approval from the Trust and the Court or the deal would fall through but our lawyer felt the Trust couldn't oppose the move. In spite of what was said to me to the contrary, no one could dictate where I wanted to live as Tom's wife and I had gathered sufficient resource material that substantiated the need for a supportive environment for both the primary caregiver, as well as the person suffering from Dementia.

As for a solid support system, my sister Norma and her family were living there and my brother-in-law Jack was the minister of one of the larger churches in Boulder. There was already a large community waiting for us with open arms. The local Catholic church which would continue to serve Tom's spiritual needs had a lay ministry which would be available to comfort him in his home when that became a necessity. And, last of all, but not least, I was now Tom's official body guardian, so I now had some voice, albeit a small one, in determining what was best for him.

As Tom's fiduciary guardian, the Trust was mandated to provide for Tom's well being and they couldn't force him to continue in an environment that was not only unhealthy but potentially dangerous as evidenced by the problems with the house in Houston. The medical documentation advised that Tom be moved to a more supportive atmosphere. His decline since the beginning of the Court action was well documented by his doctors in Houston, the clinic in Phoenix, and in daily notes I had kept on the day to day care of him.

There was also the matter of my certification as a rehabilitation counselor which couldn't be entirely ignored by the Court as giving me credibility in determining Tom's long term needs and it was obvious by now that my care of Tom and my concern for his well being was genuine as his wife. Our lawyer said if everything went according to plan there was a good chance we'd be in Boulder by September.

Tom virtually hummed through the rest of the trip home. The only glitch in the works was Tom's continuing insistence that we move immediately after closing. It was just more of the unending conversation. I kept saying we couldn't move, he kept demanding ... "Why not?"

By our return from Phoenix in June '89, we both knew that Tom was in the process of taking yet another nose dive in functioning. His increasing agitation and impatience with waiting, the deterioration in coping ability as the day ended and darkness began, the noise factors which added to his disorientation all conspired to take away what was left of a social life for us. Movies were impossible.

He couldn't sit still long enough to see one through. July 29, 1989, my birthday, would be the very last time we were able to dine out at night. We left the table before finishing our main course because he was fast approaching a full scale panic attack. Over the next two years he lost lunch and then breakfast. For a while we were reduced to a drive through window and I fed him in the car. Today he is entirely house bound.

The last of the traveling we did together was during that July as well. The trip was planned so that he could say goodbye to his brothers and as many of his friends as possible. Deep down we knew this would be the last visit we'd make to any of them as a couple. We drove because other forms of transportation were now out of the question. The tiny little cubicles on buses, trains and planes that passed for rest rooms were traps. Tom accidentally locked himself in one on a bus once and it took over half hour to get him out. He couldn't follow the directions to move the bolt. Talk about forty people on the verge of nervous hysteria as he was finally extricated from his little prison. The whole bus was aware that a grown up man had locked himself in and couldn't get out. Every head was turned in his direction as he finally came down the aisle. He made the following comment as he got himself in his seat ...

"I'd think twice about going in there. I think it was a communist lock."

Everyone laughed out loud including the bus driver who was now a half hour behind schedule. They were almost grateful that he could joke about it.

After the bus incident I didn't dare let him go into such a cubicle without me and the two of us trying to get him 'arranged' in one of those things was beyond description. However the larger men's rooms on the highways created other problems. He got lost in them which necessitated my having to ask some passing gent to please steer him out. Two or three of those incidents and it finally dawned on me that taking him into the handicapped stall in the ladies room was the only solution. It was surprising how understanding and helpful the ladies turned out to be and how undramatic it actually was. I heard this also from a friend I met through a support group a few years later. He found himself in much the same situation with his wife. There was something about seeing a man in the ladies room that brought maternal instincts out in everyone.

[However, it's still too bad the handicapped stalls aren't off by themselves in some generic little spot instead of situated in Ladies and Men's rest rooms. Most handicapped people travel with companions. Those who need assistance are always faced with that unnecessary extra little humiliation. A sink would also be nice in those stalls. In fact, I'd say the sink is a necessity.]

As for Tom's adjustment to this new aspect of life, he was true to form. It was a necessary evil and one he decided to live with. Could I do less? I adjusted.

We determined to let that aspect of the trip be an insignificant one, all things considered it was the least of the problems. The trip turned into a disaster anyway and we ended up cutting it short. I drove two days without sleep from Virginia to Texas with him hallucinating most of the return trip home. At one point I put him in the back seat in his seat belt knowing he'd never figure out how to undo it. He kicked the seat for three hours but at least he couldn't grab the steering wheel.

His confusion mounted as the trip had progressed. His tolerance for unfamiliar surroundings was eroding fast. We were faced with a different place to sleep every night, with bathrooms that had no doors and doors that couldn't hold him in the room when he was wandering. His wanderings at night resulted in towels in the toilet, curtains pulled off their rods, anything and everything that wasn't nailed down moved, knocked over, or broken. The couple of nights we tried to stay with friends ended with hasty trips to a motel. They had no idea what form his wandering could take in terms of destruction of stuff. His sleeplessness wasn't translated into just being up it was the activity and the belligerence attached to it. Friends felt I whisked him away too quickly but they had no idea what they were in for and frankly I wanted their last memory of him to be something other than that.

The restaurants on the road tended to be noisy, over decorated, and uncommonly dark at night, three things that assailed what was left of Tom's vision and hearing. One particular place had whole areas marked off with platforms and brass railings to demarcate the salad bar and desert areas from the dining areas which were defined with more platforms and rails. It was like walking into a maze. I usually requested a booth because they tended to cut down on the noise factor but the booths in this restaurant were also on platforms. Leading Tom through the maze to our table was difficult because he kept slamming into every obstacle we passed no matter how I tried to steer him. Helping him into his side of the booth was a nightmare. He kept walking into the platform, backing up and hitting it again. He couldn't get his right foot on the platform and bend his body at the same time so that he could slide into his seat. After a number of tries he finally got himself positioned so that I was able to push him onto his seat. He was by that time, annoyed and embarrassed.

It was humiliating for both of us. People were staring, some even laughing. Most assumed he was drunk. As if that wasn't enough, the table cloth and the napkins were both dark green and Tom's vision and the dimness of the room made it impossible for him to find his own napkin. It wasn't his fault that the bread basket held the only white napkin in his range of view or that he grabbed and flicked it, as he always did when putting a napkin on his lap, before I could catch his hand. The bread and rolls went flying some of them bouncing off the brass rail next to us. He just hung his head. I started to cry. I had been driving all day on half a night's sleep and I was exhausted. The waitress who observed the whole ordeal came over and placed two glasses of wine in front of us. She gently rested her hand on Tom's shoulder and said;

"I think both of you could use a drink right now ... This one's on me, honey."

Later she confided in me that her mother had died of Alzheimer's. She recognized Tom's behavior. She wondered how long my father had been dealing with it. It really bothered me that our relationship as husband and wife wasn't the obvious assumption, but then with Tom's white hair and the weight loss he looked so much older than he was. It was important to me that people knew I wasn't a dutiful daughter taking dear ole' dad out once a week to give dear ole' mom a break, I was the one there all the time. I was the only one there all the time. I was the one living this horror with him. In a way, it was as much my illness as it was his. I felt dismissed by the assumption knowing there was really little I could do about it short of wearing a sign that read ... "Me Wife ... Him Husband". One more thing to let go of.

* *People in Tom's situation don't just wake up one morning and forget who Aunt Emma is. They don't just* *wake up one morning and forget how to put a sentence together. They don't just wake up one morning and forget a lifetime of experience and love. The lights, unfortunately, don't all go out at once. People like Tom experience one of the most horrible aspects of life and death that has ever been burdened on a living soul. They experience the gradual awareness that their brain is dying and they can do nothing to stop that death, a brain assailed with images and misinterpretations and unconnected thoughts that we can't begin to imagine. If they don't know exactly what it is that is happening to them, they do know that things are different for them. They grasp at whatever they can to hang on to their dignity and their definition of who they are. They need our time, our patience and they need unconditional love. They need more than many of us thought we'd ever be able to give.* *

Much to our amazement the purchase of the house in Boulder was approved without a problem. I had all the medicals recommending the move for Tom and I had made sure he was at every Court date set whether that Court date resulted in a continuance or not. Everyone in that Courtroom, the judge included, got to see Tom in his full glory. His impatience, his inability to sit still, his anxiety, his many trips to the bathroom, the increased intensity of all of the above as the weeks passed. He had a right to be there and they couldn't tell me to keep him away. I made sure they all got to see what this so called intervention into his life to protect his interests in his estate and his life was doing to him. And Tom, made little effort to hold anything back. In fact there were moments when I wondered if he was doing some of it on purpose.

However, the court still wouldn't give us permission to move until all the estate issues were settled and we seemed to be facing one continuance after another with nothing happening. Tom took another nose dive as soon as the delays started. He became phobic about being upstairs in the house and refused to sleep in the bedroom anymore. I finally figured out that he was afraid of being trapped in a fire. We moved to the sofa bed in the living room where he could keep an eye on the front door. The upstairs bedroom at least had a door which allowed me to contain his movement on nights when he felt compelled to pace. Downstairs it was open season for marathoners. The house was one of those railroad houses with no connecting doors and with Tom on the move at night it was a vast territory to cover.

To placate his constant harping to move, I started to pack. I packed to give the impression the move was imminent and to build a walk way for him at night in case I didn't awaken when he got up. The path I constructed led from the front room, barricaded the stairway and continued through the house to the back room bathroom. Between the furniture, the boxes, and the night lights I'd placed all over the downstairs area, there was little with which he could get in trouble if I didn't awaken.

Along with the pacing at night he also developed nervous tics, little rituals of repeated movement that went on for hours on end. He started repeating words over and over and over. He got stuck on 'hello' for a while and then moved to the word 'here'. After a while he fixated on combinations of those two words all muttered while he paced from one end of the house to the other. I'd sit in what probably looked like a stupor of my own, watching him pace and pick at himself while he muttered in a monotonous drone for hours at a time.

"Here ... here ... here, here? Here ... hello? Here! ..hello? Here! ... here! *Bevaly?* ... here ... hello!"

Hang in there, Beverly!
I'm hanging Lord ... but in case You haven't noticed, my fingernails are beginning to bleed.

One afternoon a neighbor and her daughter knocked on our door. She said her daughter was going to keep Tom company for a little while and I was going home with her. She sat me down in her living room, poured me a glass of wine, and told me it was obvious to everyone how much I loved Tom and what taking care of him meant. It was a small community, things were noticed. She wanted me to know it was time to pull myself together.

"You look like hell, Beverly. You're going around town looking like a mess. I want you to start fixing your hair and your makeup before you step foot outside that house and for goodness sakes dress up in something other than those white pants and tee shirts. You look like Tom's attendant instead of his wife. You stand up and let everyone know you're still in charge of your life. If you need someone to stay with Tom while you get dressed, you call me and I'll come over. I don't want to see you looking like this again. Besides, dressing up will help you feel better. I know it's going to make me feel better."

She was right. Dressing up did make me feel better. It was time to stop feeling sorry for myself. It was time to start making some choices, and it was time to stop being a victim. So what if the money was gone! So what! I still had Tom's love, I still had my creativity, I still had a whole life ahead of me. It could be worse. We could be living in Calcutta.

Between June and August of 1989 Tom lost over 30 pounds. Except for apples and other hand held food, he had to be fed. He could still talk to me but conversation, if it could still be characterized as such, was limited to three word sentences and getting to content was like pulling teeth. He was also hallucinating again. Any reflective surface such as mirrors or windows became a problem. He seemed to get lost in them, often yelling four letter words and other diatribes in what I thought was a rather creative fashion. I wondered what or whom he was seeing. He seemed to have little if any problem getting the curse words out but then that was also a symptom of his illness. As one level of expression was lost the next lower level surfaced. It was of interest that he was still speaking German with our neighbor rather well. As for hygiene, I was now finishing his shave for him which allowed me to keep total control of the razor and his toilet problems were increasing. It was more than steering him around and arranging his clothing, he needed help cleaning himself.

God! What's next? How am I going to keep this up?
Beverly!
Yes?
Do it with love ... or don't do it at all!

There was the night I'd simply passed out from exhaustion. It was the third night with no sleep. I had sensed that Tom was out of bed and roaming through the house but I was too tired to get up. The next thing I realized was that he was gently shaking me, his head next to mine, our noses almost touching. I finally opened my eyes and heard him say ...

"Bevaly ... Bevaly ... I ... think I knocked something over."

It was one of those gestalt experiences. One of those moments when you see it all in a flash. I remembered that I hadn't screwed the top on the new gallon size bottle of Tide I'd just bought. I remembered leaving it on the vanity instead of the floor and I saw at the same time the blue foot prints reflected in the night lights, spaced in Tom's shuffling walk, through the kitchen and across the dining room floor. I smelled the distinctive odor of Tide and heard the squishing sound of Tom's feet as he padded back and forth trying to waken me. I saw the look of panic on Tom's face and the look of horror on my own. My body remembered that it had been three nights without a good nights' sleep. Somewhere from the depths of my being I heard myself groan a long tired moan.

I got out of bed and as I walked to the back of the house I knew there would be at least a half inch of Tide on the floor of the 'powder room'. Tom walked into me when I stopped at the doorway. I just stood there wondering how I was going to clean the mess up and what to tackle first. If I cleaned Tom's feet first, he'd be back in it by the time I cleaned the gook up. If I cleaned his feet last he'd be tracking it all over the house while I worked on the floor. I turned around and saw him there behind me. His head was hung on his chest and he was crying.

"I feel so dumb."

"Damn it, Tom! You look at me! I love you and you are not dumb. You are the best in the world to me and don't you ever forget that."

We just stood there holding each other for a while and then I led him back into the kitchen. I pulled out a chair, sat him in it and rummaged through the boxes until I located his wine. I opened a bottle of Beaulieu Vineyard, 1972 Cabernet Sauvignon. I took a crystal goblet from the credenza and filled it. I sat on the edge of the chair and massaged his shoulder with one hand while I kept the glass full with the other. We sat there looking at the blue footprints glistening in the night lights as we shared the wine. We didn't even feel the need to speak for a while, and then I started to laugh.

"Gee whiz, Tom, I know the floor had enough dirt on it to sod Yankee Stadium, but couldn't you think of a more subtle way to make your point?"

He started to laugh. Another crisis behind us.

━━━━━━━━━━━━━━━

August 4, 1989 Tom's neurologist ordered Imipramine raised to 75 mg in an attempt to improve Tom's sleep pattern. The 50 mg he'd been taking had done nothing. Tom was now pacing three out of four nights with only one really solid night of sleep. He was still operating on his cat naps. My nerves were so frayed that I jumped at any noise and felt dizzy and depleted. I was convinced I was going to die if things didn't change.

August 20, 1989, after nearly 60 hours with no significant sleep at all, Tom began to hallucinate actively. He got out of the house while I was in another room and was so far down the block that I didn't have a prayer of catching him on foot. I finally cut him off with the car. He was furious and not only knocked me down when I tried to get him in the car but he started running full speed down the center of the highway. A woman with a car phone hailed 911 for me and within a few minutes three police cars cornered him and led him off. He was taken to the local E.R. kicking and screaming all the way. He was in restraints by the time I arrived and he had been given Thorazine in an effort to quiet the psychotic behavior. I had specifically told the medics that he was not crazy he was mad and he was suffering from sleep deprivation. I would later realize that he had been headed towards the train station. My refusals to drive him to Boulder in response to his non ending need to state that he wanted to move ... now, made him decide he was going to go on his own. I wondered how long he'd been planning the grand escape.

The admitting doctor wouldn't let me in to see him because he was so distraught and while I filled the doctor in on the current events of our lives as well as Tom's health history I could hear him yelling in the other room. The doctor told me he was completely disoriented. He didn't know what day it was, his address, or what year it was. I explained that he hadn't known those things for the last three years. It was no test in his case. He was suffering from dementia and sleep deprivation.

When the yelling continued I demanded to see him anyway. He was yelling because he had to go to the bathroom. He couldn't relax enough to use the urinal the nurses kept thrusting at him and they wouldn't release the restraints so that he could go to the men's room. They finally agreed to let me take care of *It* myself. I closed the curtains and talked to him until he calmed down enough to recognize me. With some adjustments he was able to urinate into the 'device'. It was then that he looked at me and asked ...

"Why did I do that?"

"Beats me, Tom."

" How long am I going to be here."

"Just a few days until they get you sleeping again."

The next morning I arrived at the hospital to discover Tom had been given another dose of Thorazine during the night for combative behavior. He was sitting up but was now in a 'posy', a euphemism for restraint, which was tied to his chair. He eyes were glazed over, his mouth was open and yellow Thorazine crud had formed in the corners. He recognized me when I came through the door, but his tongue was so swollen he couldn't talk. I immediately asked to see the doctor about the medication.

It was agreed to take him off Thorazine, but Haldol was recommended instead. I voiced my concerns about Haldol and asked about trying Lithium instead. I was told that Lithium was not prescribed for people in Tom's condition. I asked what that condition was, since Tom wasn't psychotic but in the throws of what happens with sleep deprivation and the effects of his dementia. I reasoned that since Lithium is used in the treatment of manic-depressives and since his behavior seemed more like a manic attack than a psychotic one and since the side effects of Lithium are much less profound than those of other psychotropic drugs that perhaps it was worth the try. He didn't agree with my diagnosis. I'm only the one who'd been living with the situation and I'd only had twenty five-years of experience dealing with a chronic psychiatric case load, but hey ... what did I know?

They wouldn't let Tom out of his restraints unless I was with him and most of that day was involved with feeding and bathroom duty. He flatly refused to let anyone but me help him in the bathroom. By the time I was able to leave for home I was exhausted. It was the first good night's sleep I'd had in months. It was more like a coma.

I arrived the next morning to find that along with the residual effects of the Thorazine that was still in his system, Tom now had the Parkinsonian jerks and pill rolling associated with the side effects from Haldol. He was sufficiently drugged so that staff allowed him to shuffle from one end of the corridor to the other ... as long as I was with him. I had to hold him or he fell over. I found it amazing, he had 'major' medication in him, he was still on his feet, and he still hadn't slept for more than a few minutes at a time. I also suspected he'd been given other drugs in an effort to knock him out. The nurses wouldn't confirm that but they did admit he was 'difficult' during the night. I couldn't help but wonder if they'd be 'difficult' if they were strapped into their beds and had to go to the bathroom. I also knew enough about night duty to know that 'difficult' generally translated into more medication.

I also found that the nursing staff expected him to feed himself. I found Tom tied in his bed, his tray strewn with cups and plastic glasses, all of which were tipped over. The plate was on the floor and most of the food in his lap. He had tried to get the food into his mouth himself. He was a mess. When I complained, the nursing supervisor told me it was their policy to encourage patients to be as independent as possible. The phrase 'insuring their dignity', was included in the comment. I had to wonder where the dignity was in sitting in a mess with your food in your lap. I made a point of being there to feed him from that point on. One nurse aide whose grandmother had Alzheimer's was the only one to spend time with him while I was gone.

I called the doctor and described the effects of all the medication. He handed me the usual double talk saved for idiots and family members who dare to ask questions. I told him of my experience with patients on Haldol and Tom's long history of intolerance to drugs in general. (He never even took an aspirin.) I didn't see how Haldol was going to improve the situation. Tom had more medication in his system than ever before in his life and he was still on his feet. In my opinion the medication wasn't doing squat. The doctor agreed to 'get back to me'.

The next morning I arrived at the hospital to find Tom was still on Haldol and Artane had been added in an effort to counter-act the

Parkinsonian jerks which were one of the side effects of Haldol. The doctor was unavailable to see me. To make matters even more interesting he had been given Chloral Hydrate that morning to induce sleep for an EEG test. The report of that test would state he resisted sleep in spite of the medication. He was literally like a zombie.

I spent that day feeding and doing bathroom duty. He was still on his feet and he was still pacing. I was beginning to wonder if he was the incarnation of Rasputin. He had not had an entire night's sleep since his hospitalization. He was however, more verbal about wanting to go home. The doctors found that encouraging. I finally sat Tom down and told him that until he started sleeping he was not going to come home. The nursing staff informed me he slept that night. I'm not trying to attach mystical powers to Tom's ability to manipulate his environment, but there were times when it seemed exactly that. It was also obvious to Tom and me that the hospital was not a place he wanted to be for much longer.

The nursing staff were elated, I didn't tell them it was probably just his one night of sleep in his ever changing sleep cycle. He was still existing on his cat naps. I just wanted him home at that point. The hospital was totally unequipped to deal with him or any dementia patient for that matter. They had no experience with the mood swings, behavior problems, physical care needs or awareness levels of someone in Tom's situation. Their only possible solution was to treat him like a psychiatric patient. Not even the nursing homes seemed prepared. There wasn't one in our area with an Alzheimer's wing. They wouldn't have touched Tom for any amount of money anyway because they characterized him as being combative. The hospital was as glad to get rid of him as he was to leave.

In the meantime, I spoke to the bevy of lawyers now involved in dictating our lives, along with the myriad of personnel handling the Trust about what happened and told them I would now hold them personally responsible for Tom's health if they continued to delay our move. They agreed it was time to get him out of Houston. They got permission from the court to authorize our move that morning. The estate issues were still on hold, but the whole mess was going to go to court before the end of the year. We'd be back.

Tom was the next person to get the news. He was strangely quiet during our ride home from the hospital and I noticed that he was smiling. He looked like a zombie, but he was smiling. There was so much medication in his system that he couldn't stand alone without teetering back and forth. His mouth was still dry with remnants of medication drool, his fingers were twitching as a result of the Haldol and his eyes were glassy, but he managed to say as we went through the door of our house ...

"I ... waa..naa.. frummm ..."

"What Tom?" He repeated ...

"I ... waanna .... ffffrummm ...."

"Frum? ... I don't know what you mean Tom."

"Frum ... frum ..." ... he said more emphatically. He held one hand up as if to herald my attention and pointed towards his belt with the other. He took a deep breath and summoning all of what was left of his dignity ... he said ...

"I ... am ... a ... virile ... man!"

"Frum? Oh!" ... as recognition of what 'frum' meant jumped into my brain.

"You want to ... Frum!"

"God ... Yes!"

[Mother told me there'd be days like this.]

We went upstairs and showered off the last vestiges of the hospital and we made love, the first time he'd set foot in the bedroom in weeks. He had enough medication in him to stone an entire army but ... what can I say ... what a guy! We clung to each other all night, the first real night of sleep for the two of us together in weeks.

═══════════════

With help from neighbors and my sister Sandy and her husband Phil who drove in to help us pack and do the first leg of the drive with us, we moved to Boulder. I kept having the nagging feeling that somehow, in some way, Tom had managed once again to have things his own way.

What do You think?
You tell me. What do you think, Beverly?
I think he's still very much in there, that's what I think!

═══════════════

His speech was severely compromised by the medication the hospital ordered. With his neurologist's supervision I started weaning him off. It would take a month to get everything out of his system and he improved in direct correlation to the removal of that medication. The weight loss stopped but to those who hadn't seen him in a while, the change in his appearance was still very startling. We had to replace most of his wardrobe. It was less than Savile Row this time around.

The pacing would continue but he was more calm and manageable. His sleep pattern moved back to a four night cycle with one really bad night followed by a night of deep uninterrupted sleep, a pattern I could tolerate. He resumed feeding himself and except for basic care he was able to go to the bathroom unassisted once more. In fact I recall the first time he did so. I was sitting in the living room staring at the TV when Tom walked in and announced;

"Well, I ... did it."

"Did what Tom?" ... my attention suddenly focused, my body ready to spring into action, wondering what had been spilled this time.

"I ... went to the ... bath..room ... by myself."

"Gee Tom, that's great." ... as I tried to register absolute approval in his direction, overdoing the enthusiasm level just a tad. Tom just looked at me and uttered what summed up everything at that point.

"Big ... Deal! I used ... to go to ... Lon...don ... by myself."

AS TIME GOES BY

You must remember this,
A kiss is still a kiss,
A sigh is just a sigh.
The fundamental things apply
..as time goes by.

And when two lovers woo,
They still say I love you,
On that you can rely.
No matter what the future brings,
..as time goes by.

Moonlight and love songs
Never out of date.
Hearts full of passion
Jealousy and hate.
Woman needs man
and man must have his mate,
That no one can deny.

It's still the same old story,
A fight for love and glory,
A case of do or die ...
The world will always welcome lovers,
..as time goes by

words and music by: Herman Hupfeld

CHAPTER THIRTEEN

* If there is ever reason to take care of the paper work before it's too late, ours is the prime example of why it is so important. Had I had two pieces of paper, a **General Power of Attorney** *signed so that financial disposition of the marital estate could have been assumed by me, and a* **Durable Power of Attorney for Health Care,** *so that decisions about Tom's medical care could be made by me after he became incompetent, most of what happened might have been avoided. We wouldn't be involved in the sort of trust that has the autonomy this one has and we'd have paid one lawyer instead of the parade that attached themselves to us. Had Tom taken the time to draw up a will specifying his desires for the disbursement of his estate and had he provided a video record of his desires when we first married ... things might have unfolded differently. **

In 1991 the trust was formally transferred to Colorado. There is an old adage that goes ... Be careful what you ask for. I had worked very hard to get that trust account transferred. The Houston bank did not cooperate a whole lot but then the transfer would mean no one there would be able to draw any more fees once it was moved. Of course that didn't mean there wouldn't be a whole new cast of characters in Colorado to deal with. What I looked forward to was a working relationship with the new fiduciary guardian and involvement with people who had not been through a war with us. What I got was a new bureaucracy which not only seemed unable to make a decision about anything that concerned Tom's welfare without consulting a paid expert, but a bureaucracy which telegraphed an innate distrust of me, to me. I couldn't be considered an 'expert' even with my considerable experience and credentials because I was the Ward's wife and therefore an interested party in the estate, and therefore of no personal significance. It was an interesting dichotomy since I was also the guardian of Tom's body. Instead of working with me to provide some level of dignity to our bondage to a system we had no need of, but one to which we were inexplicably tied, I faced what I felt to be an adversarial and often punitive response to my requests to meet our daily living needs as they changed.

A temporary budget was set as soon as the Colorado Trust took over, based on expenses from our first year in Boulder, a year that saw some improvement in Tom's care needs and therefore an actual reduction in medical costs, a year in which little travel was done, a year in which expenses on the whole were fairly low. The permanent budget was to be set within six months after the Trust was officially moved to Colorado and was to reflect a truer appraisal of actual expenses with assumption of future increased needs as Tom's illness progressed. It was closer to a year and a half before the permanent budget was set and during that time I was kept to the original temporary agreement, while our actual expenses continued to mount most of which were charged on Visa and most of which were characterized as my debt because they were over the 'budget'. A debt I had no way of paying off as long as I was taking care of Tom 24 hours a day and unable to work. A debt that couldn't be paid off out of the monthly allotment I received for Tom's care without misappropriating those funds for the purpose of paying 'my debt'. An interesting dilemma.

There was no allowance made for changes in Tom's care needs or mine and the trust seemed unwilling to accept that changes in Tom's condition happened over night or that accommodations for those changes had to happen just as quickly. It took two weeks to get permission to purchase a recliner for Tom after one such change, a purchase I characterized as equipment, a purchase the trust characterized as furniture, wherein laid the problem in communication. Two weeks might not seem like much of a wait, but given the impact of the reason for that chair on both Tom and me, it was a small eternity.

One day, during one of Tom's passes through the house he went to sit down and instead of bending at the waist, he stiffened and fell backwards. Fortunately I saw it happen and managed to catch him just before his neck hit the back of the sofa. He had lost the process involved in sitting or lying down on his own in that one movement. From that moment on I had to stand over him and guide his body into a chair or bed. The problem was compounded by our sofa having a low back which left Tom's neck and head unsupported. He couldn't just slide down to a more comfortable sitting position without ending up on the floor. Lifting him back on the sofa was like trying to move a beam around. His rote memory of those movement patterns was gone. He could no longer figure out how to position his hands or feet under him or how to shift his weight in order to stand. He couldn't follow any spoken directions, and it was impossible to place his limbs into position to help because his brain wouldn't allow him to cooperate. I had to roll him on to his stomach, place both my arms around his waist and lift him, butt up first, until one of his feet or his knees touched the floor and then he was sometimes able to hold his weight. By holding him and bracing him with my body I'd eventually straightened up his torso long enough for him to find his balance at which point he'd immediately begin to pace again. From what I observed, he had lost all connection with his body. He couldn't even figure out how to swing his body into bed without help and so I'd have to hold one hand behind his head and swing his legs with my other to get him to lie down.

Compounding the problem was his continuing constant need to pace. I'd often just get him situated on the sofa (or in bed) when the urge to move took over and he'd stand up, which he could still do on his own, to resume pacing through the house. Five minutes later I'd have to repeat the whole process of getting him down again. His gait had already taken on the shuffling aspect so many late stage people develop so he was always in danger of sliding down along a wall when he paced. There were days when it seemed all I did was seat Tom or pick him up off the floor, and nights and nights without any real sleep for me. Our situation was one that needed immediate attention.

[Tom's ability to stand up and walk without help continued until June 1993 and then that was thankfully gone. I say thankfully because once he became immobile, life got much easier on me and those who were helping to take care of him. Once he was situated in his recliner or his bed he was there until we moved him. The stiffness that began the day he fell into the sofa would increase as his illness progressed until his body actually started to constrict, his hands arms and legs curling inward.]

Once our aide left our home afternoons I was entirely on my own to face yet another developing aspect of Tom's illness. The "Sundowning" that began while we were still living in Houston had now escalated to epic proportions. As a result, early morning was his only best time. As the afternoon wore on and evening arrived he became less and less adept at everything and increasingly more active and belligerent. Since I was the one there alone with him during evening periods, I was the one who faced most of the problems.

The recliner held the promise of providing both support to his back and head and a more confining place where he might actually be forced to sit still for a while. Once in a reclining position, it wouldn't be as easy for Tom to figure out how to kick back the foot rest while simultaneously bringing the chair up to a sitting position without help. I was relying on his being unable to learn the new movements involved to get out of the chair a notion that actually turned out to work. He'd become so preoccupied with trying to get out of the chair that sometimes the compulsive urge to move would pass before his feet hit the floor and he'd just lean back and sit until the next urge struck. He'd repeat that pattern several times before actually making it to his feet. Sometimes I'd get a whole 10 or 15 minutes without seeing Tom's ever moving body flitting through my peripheral vision.

[One learns to appreciate the little gifts in life.]

It seemed obvious to me that a reclining chair was an essential standard item for in-home care of an Alzheimer's patient. I know our doctor did. She thought it was unheard of to have to write a prescription for such a thing. It was unheard of but something I could have lived with if getting the prescription had been the end of it. It wasn't. I now felt I was involved in hoop jumping just for the sake of seeing how high I would jump. I dropped off photos of Tom and the sofa with a detailed description, in writing, of the events leading to the request for the chair and signed it with all my professional letters after my name. I was beginning to get very mad. The more I felt as if I was being jerked around, the more I dug in my heels. My increasingly frantic phone calls to the trust resulted in my being told I would be notified when a decision was made.

[A decision to 'what', not buy the chair?]

I threw my back out trying to move Tom's dead weight myself while I waited for approval to buy the recliner. After I threatened to take the issue to the Court for a decision, I was then told to go ahead and charge the chair on our VISA. That charge then hung on the bill gathering interest charges for a year before the bank finally paid it. When I voiced ire at the trust allowing that purchase and other expenses resulting from my back injury to just hang unpaid and gaining interest charges on the Visa, I was told I had gone over the monthly allotment for medical expenses and those fees were now my problem as well.

We have to keep in mind here, that I wasn't working, I had access to no money except for a monthly allotment that had been budgeted to cover living expenses only, living expenses that averaged the previous year's utilities, gas, clothing, food, entertainment, adult diapers, hygiene products, and respite companion, all of which were much below what this year's expenses were going to be because of Tom's increasing needs. For one thing he now needed a certified aide which was much more expensive than a respite companion and his hygiene and adult diaper needs were escalating. There was no allotment for my personal use except for clothing and food. That means I had no personal spending money of my own. I felt as if I was entering into a new form of slavery and facing personal debt as punishment for having seen Tom through his illness. Some might call that unnecessary emotional stress. I called it torment. The trust called it doing their job to protect the estate for Tom's benefit. The fact that Tom's well being depended on my mental and physical health didn't seem to enter the thinking process.

The back injury I sustained left me unable to even walk or stand without pain. I had resorted to ordering food delivered to the house, another additional expense, because the continuing need to still move Tom around in the aide's absence left shopping for groceries and cooking and cleaning almost impossible. If Tom slid off the sofa, there was no one to help him stand except for me, a situation that kept exacerbating the back problem and one that interfered with any real healing for months. Meanwhile all the charges where accruing on the Visa bill. I was totally at the trust's mercy with decisions that seemed arbitrary in nature and I had Tom at the worst part of his illness to deal with as well. My grief over his losses and the fear that consumed my being during that period cannot be expressed in words.

My attempts to enlighten the trust to my needs as Tom's caregiver and wife often resulted in my breaking into tears. Tears that reflected my frustration, my lack of sleep, and the ignominy of having to beg for every nit picking thing I needed for our survival. I can only speculate about the impression I made after all of the above took its toll. My tears had to have been an indication of emotional overload by them. My anger had to have been an indication of displaced aggression. From this point of view I doubt if anyone in the trust felt I even had a reason to be upset by our situation. But there were days on end when I felt nothing but despair at the thought of having to ask the trust for anything. I stopped going for treatment on my back because I had no way to pay for it and I wasn't getting anywhere asking the trust to honor those fees.

Thank goodness for the women's spiritual group I attended in my church. I got to spend time on a weekly basis with forty women who represented a cross section of every stage of life from young mothers, to grandmothers, from professionals to home makers, from those physically fit to those facing terminal illness, all of us working together to make sense of our lives. Had it not been for their support and their prayers I don't know if I could have survived the emotional trauma I felt during that period. All my energy was being depleted and it wasn't because of Tom's needs, which where reason enough. It was from the constant reinforcement I got from the people who controlled our lives that I had no worth.

My personal conversations with God increased until I finally figured out that nothing that was happening had any reality in my life. None of it reflected on who I was in my core. It wasn't until I was able to get out of feeling victimized that I was able to take charge again. And I wasn't able to do that until I decided that I was not someone to roll over and play dead and I was not about to start now.

However, when it then became apparent to the trust that I wasn't going to go away, they hired a private case management team to 'assess Tom's care needs'. The resulting report was so slanted against me I almost laughed when I read it, except it wasn't funny. I interpreted it to be the first step towards having me removed as Tom's plenary guardian and my input as his wife and primary caregiver further diluted. It characterized our marital relationship as "symbiotic, enmeshed and overinvolved", to the point where I was

"... furthering Tom's dependency on her, and to a degree making it difficult for other caregivers to fully meet his needs."

This was written in spite of the fact that Tom was now bedridden and unable to voice any objection to care no matter who was doing it and I now had a full time aide working in the house with Tom, an aide they met and evaluated, an aide who seemed to have no problem working with Tom or me for that matter. The report also underplayed Tom's neurologist report which stated that he was in the very best care situation he could possibly be in. It also very conveniently neglected to mention any of my considerable experience and training, which I might add was more considerable than that of the people writing the report, or that the way in which Tom's care had been set up was not only adequate, it was a model for how to work at home with a mid-late stage Alzheimer's person. A model later incorporated into a presentation made to the Alzheimer's Association for training purposes for other long-term caregivers.

I felt that I was faced with an immovable object, a wall that ended up costing my sons thousands of dollars in legal fees on my behalf. They got so tired of the emotional torment I faced dealing with this guardian of the money, while noting Tom's increasing care needs, that they hired an attorney to take the trust on. More money was changing hands but at least I didn't have to deal directly with the trust anymore. It was nearly another year before a fair agreement was made regarding the budget and my role as Tom's wife and caregiver and I finally entered into a working relationship with the trust.

Tom once said to me that bureaucracies breed people who function out of fear. Basically they fear having to admit they've made an error so they avoid doing anything that might result in an error. Unfortunately, they also spend an inordinate amount of energy covering up the errors they do make. They hide behind rules and regulations and use them to justify inertia. There are two groups of people they never take on, those

*who have so much money they can't be affected by little
power trips, and those who have political clout.* *

I'd like to say that becoming an advocate for increased public
awareness of the long term care needs of people with Alzheimer's
Disease, and a self appointed spokesperson on the impact long term
illness has on caregivers was a conscious decision I made at that
moment, but the truth is my advocacy resulted out of a desperate
need to find a way to reclaim my life, a need that started the day we
moved to Boulder. I kept asking myself, how would Tom handle
this guardianship thing? He certainly wouldn't respond with anger.
He would respond with action. As for my situation, I had no
network of friends or colleagues in our community and Tom's care
needs kept me conveniently isolated and chained to our home.
Everyone who had power in our lives treated me as if I was no one
to acknowledge. I may not have had any money, but I have always
been a fast learner. I reasoned that I needed to find a way to
empower myself, and I needed to do it for reasons that had to do
solely with my sense of myself as a human being.

I started by joining a support group which led me into doing as
much volunteer time for the Alzheimer's Association as I could
spare. I gave speeches and wrote articles for them, one of which
was subsequently included in the Congressional Record. I was sent
to Washington DC, three years as a delegate to the Alzheimer's Association's National Public Policy Forum. I was appointed by
Governor Romer as a participant in the 1995 White House
Conference on Aging. I joined the Community Eldercare Coalition
of Boulder County where I was able to network with political,
public, private and volunteer groups dedicated to long term care
issues of the frail and elderly. I was named to the Board of the
Colorado Respite Care Coalition. I am active as an advocate for
Alzheimer's families. As a result of my growing reputation and my
presence being made in my community I was asked to become
editor of Care Connections Newsletter which is the only publication
I know of that specifically targets caregiver needs and matches
those needs with services available in their community. Our
circulation, after only 6 months in operation, reaches over 2,500
county residents and numerous others across the United States. I
have been published in newspapers, including the New York Times
and I feel as if I am just getting started.

If nothing else happens, I have already paved a possible career for myself in the field of long term care, bringing with me the combination of professional experience and the intimate hands on knowledge that caring for Tom gave me. I also found that advocacy gave me a legitimate focus for my anger and frustration, the value of which cannot be underestimated. And that focus is to improve government and public awareness of caregiver needs so that what happened to me won't happen to others. As for the trust, I had made a point of documenting everything as things started to unravel, a habit I learned to cultivate while working for the mother of all bureaucracies, the State of New York. The trust finally realized that I was not going to go away and I was not going to accept patronizing, jerk-off answers to my requests. Sooner or later they were going to have to deal with me on an equal basis. Also, I don't think my advocacy went totally unnoticed.

All I ever really expected was to be treated with dignity and with some regard for my experience and my desire to give Tom the best care possible. I never asked for anything outrageous in the first place. It was time to put it all behind us and get on with our lives.

Please ... help me put it behind ...

Boulder offered us a fresh start. It was in Boulder that Tom's B12 deficiency was discovered. His internist asked if Tom's hair had turned white at an early age noting a correlation between early graying, light colored eyes and B12 deficiency. Tom's hair had turned white in his late 30's. Tests confirmed the suspicion. Somewhere along the way his system had stopped absorbing that vitamin. I had been giving him all the B's every day, but his body had simply flushed them out. The deficiency could have resulted in the Alzheimer's like symptoms that began to escalate when we married. He started injections immediately.

The change was remarkable. Aside from the obvious improvements in speech and thought process, we started laughing again. He joked with the nurses and doctors as well as the lady who served us breakfast on her roller skates every morning in the local '50's diner. We started making love again, something he felt compelled to share with his neurologist. She smiled ...

For a while I actually hoped it was all going to go away. To share real conversations again was nothing short of bliss. The improvement continued over the next few weeks and then leveled out. He held on to the improvement until the end of the year at which point he started to fail. It was during his series of shots that I learned how routinely the test for B12 deficiency was given in suspected dementia cases because it is a treatable condition and how blatantly absent it was from Dr. P.'s results. Every doctor who saw Tom after Dr. P's examination scanned the results looking only for the obvious negative responses on the printouts. I doubt if they even looked specifically for that test, assuming it had been given. It was a couple of days before I allowed the ramifications of that thought to sink in. If the final blow in Tom's deterioration was the B12 deficiency then what had happened to him was all the more pointless. Somehow my cavalier joking about Dr. P.'s initials fell flat this time around. With one wave of his arrogant arm he condemned both Tom and me and in some ways every member of our respective families.

Doctors were hard pressed to explain the rush of improvement and why it didn't continue. Perhaps too much damage had occurred and his brain was just unable to recoup. Perhaps another process such as early onset Alzheimer's had now taken over. Perhaps he was just unfortunate to have had a series of traumas which as individual afflictions could have been compensated for, but in combination caused his brain to overload and literally short itself out. Perhaps, well, nobody seemed to know or would know until an autopsy could be performed.

[In March 1995 a study was cited that linked early onset of Alzheimer's disease with the gene apo-E4 and closed head injury. Research is in the early stages regarding this issue, but it may ultimately answer why what happened to Tom happened.]

Whatever optimism I felt at Tom's initial surge when the B12 shots were started was followed with sheer despair as he began to slide. He gave up. He told me to let go of it. What was done was done. I was unable to let go of any of it. I suppose my behavior for the next few months could only be described as desperation. For me it was the last ditch effort to help Tom focus his energy and give him something to grasp at. I wanted him to pull a miracle out of his being and come back to me while he was still capable of thought. Since conventional treatment had nothing to offer us, we were now back to holistic practitioners and prayer.

Tom couldn't lie still long enough for acupuncture treatments any more so they were out. I turned to a chiropractor/healer who saw Tom every other week for body alignments and energy boosts. There was marginal short term improvement in coordination. I started feeding him a herb concoction three times a day that had the intrinsic value of brown sludge but which was reported to improve body chemistry and balance. He took it dutifully for several weeks and then refused it any longer. I was operating on the belief that healing had to come from within Tom and it really didn't matter what triggered his ability to focus as long as he believed in it and wanted it.

One healer commented that Tom's energy field was severely depleted. She whooshed him several times but felt there was little response. She refused payment of her fee, offering that Tom had made a choice and she couldn't help him. Tom said he felt lifted by the experience and had seen an image of his mother happy and waiting for him at home in Philadelphia. From this perspective there were more than a few hints floating around that day. I ignored all of it. I even considered asking the Catholic Church to do an exorcism but couldn't decide how to word such a request and decided to have a glass of wine instead. The notion passed.

Tom went along with it all but looking back on it, he was waiting for me to get it all out of my system and finally accept the inevitable. Finally in May 1990 he put a stop to it all. We were only four years into our marriage and he told me he wanted to die and get it over with. He was tired. It wasn't the life he could stand living anymore. I didn't have time to get depressed because things started happening at bullet speed again. Perhaps that was Tom's plan, to keep me so busy I couldn't interfere with letting him go. The problem was that he had married the second most tenacious person on earth, he, being the first.

[As for his death actually following his decision to let go of life, that was five years ago and he is still surprisingly healthy for someone in his present stage of Alzheimer's Disease. So letting go isn't all that easy.]

By late June 1990, he'd lost another 35 pounds, he'd stopped sleeping again, the hand rituals and the perseverance with his speech were back in full bloom and he was actively hallucinating.

When he became so violent I was in danger of being hurt I was forced to call the police. He had wrecked everything he could get his hands on in the house and was kicking the walls in the bedroom when the police finally arrived. I was covered with black and blue marks from accidentally getting in his way and was suffering from sleep deprivation myself by then. It may be significant that he chose a time to do this when my entire family was out of town. My sister and her family were on vacation and both my sons, who had since relocated to Boulder to be near us, were back east visiting their father. There we were ... just like the good old days in Houston ... the two of us alone in hell. He spent the next two weeks in a neuro-behavioral institute, this time under the care of doctors still capable of original thought.

Thankfully, he had started sleeping again by the time of his release and the weight loss stopped. He was down to 124 pounds. The doctor had no explanation for the weight loss because Tom's eating pattern had never changed during the entire episode. He offered that in cases such as Tom's, a sudden profound weight loss for no organic reason sometimes happened. Four weeks of constant frenetic behavior and no sleep, seemed reason enough.

Several months later his neurologist and I agreed to take him off all the medication that had once more crept into the picture. Tom was one of those people for whom medication solved no problems. If it worked, it worked for only a few weeks and then his system over rode whatever it was doing. Sleeplessness would be the first indication that things were changing again. Combativeness would follow in direct response to lack of sleep. All of it conspired to deprive me of sleep as well. As behavior changed, medication was added to and doses increased because it was assumed the behavior had become more overt and not that the system was rejecting the medication. Tom's needs aside, I was the one at risk had the assumption been correct. I had seen what an adrenaline surge could do to a psychotic patient and how many aides it took to bring that patient under control. It was a valid concern. Six months after his hospitalization he was on four different medications, he was still sleeping erratically, he was still prone to combative episodes and he was now also walking into the walls.

Since I was willing to monitor the removal of his medication at home and willing to take the chance that he might also erupt, his neurologist agreed it was time to get a base line of his functioning without medication clouding everything up. It took four months to wean him off everything. He again improved as each medication was removed and has been off all medication since then. It was apparent that the sleep problems were just a fact of life and as long as they approximated any sort of pattern, I'd just have to learn to live with it. There was no magic pill.

The positive thing is that he was no longer walking into the walls and I took off the bubble wrap I'd put on all the corners and door jams and he no longer had to wear his Stetson indoors. I had considered getting a helmet for him when the wall banging started but it would have looked ridiculous on him. As it turned out, simple is always better. The Stetson he already had in his hat arsenal worked wonderfully. He was signaled to back off as soon as the brim touched the wall and aside from keeping his head cushioned, the hat gave him a certain look of dash.

[I always tried to help Tom maintain his quota of dash. He was a fastidious dresser, and I did my best to keep his appearance up to par regardless of how he deteriorated. To this day I pick the colors that look best on him and I surround him with the things that serve to enhance him as the person he was. What can I say? He is still Sean Connery to me.]

At least our home was looking more normal again. However, Tom was now officially into the last stages of what was now being called Probable Alzheimer's Disease. The deterioration would continue in it's downward spiral, and it would be unrelenting in terms of its impact on me.

Today he is looking more and more like that man we saw in the nursing home in Houston. He is now in a wheelchair and like that gentleman, his jaw sometimes locks open leaving him caught with a most horrifying expression in his eyes. Sometimes a touch on his face is all that's needed to allow him to relax the muscles that hold him prisoner. To demonstrate just how dramatic the deterioration could be, he walked into his room under his own power one evening and woke up unable to even sit up without help. He had not had a stroke.

It now takes two of us to get him dressed, showered and into the living room, even with a wheelchair. He is unable to assist in any movement. His body stiffens and it's as if he grows roots down his back which triples the amount of weight we have to shift. The body no longer bends normally and his arms and hands have started to constrict. The recliner, the trust was so reluctant to approve has been a life saver. The chair conforms to his body and it enables me to keep him in the living room instead of confined to the bedroom. As physically demanding as this new development is, life is actually somewhat easier and more predictable for me as long as his attendant is available to help move him. It's also a quieter life these days. When he was still able to move about on his own there was always the danger of falling and being hurt and there was also the constant pacing, the repetition of sounds, and the constant twitching to deal with, and the prowling around in his room night after night after night.

That period of his life started in February 1989 and lasted until August 1993, four years. It stopped when he became bedridden. There was always some part of his body in motion during that period. In varying degrees of intensity it was non stop. Some of it took on a ritualistic nature, patterns of body movements and facial distortions that seemed to follow some unwritten rule, one action automatically triggering the other. Some of it just compulsive, unrelenting pacing.

During one phase he systematically picked all the buttons off his shirts and jackets because he was constantly trying to button them. A phantom remnant of a memory, but not the entire memory. The sound of his finger nails rubbing on fabric was unbelievable. When I started putting turtlenecks and overhead sweaters on him, he picked holes where buttons should have been. One day he stopped the assault on the shirts and moved to his trousers. He went through six pairs of pants in one week just digging at his pocket with his right hand. Putting a mitten on that hand finally slowed the destruction down.

There was a time when I wondered if his entire body was covered with velcro because there was always something attached to him as he wandered from one end of the house to the other, and there was always something in his hands that got dropped and tripped over if I didn't retrieve it fast enough. Considering his visual problems it was amazing how he zeroed in on the one thing I left in his reach, coming sometimes from the far corner of the house to snatch it. It's as if it was the only way he could let me know he was still in there. It was an act done with a combination of achievement and contempt written on his face, as if to say ...

"There ... you didn't think I could do that!"

One would think as his deterioration progressed that what was lost was now lost forever. Not so. Little abilities appear and vanish just often enough so that I have to wonder what is still working in that brain of his and fear that his ability to integrate input is far clearer than his ability to formulate output. To be trapped in a brain that accepts information but then refuses to do anything with it ... there are some things worse than death.

It's not a pretty picture, is it?
No, but it's real. How do you feel, Beverly?
So far so good, Lord! It's amazing how content I feel about Tom. How much I love him. How much I still love him.
You're doing OK, Beverly.

Long after he was unable to construct sentences he'd answer clearly to direct questions that required either a yes or no. "No" was the last word he was ever able to use consistently, something that was of no surprise to anyone in his family. And for a long time, he'd answer to questions directed at others in the room or on the television set. He still responds with a noise when his name is mentioned. At this point, even no, has faded from his ability to communicate. He engages in what sounds like conversation, much the same sort of sounds my young grandchild makes now that he's beginning to recognize and enter into speech. The inflections in Tom's voice, the pauses, and the expressions on his face register fear, humor, pain and on occasion, deep sadness. Mostly he sleeps or stares.

I remember an incident that happened shortly before Tom stopped walking. My son stopped by to share lunch with me before going on to his next job and to check in to see if I needed help with Tom. As soon as Tom smelled the food he started following us around the house. He had just finished a huge lunch so I knew he wasn't hungry. Finally he just started ranting at me ...

"You ... you you you ... and you you ... and you you you ..."

And on he went, shaking his finger in my face. Tom was upset when my son arrived and it wasn't because he was hungry, he was upset that I was talking with someone other than him and I was laughing, and more importantly, neither of us had included him in our greeting to each other. He had been left out. Of course, neither of us realized that's what was happening. Tom was at the other end of the house when my son arrived. My son who was feeling very uncomfortable, started to laugh out of nervousness and because of the bizarre scene that often happened when Tom went into one of his tirades, at which point Tom spun around to him, pointed his finger at him and said most intently ...

"... and you! ...Worse!"

And my son responded, as we both recognized the completeness of Tom's choice of words ...

"Gosh Tom, if I'd have known you'd wanted a hamburger I'd have brought you one. It's Mom's fault ... she told me you already ate. I won't forget you the next time, Okay?"

And he patted Tom's shoulder at which point Tom grunted and moved back into his pacing pattern, stopping only for a sip of my soda as he passed and to accept a french fry from my son on the rebound. As if to say ...

"I'm still here damn it!"

And so, Tom was still making his presence felt even at that late stage. He hadn't been able to pull my name from his memory for over a year at the time of that incident, but just when I thought he didn't even know who I was anymore, he touched my hand as I was putting him to bed one night and said very clearly with tears in his eyes ...

"I love you".

I can't tell you what that meant to me. He has not spoken an intelligible word since that night, but there are times when I still recognize the words in his eyes. They tell me the personality, the essence, is the very last thing to go. From my experience I can only affirm that observation. Tom's essence remains very much in view. But then, I choose to continue to see it.

As for my communication attempts with him, I operate with the knowledge that Tom read body language better than most of us read words. I assume he still has that capacity even if the odds are that he hasn't. I don't over explain to him what is going on, but I try to treat him with the same acknowledgment I'd give anyone else in my presence. It is sometimes a battle to keep that awareness in focus when he seems to have gone elsewhere in his mind, but then he still has ways of letting me know when he's back.

I've tried to keep his life as normal as possible honoring the second promise I'd made to him in Houston, the first being our marriage vows, but changes have been inevitable and none of them came easy. Even the simple things like removing pictures out of his walk area held an aura of giving in to the illness. I found the *little deaths* weren't just limited to Tom's skill levels. They found their way into every corner of our lives.

Tom's constant pacing and activity at night often forced me out of our queen sized bed and across the hall in my ever increasing quest for a good night's sleep. I had put a feather mattress on it hoping the softness would encourage him to spend more time in it, and for a while it did help a little. On good nights I could still crawl in next to him and at least pretend things were somewhat normal. I eventually added an egg crate mattress on top of the feather bed to lessen the chance of him developing bed sores once he became immobile. Then I added the down comforter and he was literally sleeping in a cloud of down at night. Too many bed covers created major problems. He was constantly tangled in sheets and blankets. Half of my night was spent unwrapping him every time he turned over. The down comforter was heavy enough to stay in place on the nights he was active without getting tangled in his legs and it didn't impede his compulsive need to get out of bed on his own. The comforter also eliminated the need for a top sheet which was just another booby trap and one less thing to untangle from his legs.

That arrangement worked well until he became immobile and then lifting him in and out of bed became extremely difficult. No one ever told me about the stiffness that might set in as yet another of the late stage symptoms. Something else I got to find out about and learn to deal with on my own. It became impossible to lift his arms to dress him without exerting tremendous strength. I couldn't lift his head high enough to get my arm under it to hold him without straining.

As much as I dreaded getting a hospital bed, the time arrived when it was the only choice to make. At least the hydraulics of the bed could sit him up and lay him flat without my needing an aide to help. I was plunged into depression over the prospect of that metallic, cold, electronic monster invading our lives. It was a symbolic expression of yet another failure for me and further isolation from Tom. And even though the reality of that bed made life easier on me and Tom, and I now wonder why I fought getting it for so long, it changed what was left of our life together. I always started our nights together in bed moving into the other room if he got active, and nights when the twitches that had taken over his body were less pronounced I stayed the entire evening. There was still something valid about sharing our bed and waking together. Our bed was the last normal thing in our lives that was left to share.

The day the hospital bed arrived I stood at the entrance to the bedroom staring at it for the longest time. I found myself pulling the queen sized feather mattress, which was planned for storage, up on top of the hard, plastic covered twin mattress on the hospital bed and standing back to survey it's placement. The extra width flopped over the bed rails almost covering them. While still unaware of what I was doing I then reached for the queen sized egg crate mattress and placed that on top. I then covered both the mattresses with a beautiful teal green queen sized flannel sheet, threw the queen sized down cover on top, added a throw on the back to cover the metal legs and wires and rails and finally realized what I was doing. I wasn't just making the bed comfortable for Tom, I was trying to cover it up altogether, as if covering it up with down and foam and draperies made it into something other than what it was.

> * *That was a lot like ordering a casket that has carry slots instead of handles, on the outside chance that it will be mistaken for a very large hope chest.* *

But like all the other landmarks I faced as Tom continued to deteriorate, I managed to get through that one too. It was just another one of those *little deaths* reminding me that the main event was still waiting down the pike. The changes never got easier, no matter how hard I scrambled.

During the transition from the mid to late stage of Tom's illness, our bedroom became the safe room in our house with only the bed and a dresser left in place and wall to wall carpeting with double padding on the floor to cushion falls. Overhead track lighting was installed which worked with a dimmer switch in order to keep a low grade light on nights he felt compelled to pace. All wall plugs were covered and all lamps, pictures, mirrors and anything that might catch his attention or be potentially dangerous were removed. I played soft music through the baby monitor.

The safe room also served the purpose of allowing Tom a place where he could pace safely while I napped and a place where he could go when he was agitated without danger of getting hurt. The lack of stimulus in that room tended to dissipate whatever it was that had him in a rage because there was nothing in there to distract him. He even seemed to like the quietness of that room, often seeking it out on his own during the days when he was still walking on his own. It was also a place where I could put him when I needed a few minutes to step away from all the activity his body generated. It never seemed to take more than fifteen minutes of quiet for either of us to rejuvenate ourselves.

The period in his illness that necessitated this room was the hardest on me. It was like having a six foot toddler on my hands. Nothing that was within his reach was safe. Having had the recent experience of watching my grandson move into the terrible two's, the activity of which was so much like Tom's during that period of his life, gave me a new appreciation for what I had been dealing with. It was the same energy, the same constant movement, the same ability to get into everything especially things I thought I put out of reach.

On bad nights when he was 'up and moving' I slept across the hall, or tried to, with an infant monitor on my bed table and ear plugs in my ears to blot out the noise he made, an interesting conflict of ideas now that I think about it and one that never really worked anyway. Tom's ability to get my attention far outweighed anything I came up with to find quiet. Rattling the closet doors was his personal favorite. I was actually desperate in my need for sleep. While Tom had no trouble getting out of bed he was totally unable to get back in bed without help. So, no matter how much my body ached for sleep, I was up at least two or three times a night to assist him or know that if I didn't hear him moving via the intercom, he was frozen in a standing position staring at the bed or the wall or the window unable to move in any direction without help and probably fearful as well.

Before I set the room up I had no peace and no break unless I physically left the house and that necessitated having someone else watch Tom. His constant movement, the ritualistic noises he made, the inability to watch a television show without his body moving back and forth in front of the screen was unrelenting. I often felt the need to scream. Sometimes I took a shower and did just that.

Sometimes I went outside and raked leaves. That room made the difference between being in control and feeling victimized.

However, even with all the accommodations his wandering imposed, our home remained a home. An area from the bedroom through the living room was defined with furniture and bungie cords where Tom could pace all day long with open access to his room and still have visual access to the rest of the house. Pictures were removed from his walk area and rehung out of reach. The kitchen was completely off bounds but a bungie cord across the doorway still allowed him to watch me cook. Amazingly a simple bungie cord became an adequate deterrent to keeping him out of rooms. He'd lean on it, feel the bouncing movement and move on. Gates were a royal pain in the neck and he just kicked them down anyway. It never occurred to him to bend down and go under the cord and he never tried to unhook it, although he did learn to thwang it when he was annoyed.

His bathroom became accessible to him only with supervision from the moment he was unable to distinguish hot from cold in the faucets. The shower has a hand held nozzle with a water flow control button and an eight foot hose to facilitate easy reach whether he's sitting or standing. Thanks to my sons, the bathroom was completely modified to meet his needs and there is a drain in the middle of the floor to enable me to simply hose down the room after we're finished, a foresight that greatly eased the present hygiene problems we face now that Tom can't walk or stand without help.

He became completely incontinent by 1990. We were lucky again. The level of intimacy the two of us enjoyed with each other allowed an easier transition for us as his needs changed. The crossing point for both of us occurred when I realized he wasn't cleaning himself properly. I took the practical approach and offered what I saw as the only alternatives. Either he let me help, or someone else was going to have to help, or he'd end up dying of filth. Tom was pragmatic as always. As for my attitude towards doing 'it', I could see only four choices. I could choose anger, disgust, benign complacency, or love. I made the conscious effort to choose love. Assuring him I could also do this for him without revulsion or personal pain made the transition a lot easier for him and for me. Just to demonstrate that moments of tenderness were possible in what had to be thought of as an impossible breeding ground for such moments, I'll never forget the following incident ...

Tom had contracted a stomach virus which brought with it all the horror one can only imagine in the care of someone with the combination of motor control and reasoning problems Tom had. If there is hell on earth, diarrhea in a late stage Alzheimer's person is it. If there is a heaven, it only lasts 24 hours. Given my state of sleep deprivation and the physical energy it took to handle Tom's relentless need for help, I was at my wits end as we once more made the trip to the bathroom with pajamas that had to be changed and floors that had to be cleaned. I wanted to scream I felt so tired, and used, and spent, and unappreciated. And poor Tom. He was just responding to being sick and anxious from all the activity surrounding that night, getting more and more combative as the night wore on and as my own anxiety level increased. I remember steering him one more time into the bathroom and out of desperation, (I don't where the words came from,) I uttered ...

"Thank you, Lord!"

And Tom responded ...

"Thank you for what?"

"It could be worse, Tom."

"How?"

"I might not still love you as much as I do."

He turned his head towards me and said ...

"You still love me?"

"Of course, I love you."

"God, I love you too." I saw tears form in his eyes and he continued ...

"Bevy!"

"What, Tom."

"Thank you."

The evening became one of sharing the absurdity of what was going on in our lives and one of reconnecting to each other. And it was a sort of turning point for me. I stopped feeling victimized by what Tom's care needs meant by simply moving out of anger and into love, realizing in the process that it was as easy as making the choice to do so. I had two choices in attending to Tom's needs and that was to do them happily or do them mad. Either way, they still had to be done. And I realized something else, I realized how much Tom still needed to be loved. After all, what were we actually dealing with? A little poop between lovers wasn't really that much of a big deal.

Figuring out the logistics of taking care of those needs was not that easy however. This area of care is singularly the one thing no one wants to talk about. In fact, it is the best way I know to clear a room. I will never forget the first time I went to buy a bag of adult diapers. I stood there for twenty minutes staring at a wall of products. I was so upset and embarrassed to be even seen standing in that area of the store that I was unable to integrate the directions on the packages or make any kind of decision as to what to buy, but then I still cringe a little when I buy feminine hygiene products. The sweet young thing who was stacking the shelves just looked at me blankly when I asked her if she knew anything about those things. It took three visits (in different stores) before I finally made a purchase. It took months to set up a system of utilizing the various products efficiently, a system that combined certain items with other items in order to keep Tom as dry as possible for as long as possible without overtly invading what was left of his modesty.

The task of keeping the bed and the rest of the house protected without putting up a neon sign that screamed -- *Incontinence Lives Here!* -- was part of the challenge. I found that once again, simple was better. By using common sense, a little imagination, and shopping for usual items to do unusual things, the house never took on the aura of a nursing home even during the worst of it all.

I had read most of the usual books on Alzheimer's Disease by then, but frankly speaking, they didn't begin to fill the needs home care imposes. They were particularly useless when it came to talking about incontinence. It was as if limiting liquid and regulating food intake was all there was to it, as if behavior modification could actually make a difference over the long haul for any dementia patient. How do you make sure someone goes to the bathroom 'before' going to bed? Those writers have never had to deal with trying to tell an Alzheimer's patient to do anything that isn't already their idea. They treat incontinence as if it's something that can really be avoided if you, the caregiver, scrambles fast enough. It is still the great taboo. Handy little hints like putting labels on doors and hiding toilet paper because it usually ends up in the toilet, and expecting the Alzheimer's person to clean themselves and use 'those things' themselves, is not facing this problem. One woman I met in a support group told me she found her mother wearing an incontinence pad on her head. Another set the dinner table with them. One thing was certain, by the time Tom needed those things, he was past the point of knowing what to do with them.

Those same books also describe the last stages of this illness in terms of a return to infancy for the demented person and at the same time are devoid of the most basic information necessary to deal with the hygiene problems that infancy stage imposes on the caregiver and the person suffering this very last bastion of control in their lives. And trust me on this, the patient in varying degrees of awareness must be filled with fear, anger, revulsion, and a sense of loss over the inability to put it all together anymore or do anything about it. Why else is soiled clothing hidden so frequently? Why else are waste paper baskets mistakenly used as toilets? They are vainly trying to do it on their own, that's why.

This is the most obvious barrier to home care that exists in my opinion. It isn't just the practical information about what to use or how to use it, it is the recognition of the emotional upheaval it causes the caregiver and the loved one. It's everyone's nightmare come true. It cuts deeper into our psyche and taps primordial fears and feelings in ways no other event in our lives can with the possible exception of facing death itself. After all, toileting ourselves is one of the primary focuses of our first years of life and our first major test as social beings. Becoming continent is a matter of pride, confirmation of our intelligence and the first example of outstanding achievement by which parents measure their success and ours. The basic function of relieving ourselves is then placed behind closed doors and spoken of as little as possible for the rest of our lives.

The only other time any of us focus on the goings on of our bodily functions, if we're lucky, is the right of passage we as women face when our periods start. We all cope since there isn't any choice in the situation, some of us with as little information as a bag of Kotex thrust in our direction. Unfortunately, dealing with incontinence in an adult seems to be left to much the same sort of muddling around also with little choice in deciding to cope. When it happens it has to be dealt with. However, given the way these products disappear from the shelves when a sale is announced in the paper tells me there are vast numbers of us out there doing just that. Coping!

I decided that next to food, water and air the thing we value most is being clean and dry and warm. These are basic needs that are as true of our older frail loved ones as it is for our new born babies and if memory serves me right, by the time I was clean and dry after the birth of my first son, having been told I couldn't sit up after the spinal I'd had and then left on a gurney in a hallway for what seemed like hours. I wouldn't have cared if Arnold Schwarzenegger had appeared in his terminator suit to do it!

However, incontinence in Tom did bring with it another set of considerations that aren't faced with a new born or a disabled young adult who still has their thinking process and their lives ahead of them. For me, it was the final recognition that this illness was actually going to kill Tom and my first realization that he had no part in the choices anymore. Tom was not going to be able to give me permission to take charge of this situation. Diapering him was something I had to come to terms with. The trauma was mine, not his. It was my reticence, my fears, my attitude that had to change, not his. I honestly believed that diapers would be the final straw in my ability to take care of him at home. I was wrong. Nothing is ever as awful as you imagine. Managing it all came down to attitude and organization. They have actually been easier to deal with than constantly doing the race to the bathroom bit, which was far more demeaning and much more traumatic on both of us than diapers have ever been. All Tom would know is that he didn't have to worry so much any more, he was dry and clean, there was another piece of clothing in the dressing drill and most of all, he was still loved. The plus for me was that structure was back in our lives. Never underestimate the value of structure. We could now take those drives again, and eat out again, and go for walks in the park again without fear of the unthinkable. In retrospect, I waited too long to make this decision fearing his adjustment. In reality, his transition to diapers was far less traumatic for both of us than making him give up driving.

I faced three years of his constant railing against that loss. In some ways he went through all the stages of dying on that symbolic level. He raged against it, he cajoled and bargained, he prayed to God and he accused me of belittling him. The basis of most of our arguments evolved out of his demands to drive and my refusal to let him. Reasoning with him was truly a waste of time. Calls for help from his family didn't work either, they had no more control over him than I had on this count. How do you tell a parent he can't drive any longer? Well you do, but you aren't exactly thanked for the information. I finally reduced my side of the arguments to the word 'no'. It was short, it was simple, and it was definite, not that he paid even slight heed to it. He might back off but that was only so he could reconnoiter and launch an attack from yet another direction. He must have been hell to work for at times.

As for my meeting the barriers to his care, most of it was flying by the seat of my pants and most of it was playing catch up. I'd see signals that things were changing and start considering ways to compensate. Most often by the time the changes happened I already had a tentative plan in shape but the adjustments always took time. I felt very frustrated most of the time.

I became an observer of Tom's condition and through those observations I reasoned that the world as we see it, hear it, and feel it, is not necessarily the world of the Alzheimer's brain. Trying to keep someone afflicted with this illness confined to our world only increases their problems. Nothing can be taken for granted in their world. For example, walls and floors aren't necessarily square or flat. A change from carpeting to a hard tile floor sends all sorts of information on texture, color, depth perception and temperature to the brain, information that can be misread in many ways. A scatter rug in the middle of a hallway might actually translate as a hole in the middle of the floor. Patterned wall paper may seem to make the walls move or appear transparent so that they no longer offer clues of boundary. Patterned sheets on the bed may be part of the reason bed time is so traumatic. How does the Alzheimer's brain distinguish the dinner plate, from the place mat, from the table? One woman I know told me her father's eating habits improved once she removed the floral table cloth from the dinner table. She realized he was trying to avoid placing his glass on the flowers thinking they were real.

A noted neurologist here in Denver once remarked to me that the difference he saw between Alzheimer's and other dementia patients was that the Alzheimer's patient needed to constantly redefine his surroundings. All that reaching and touching and shuffling was their way of identifying their boundaries, and since their memory couldn't hold on to the information it received, the process had to be repeated over and over. Keeping that statement in mind suddenly explained so much of what I had characterized as involuntary movement. Perhaps there actually was purpose to all of it.

I tried to imagine what an Alzheimer's brain went through trying to identify, interpret, and channel the cacophony of sounds that entered when it had lost the ability to do so. I realized their ability to distinguish one sound from another is often so impaired that one voice is lost in the sounds of others talking, the noise on the television. I tried to imagine how an Alzheimer's person interprets the noise that happens in the bathroom with hard tile walls and floors and the shower running full blast and a caregiver talking loudly in order to be heard over the running water.

They interpret the caregiver's raised voice as shouting. Their clothes are being taken off and they interpret being moved under the shower as being shoved and manhandled. On top of that they are suddenly sprayed with water which may or may not be the temperature they can tolerate because sense of touch and temperature is also impaired. Strangers are crowded into the room with them and they can't tell if they're being observed or threatened or ridiculed. They have no way of knowing those aren't other people at all but reflections in the mirror on the bathroom wall. They must feel terribly violated. They are bombarded with so many variables that it must at times seem like hell, and we wonder why bath time is traumatic. Better yet, we complain that the patient is combative.

The average person has no way of seeing the ramifications of this aspect of dementia which is why I urge people facing this illness with a loved one to step back and try to put themselves inside that person and view the world through their eyes and ears. Simply turning the bathroom mirror to face the wall and keeping my voice as soft and as assuring as possible alleviated most of the combativeness I was having to deal with at shower time. Reasoning why Tom tended to plant himself at the threshold resulted in my awareness of the barrier the white marble slab between the bedroom and the bathroom presented and the effect the change in temperature and texture caused him as he stepped from the carpeted floor to the hard cold tile floor in his bare feet. Nothing I did could coax him to move either foot forward or backward once we reached that barrier. He'd stand there teetering back and forth getting increasingly more frightened while I tried to force him into the room. Those moments were usually impacted by the need to get him out of soiled clothes.

Letting him be and coming back to the situation later was not an option. Laying a solid color towel on the floor from the bedroom to the shower stall created a solid bridge upon which Tom could walk. Facing him and holding both his hands while I backed over that bridge and into the shower stall showed him that solid footing was in front of him. The key was not that he figured it out, the key was that I became sensitized to those types of perceptual problems and found ways to work around them.

Something else significant happened to me as Tom deteriorated into the last the stage of his illness. I was forced to accept responsibility for Tom's life, something I had fought doing under the premise that I was preserving his dignity. Dignity is a relative term that is often confused with insisting on behavior that isn't possible anymore. There is no dignity in forcing someone to eat unaided when they no longer can. There is no dignity in forcing them to make decisions when they no longer can. It took five years of our marriage before I realized the decisions were no longer his decisions, or our decisions, the decisions were mine. The amount of time and effort it had taken to keep him a part of that process was beyond reason by then. I didn't need permission to take him to the doctor anymore. I didn't need to get approval to alter the furniture layout or remove pictures he liked out of his reach. The relief I felt when I finally accepted the tasks at hand as mine cannot be put into words. It was when I took my own life back.

It became a matter of making life as simple as possible for myself in order to survive. It was the time when my decision about nursing home placement was made and when my commitment to Tom was examined and put into perspective. It was when I started to examine my needs and when I started thinking about my future, a future without Tom. Had I been unable to make those choices, either through lack of recognition of the need, or money, or circumstance, I might be in a very different place than I am today.

I was also lucky. I had health and relative youth on my side. Tom and I were only eleven years apart and we were both young by Alzheimer's standards. I also had height and weight on my side. Had Tom been taller or heavier I might have found myself making a very different choice about home care given his tendency towards combativeness. There were also other intangibles. I grew up knowing all my grandparents died in their own beds. I'd watched my aunts and uncles and cousins surround the elder members of our extended family with love, respect and care. I knew it could be done. In my mind's eye it was a given, much the same way nursing my sons had been a given during a time when hospitals and nurses considered that act the bother to end all bothers. There was no one to encourage me then and there was no one to encourage me now.

All discussion about Tom's care, except for a few enlightened individuals, revolved about how soon I could get him into nursing home care. Why would I want to take care of him at home? Why do this? What was wrong with me? I hardly even knew the man. I should feel cheated and angry. Why make such a needless sacrifice? Why was I still smiling?

For the longest time I thought I was the only one in the world making this choice. Given the level of isolation this illness imposed on me that wasn't an unexpected assumption. Given the level of tenacity that was also a part of my character, the more discouragement I received, the more convinced I was that I could do it. I was also not without resources. I was insightful enough to realize a creative effort was still a creative effort regardless of the material at hand. Instead of choreographing a dance, I was choreographing our lives. I chose to view my role in Tom's life from the most positive place I could find. I'd also had twenty five years of professional experience solving care problems for others and altering home environments for the handicapped, so I wasn't intimidated by the impact of Tom's needs.

Most of all, I have a firm belief in a Universal Power and my ability to tap into that Power for strength and purpose, and I had a family that never once in my life told me I was incapable of doing anything I decided to do. In some ways, my entire life had been spent preparing for this challenge. If there was anyone who could handle this situation it had to be me. I was lucky in all those ways. I was lucky in another way as well. I'd had Tom as my mentor.

Tom once told me that being successful had very little to do with doing what you like in life. Being successful had to do with liking what you did. Tom lived by those words. I saw it in the life he led before we met, I saw it in his work with the homeless and at church, and I saw it in the way he related to everyone around him. I saw him approach everything he did with the same modus operandi and intensity. He found a way to treasure every life experience he had. If there was any tribute I could give him it would be to learn that lesson. I decided to look for and treasure the good still left in our lives. Besides, we were still newly weds, what was I to do, stuff him in a corner some where, let the marriage whiz by and have no memories? I had to trust that everything happens for the good and I was learning to believe those words. I managed to reach a state of acceptance and peace about our life together. That doesn't mean that life became easy for me, but it is easier. It has never stopped being work though.

I remember staring at him one day, noting an intense sense of sadness deep inside of me. I saw the weight loss, the vacant look in his eyes and the constant twitching of his hands as he moved back and forth through the rooms of our house. I suddenly realized I couldn't remember what he looked like when we met. The pictures came out that day. I've peppered our environment with pictures of Tom at various stages in his life and pictures of the two of us, pictures of us when we first married with his arm around me and mine around him. We are smiling in those pictures and there is a spark in his eyes in those pictures, that I recognize and remember. I have chosen to keep the image of who he was in view at all times. It may have no meaning for him since he can no longer focus on anything as abstract as a photograph anymore, but it helps remind me of why I'm here. I suspect they will come down when I'm ready to let him go, and after a while some of them will reappear again after he dies.

I suppose it would be superfluous to say I often feel cheated and envious especially when I see older couples in public sharing their lives and I know that couple could have been Tom and me. Those are pointless digressions and they are digressions I fight to stifle. There is no point in feeling sorry for myself and I refuse to see either Tom or myself as victims. Neither one of us saw this break in life as some form of senseless retribution. As a friend of mine from a support group said, it was a rotten break and that's all it was. All things considered we'd have preferred the life Tom had before all this happened, but this was the life we got and we tried not to miss the opportunity it offered us. We were successful in reaching each other and taking the best we had to offer each other. We squeezed more into the years we had than many have in 25 years of marriage. I have valid memories of Tom, memories that will carry through with me to the end of my life and I know I did the very best for him I could do.

If there is any continuing speculation on my part as to why this had to happen to us, it is to consider that perhaps it was just Tom's time to let someone else take care of him. Perhaps it was just his turn to be touched and cooed over and simply loved and that is what I do. I hold him, I touch him and I caress him. I found that he tended to settle down easier if I stayed with him in his bedroom and held his hand for a while. I have, on occasion, crawled into bed with him and held his hand the entire night. Waking together still serves a purpose for me and touch seems to give him a sense of security and comfort. I guess I'm still his life line to reality. I also believe the touch is as valid for him as it is for a newborn baby. We don't require response from newborns but we hold and caress them and love them anyway. I no longer require response from Tom. Even though it appears to be a one way street these days, the touch is still valid for me. It is a continuation of the physical relationship we once enjoyed. It's different, but it's basically the same. I still feel the same. I still feel warm and close to him. At night when I check in on him and see his legs drawn up like a baby's, I kiss him on his forehead the way one would kiss an infant and I give him a silent blessing. I tell him every time the words fly through my brain that I love him and I am here for him. He is still somebody important to me, his illness didn't diminish that feeling in the slightest. The unexpected boon of all of this is that by reinforcing my love for him I inadvertently turned that love back onto myself.

This book started out being our story, but the reality is that it ended up being mine. I will never be the same as a result of this experience. Something unexpected happened to me as a result of the journey Tom and I embarked upon when we married, because I am a more centered and complete person for the experience. Having learned what it feels like to love Tom in this way has helped me recognize those same feelings towards the people I care about in my life. It has opened the possibility of someday being able to transfer that oneness to all the others who cross my path. I see a long road ahead of me, but I also see that it is a possibility.

..........and people wonder why I am still smiling.

This much I do know ... the touch of him is just as meaningful to me as it was the day we met, and kissing him and being kissed by him is just as sweet, and when he connects and finds the humor and his face lights up and he smiles, well, who can possibly describe the feeling I feel. He might leave this world having no recognition of me and with no memory of anything or anyone else but he will not leave this world unloved. The trap, if one needs to see this relationship as such, is this: I still know who he is, and I know myself too well to let it not matter!

When people venture to ask if Tom would do this for me, my only reply can be that it really doesn't matter what Tom might have done if our situations had been reversed. In the final analysis, it's how I faced the challenge that mattered, not the hope of being paid back on some esoteric level somewhere in the future. If there was no God, no promise of a life after death, no retribution for bad deeds and no reward for a life well spent, would it change how I must behave towards others? I think not. If asked if I would do this all over again, I have to say that I wouldn't have missed Tom Murphy for the world. He's given me more than anyone could have imagined.

I'LL BE SEEING YOU

I'll be seeing you,
In all the old familiar places
That this heart of mine embraces,
All day through

In that small cafe
The park across the way
The children's' carousel
The chestnut tree, the wishing well.

I'll be seeing you,
In every lovely summer's day,
In everything that's bright and gay,
I'll always think of you that way

I'll find you in the morning sun,
And when the night is new,
I'll be looking at the moon,
But, I'll be seeing you.

words by: Irving Kahal   *music by: Sammy Fain*

EPILOGUE

For most people, mourning begins when their loved one dies. For those of us dealing with long term illness, such as Alzheimer's Disease or Parkinson's Disease, or MS, the mourning starts long before the dying happens and caregivers are forced to experience that dying in bits and pieces over an indefinite amount of time. Those of us who have dementia to deal with as an added aspect of our caregiving, share the unique task of mourning the death of the memories we once shared with our person, because dementia effectively locks us out of their inner life. Ultimately we mourn the loss of the relationship because whatever it was, it will never be the same again. When books describe Alzheimer's Disease as the mourning period that never ends they hardly begin to scratch the surface of what that means.

Compounding the constant sense of loss that permeates the process of caring for such an individual is the physical drain that also must be dealt with. The two greatest enemies that physically bombard these caregivers are loss of sleep and lack of respite care so that they can get away from the constant stress. More Dementia patients than not, have severe sleeping problems, problems that keep them up for nights on end. As a result of Tom's wakefulness at night, I didn't have a normal sleep life for over 4 years. That was over 1,460 nights without restful sleep. Its not a simple case of moving into another room and shutting the door. Their coordination and vision problems present a constant danger to them, so they must be supervised. Rarely are they quiet during those nocturnal wanderings. The end result for the caregiver, and whomever else is in the vicinity, is sleep depravation.

One caregiver told me that her grandmother rapped on the walls all night long repeating the *"Shave and a Haircut, Two Bits!"*, pattern, over and over. However, she neglected to finish the *"Two Bits"*, part of it, leaving everyone in the house hanging and waiting for the last two raps. After the first few rappings, which were followed by the screaming silence of those two missing raps, the entire family, in their various rooms, would methodically bang on their headboards with a fist, flop a foot on the floor, or slap a hand on an end table just to finish the 'two bits' part of the pattern. It was a unique sort of torture that they all laugh about now, but which drove them crazy for months.

Lack of sleep clouds the mind and thinking process in ways you cannot imagine unless you've been through it, and not having a respite break can actually make you crazy after a while. As much as you might love the person, being trapped with them 24 hours a day, day after day takes an insidious toll.

Dementia is a disease of continuing changes and the demands of dealing with those changes start the moment the diagnosis is made. For the caregiver, that is also the day mourning begins. Facing the initial diagnosis means facing a death sentence, an interminable death sentence, and even though most of us hope and pray that this horror is not going to win out as we live through the early stages of this illness, the time arrives when all of us realize there is nothing that can be done to stop its relentless destruction.

As we accept the cruel fact that death is going to win out we then find ourselves in yet another quagmire of confused emotions. We get to deal with the guilt associated with accepting that knowledge and making the decisions to get on with our lives while our loved one is still alive. On some levels we feel as though we are abandoning them even though we know we are doing everything in our power to be there for them. The planning that's necessary for the caregiver to say their goodbye while their loved one is still able to participate in the act is unique in grieving. For the effort, they get to face the loneliness of loving and caring for a person who can express little back as the illness continues to claim them, and it does claim them.

Rarely does anyone ever talk about the loneliness of that vigil. Days and nights that stretch into years, with no one to share your life while you watch over someone else's. It is a singularly lonely experience with one sided conversations, one sided expressions of love, one sided laughter as you try to find some humor and sense to life, alone with someone who cannot give anything much back.

But, as difficult as overcoming these barriers are, life does go on. The flashes of grief come and go, because it is physically impossible to mourn continuously for any length of time, and the day-to-day decisions must be made by someone. I found as a result of my involvement in the support group system, that eventually, most of us take the bull by the horns so to speak and just do what has to be done.

The crossing point for me happened when I realized the time had come for strangers to help take care of Tom. He could no longer accompany me on errands and he couldn't tolerate going into restaurants anymore. God knows I tried to keep the world open to him for as long as was humanly possible. I needed to find someone to stay with him in the home while I left. I expected that to be a monumental task and again, I discovered the fear of making the decision to hire someone was harder than actually hiring someone. People are out there who do this sort of work and finding them took a little effort but the effort made a difference in my quality of life as much as Tom's. I wasn't the only one who needed a break.

The first few weeks I hovered, never leaving the house for more than an hour or so until the woman I'd hired told me to get out of her sight and let her do her job. Psychologists refer to this phenomena as 'separation trauma'. I felt much the same way I'd felt leaving my first born son in day care when I returned to work. However, life's demands being what they were, I didn't have much choice back then and I forced myself to make that adjustment. Reason dictated that I didn't have much choice now. However, as much as I knew I had to take this step away from Tom as well, I also knew that stepping past that barrier meant I had also started to say goodbye to him.

Taking hold of my life again was not easy. I'd become so used to having Tom with me everywhere I went that even going for groceries without him was difficult. There were other issues. Sooner or later I was going to have to look for work if only to support myself after Tom died. I needed to start some serious planning for my future. A job at that time was out of the question since just leaving the house was an effort for me, and Tom still wasn't sleeping, so I always felt exhausted. Just getting myself out of the house and breaking the isolation that had taken over me had to be the essential first step.

I'd heard about a six hour symposium the Alzheimer's Association was running in Denver by accident, a brochure someone handed to me after hearing Tom had Alzheimer's Disease. I sent in the application and then spent the next few weeks talking myself out of going. I literally had to talk myself through the drive there and force myself to go in the door. I remember thinking, "If they've lost my application, I'm out of here". I almost drove out of the parking lot without even attempting to park the car. It was the first time I'd gone anywhere without Tom for more than two hours in over three years. I left that symposium stunned.

It's title was *Obstacles To Caregiving: Confronting the Issues*, and the keynote speaker was Lisa Gwyther, the Director of the Duke University Center for Aging Family Support Program. It was when I learned that over 80% of the people with this illness are cared for at home by one other person. Only 5% of people 65+ actually find their way into nursing homes, 3% of whom have memory disorders. The rest are cared for in supported living arrangements with a combination of private and family care. Most caregivers keep their Alzheimer's people home for years before making the decision to place them in a nursing facility. However, vast numbers are maintained in their own homes until they die. From onset of symptoms, Alzheimer's Disease can last anywhere from 3 to 20 years or more. It always ends in death.

Where were these caregivers? Obviously, large numbers of us were somehow muddling along. I looked around the room and noticed very few of us there were from that 80% category and then I realized, most were probably home taking care of their person with little opportunity or energy to get out let alone attend a seminar. I remembered not being able to leave Tom alone long enough to attend a support group while I was in Houston and how trapped I felt. Thoughts began flying through my mind and I found myself actively participating in the discussion groups realizing I had a lot to offer in terms of my experience both as a professional and as a person with an inside view of what the caregiving experience is first hand. I was one of those 80% who had made it out. I remember hearing my voice constructing sentences that made sense and seeing heads nod in agreement at what I had to say. I remember hearing that voice in my head saying ... *You can do this!*

I left with a vague plan. I needed to reach the people who weren't there. I needed to find out how they were. I needed to share my experience. I needed to be voice for them as well as for myself.

I discovered, as I started meeting others like myself in my support group, that I wasn't the only one still smiling. I found a sense of acceptance and peace in many of us who reached the last stages of this illness with a loved one and a sense of strength in them that I couldn't ignore. One man told me that once he got past the shock, the denial, and the anger when his wife developed Alzheimer's, what he found waiting for him was a profound sense of having experienced a blessing as a result of his caring for her. This illness forced us to test our mettle whether we liked it or not. Many of us also found a sense of priority in our lives quite different from the one we might have recognized before Alzheimer's entered the scenario.

Those of us who have faced this illness head on know that survival is not only possible, it is also possible to think well of yourself when it is over. This experience gave me the opportunity to look deeply into myself and explore issues I thought were light years away and to open my eyes to what really matters. And over the past few years the vague plan that formed as I left that first symposium has evolved into a mission. A mission to increase awareness of caregiver needs, and to work as an activist to improve the care of and attitudes towards the frail elderly in this country.

Those of us who take on the challenge of caring for someone with dementia take on more than just the full time care of someone we're supposed to love. We take on all the nuances of rejection our loved one receives from those around us and we take on a job which has little reward or thanks inherent in its pursuit. However, I believe those of us who do it successfully have a basic ingredient that allows us to greet our loved ones with sensitivity instead of dread, and I think it is resiliency. Some of us are more resilient than others. I have come a long way since my life with Tom started. I believe those of us who take on the task of seeing someone through an illness like Alzheimer's Disease do so because we can. Those who don't probably shouldn't. And those who don't must not be faulted because they don't. It does mean however, that other avenues of help must be developed when those you counted on aren't there, and the keyword is *"help"*. No one can survive this illness as a caregiver alone. Take it from someone who knows! There are certain basic truths caregivers must come to terms with as they grow into the job of caregiving, truths that aren't inherent in our makeup, truths that aren't easily accessible to our learning process, truths that surface only if someone going through this illness can pass them on to others.

It took me nine years of a marriage, a lot of trial and error and much introspection before I was even able to look closely at what had transpired during Tom's illness and to us both as a result of that illness. It took a great deal of spiritual work to make sense out the ditches I fell into as I dragged myself through more bouts of grief and anger than I care to remember. Grief over my loss of Tom, grief over the loss of our relationship, grief over the feelings of abandonment, grief over accepting Tom's constant continuing deterioration and facing what will be his eventual death. It took work to find the place of contentment and peace I now carry along with a sense of a job well done. It was a long arduous road that carried me to the basic truths I came to recognize as a result of the above and they are these ...

1. Learn to ask for help. Caregivers are in charge of two lives, theirs and their loved one's. In order to be a help, you must first learn to help yourself. **Mind reading does not work!** Learning to say no, asking for what you need, taking a break from the responsibilities to rejuvenate yourself are vital skills that often must be learned. Start by getting yourself to a support group. Your teachers are those who've already been through it, and the social bond that develops is vitally important to your sense of well being.

2. You must not waste energy when people you feel you should be able to depend upon aren't there. Not everyone is able to handle the aspects of a long term illness. Your energy should always be focused on meeting your needs as well as your loved one's and if family and friends can't fill the gaps then you must learn to reach out to

other resources as the only other alternative. And if I seem to be repeating myself, its because this bears repeating. **No one can do this entirely alone!**

3. You can never build your strength on what others think of you. You have to find valid reasons that are self generated and allow yourself to feel that strength.

4. Feeling sorry for yourself never helps, and seeing your loved one as a victim only empowers the illness. It does nothing to aid your self worth or theirs.

5. Abe Lincoln once said ... "Most folks are about as happy as they make up their minds to be." As hard as this is to believe, joy can exist in almost any circumstance. I, and many others I've met, find that it's the love we experienced that lasts in our memories and not the horror. And this was true of every stage of Tom's illness I encountered with him. As new challenges were faced, the old ones were filed away as having been successfully met.

6. Never underestimate the value of unconditional love as the greatest power tool available to the caregiver. The giving of love freely to an individual who is less and less able to commend you for your efforts is a gift in its finest sense. It enriches the giver in ways you cannot know until you do it.

My first grandchild was born in the winter of 1993. I look at Alex and I see this wonderful child developing and growing and know all the promise that exists for him. I look at Tom and see someone at the other end of the spectrum and yet both are sharing a commonality. Alex and Tom do many of the same things when they're hungry or uncomfortable or tired. In fact Alex seems to be developing awareness and abilities in the same order in which Tom lost his. Perhaps death *is* merely the opposite of birth. It occurred to me as I observed these two precious beings in my life that there is no reason for my feelings towards Tom to be any different than my feelings towards this child. Both deserve the same regard and attention and neither is more valued because one is at the beginning of his life and the other is nearing the end.

I decided to embrace this last experience of our marriage as a special and sharing thing for both of us. Why should I face Tom's eventual death as a burden? Who said it had to be burden?

As I struggled to answer those questions I discovered what unconditional love is really all about. It is that state of being when you no longer see just the body before you. You see the essence of that person and in your eyes it is all good. Being able to see Tom in that light allowed me to face anything the future had to offer us with dignity and on some levels, actual joy.

That joy doesn't alter the fact that I am caught in the midst of a death watch that might last years more. It's the uncertainty of when it's going to happen that wears me out, not the eventuality of the event. I find myself waiting for the inevitable and wondering whether it will be pneumonia or an inability to swallow that finally does him in. I now have hospice to help me through the process but I still pray every night that God will grant us as easy a time as possible. All I can do is give it up to the Universe and hope that I will once again be able to face whatever that future offers us.

When he finally dies, they say, the mourning will have already happened. I tend not to believe them. It can't be that simple. Life without Tom, that's something I have yet to discover. The years of our marriage flew by so fast and furiously that at times it almost seems as though it didn't happen at all. I dread having the memory of him fade away. I can't imagine that his death is going to be easy in any sense of the word.

I think people like me have been written off in the grieving department. Because the illness lasts so long we are expected to be relieved when our loved one dies. I remember reacting to the loss of my friend Irene's father and feeling almost envious that it was over for her. It was far from over for her. Its been two years and she and her family are still dealing with it. The level of involvement in the day to day care of someone like her father and my Tom, fills every moment of your life and then they're gone and there's all that time to fill. Those of us who care hand and foot for such a person have a particular sort of grief to work through. I think most of us are left hanging the way our men and women returning from Vietnam were left hanging. They were expected to be happy it was all over with and get on with their lives especially since so many of us at home felt it wasn't *our kind of war*. Most never got the chance to resolve the horror and too many suffered emotionally as a result.

I have been through such a war. I have been assailed and demeaned and battered emotionally and physically. I am constantly subjected to professionals and acquaintances referring to the caregiving of an Alzheimer's loved one as a *burden* instead of a *challenge,* and I hear phrases like *co-dependency,* and *martyrdom* and *needless sacrifice* used as though those of us who face the challenge are emotionally deficient in some way. After all, who in their right mind would 'sacrifice' their time and effort to do this in this day and age? Those of us trying to make care decisions need realistic options and help in wading through our feelings and fears, we need practical ways to deal with the changes we face, and we need a break once in a while. A simplistic assumption of caregiving being too hard to do is no help, it only undermines unspoken needs to try, and it fosters a negative attitude before anything positive can be felt.

How many times have I said to those I meet who register surprise when I tell them yes, Tom is in the last stage of this illness and yes, he is still in his own home, who then need to ask ... "Why?"

> a. *Because caring for him now is actually easier than it was two years ago. I've already been through the worst of it. Why pay a nursing home now when the hardest part of his care has already passed.*

> b. *I finally have a routine I can depend on and one that works for us. From here on it is just a matter of loving him and having the help I need to physically move him and wash him.*

c. When I feel the urge to tell him I love him, or kiss him, or stroke his head or tidy his surroundings all I have to do is cross a room. I don't have to block out time or drive half way to kingdom come in order to do those things.

d. I want him to die in his own bed with me there to hold his hand in the serenity of our own home.

e. I was physically and emotionally able to do it.

f. All of the above ...

I am tired of justifying why I have Tom home. I don't see my care of him as a sacrifice in the negative sense of that word and whether my act of being there for him is seen as a gift or a burden is really a matter of how I view the choice I made. I have not been endowed with some special corner on the caregiving skills market. When well meaning friends and relatives offer that they don't know how I do it, I can only reply ...

* *No one knows what they can do until they have to do it.* *

All of us have choices to make and commitments to keep and all of us have the right to make those choices, choices that are more easily made if the right information is available and help is attainable. I can't imagine that any of us would actively seek this sort of challenge out if we didn't have to. As for me, I'm just trying to live the life I've been given as happily as possible and with as much creativity as I can muster in spite of circumstances that test the limits of human ability, emotional strength, and spiritual resolve.

There is no denying that caregiving takes a toll and no one can understand the toll taken unless they've been through it. If there is any such thing as a two person illness, seeing someone you care about through dementia is it. I watched my husband impaled by his losses and felt every one of those losses twice over because I felt for him as well as for myself and I was so isolated that even the sharing of my loss was denied me. I have been through a war and I want the recognition of having survived that war. I want my parade when this is over. I don't want to hear that I should be relieved. When all is said and done I will still miss Tom, I will miss everything we missed, and I will cherish every moment we didn't miss and everyone needs to know that.

Some years ago I attended a seminar run by Dr. Elisabeth Kubler-Ross. I was finishing up my master's degree and I was considering the possibility of specializing in grief counseling at the time, something I reconsidered and ultimately rejected as requiring more emotional energy than I could afford to give. Little did I know what part those studies would play in my life later on. I remember being so impressed with that woman's dignity and her ability to express the deep emotion so much a part of her, and to not be ashamed of that emotion. She let the tears flow down her face as she spoke and why shouldn't they flow? She was talking about the moment of truth people who are facing death have and she was talking about sharing that moment with them. Her tears were both natural and appropriate. It was a highly charged experience for all of us in that room. Her stories were heart wrenchingly beautiful and painfully explicit at the same time. By the end of the day I was exhausted, as were we all. Her closing remarks have remained etched in my memory.

She spoke of the need each individual has to define their own image of death before acceptance can happen. She said it is the one constant that everyone goes through and whether that image includes the concept of heaven, or reincarnation, or something as abstract as a spirit rising in the form of a cloud, the process has to occur if any level of peace is to happen. It is only through that sense of peace that those of us who are left behind can finally let go of our loved one and get on with life. Sometimes it is the one last step that allows our loved one to let go and die.

As I started to prepare myself for this final test I found myself listening more and more to the nostalgic channels on the radio and dragging out my Ella Fitzgerald and Big Band records. It is no accident that the songs that began each chapter found their way into this book. They are our songs, Tom's and mine. They were as much a part of Tom's history as they were mine and the lyrics speak of a time when romance and love and commitment were expected. That we chanced to meet long after those songs drifted into the recesses of our memories is a moot point. The important point is that they were always there as if we had grown up on them together. I have chosen to make them the expression of the life we shared rather than dwell on the present that is our reality. I have chosen to grasp on to an image of a better place, a place where Tom and I can pick up where we left off and finally, fly together. This was after all, a love story.

Thanks to Fred and Ginger and Radio Pictures, this is my image ...

....the scene opens............

* *A handsome gentleman in white tie and tails is at a gaming table. He is surrounded by beautiful women. He has been winning and winning high but it is now obvious his luck has turned. He loses roll after roll of the dice and finally with all of his money gone, he pulls out his gold cigarette case, he looks at it for a moment and then cavalierly tosses it on the table. He loses it in the final roll. In the end he is standing there alone, for as his luck changed, one by the one, the ladies and the gentlemen have turned their backs on him and walked away.*

The scene changes to the deck of the gambling ship where he now is quite alone. Others who were at the table with him now ignore him and move away as he approaches as if his mere presence will bring bad luck their way. He reaches into his pocket and removes a revolver and is about to place it next to his temple when he spies a woman walking slowly and steadily towards the rail. She doesn't see him. She doesn't seem to see anything. She is as if in a trance. She stares at the water for a moment and then steps up on the rail.

He leaps to her side and pulls her back. She resists him at first but then he reaches into his pocket and shows her his empty billfold and smiles as if to say I understand more than you know.

The orchestra has begun to play a soft haunting melody as this scene unfolds. It gradually becomes more and more a part of the action until it is so pervasive and so much a part of the scene that it can no longer be ignored.

As the music swells in volume and intensity and as if on cue, the gentleman moves around the woman. He places his arm in the small of her back, she resists slightly but the music is too compelling and he is too entrancing and she is swept up into the dance.

The music is hypnotic and they are totally enmeshed in it's rhythm. They sway and turn and pause and move again, ever in each other's arms, ever in time and attuned with the music. He lunges, his arm holding her as her back arches, her hand brushing the floor ever so slightly, her hair touching it as she is caught once more in his arms and swung into the air where he catches her in a tight embrace. And finally, with his body pressed behind hers, his head next to hers, his cheek touching hers, they pause, they throw their heads back in one last defiant move and with their legs lifted and posed as arrows ... they leap together into their destiny.

.........it's all in the dance!

STAGES OF SYMPTOM PROGRESSION IN ALZHEIMER'S DISEASE

Symptoms of Alzheimer's disease generally progress in a recognizable pattern. These stages provide a framework for understanding the disease. It is important to remember they are not uniform in every person and the stages often overlap.

First Stage 2-4 years leading up to and including diagnosis:
Symptoms -
- ◆ Recent Memory Loss
- ◆ Progressive forgetfulness; difficulty with routine chores
- ◆ Confusion about directions, decisions and money management
- ◆ Loss of spontaneity and initiative
- ◆ Repetitive actions and statements
- ◆ Mood/personality and judgment changes
- ◆ Disorientation of time and place

Examples -
- ◆ Forgets if bills are paid
- ◆ Loses things and/or forgets they are lost
- ◆ Arrives at wrong time or place
- ◆ Constantly checks calendar
- ◆ Forgets frequently called phone numbers

Second Stage 2-10 years after diagnosis (longest stage):
Symptoms -
- ◆ Increasing memory loss, confusion and shorter attention span
- ◆ Difficulty recognizing close friends and/or family
- ◆ Wandering
- ◆ Restlessness, especially in late afternoon and evening

- Occasional muscle twitching or jerking
- Difficulty organizing thoughts or logical thinking
- May see or hear things that are not there (Hallucinations)

Examples -

- Sleeps often - awakens frequently at night and may get up and wander ("Sundowner's")
- Perceptual - motor problems - difficulty getting into a chair, setting the table
- Can't read signs, write name, add or subtract
- Suspicious - may accuse spouse of hiding things or infidelity (Paranoia)
- Loss of impulse control - may undress at inappropriate times or places
- Huge appetite for junk food - forgets when last meal was eaten; may lose interest in eating

Third Stage 1-3 years

Symptoms -

- Unable to recognize family members or self in mirror
- Loss of weight even with proper diet; eventually becomes emaciated
- Capacity for self-care diminished
- Oral communication disappears, eventually becomes mute
- Tries to put everything in mouth; compulsion for touching
- Bowel and bladder incontinence
- May experience difficulty with swallowing, skin infections or seizures

Examples -

- Looks in mirror and talks to own image
- Needs total care with bathing, dressing, eating and toileting
- May groan, scream or make grunting noises
- Sleeps more, becomes comatose, eventually dies

Source: Adapted by the Alzheimer's Association - Detroit Area Chapter. Credit Lisa P. Gwyther, MSW, ACSW.

Functional Assessment Staging (FAST)[1]

Stage 1 No difficulties, either subjectively or objectively.

Stage 2 Complains of forgetting location of objects; subjective word finding difficulties only.

Stage 3 Decreased job functioning evident to co-workers; difficulty in traveling to new locations.

Stage 4 Decreased ability to perform complex tasks (e.g., planning dinner for guests, handling finances, marketing).

Stage 5 Requires assistance in choosing proper clothing for the season or occasion.

Stage 6a Difficulty putting clothing on properly without assistance.

Stage 6b Unable to bathe properly; may develop fear of bathing. Will usually require assistance adjusting bath water temperature.

Stage 6c Inability to handle mechanics of toileting (i.e., forgets to flush, doesn't wipe properly).

Stage 6d Urinary incontinence, occasional or more frequent.

Stage 6e Fecal incontinence, occasional or more frequent.

Stage 7a Ability to speak limited to about a half-dozen words in an average day.

Stage 7b Intelligible vocabulary limited to a single word in an average day.

Stage 7c Non ambulatory (Unable to walk without assistance).

Stage 7d Unable to sit up independently.

Stage 7e Unable to smile.

Stage 7f Unable to hold head up

[1] Reisberg, B. Functional assessment staging (FAST). Psychopharmacology Bulletin, 1988; 24:653-659.

STAGES OF DETERIORATION[1]

STAGE I. FORGETFULNESS STAGE
Only apparent to client or possibly family
Financial matters once handled well, no longer
Covers up
Denial
Changes in social behavior

STAGE II. CONFUSIONAL STAGE
Definite impairment
Severe forgetfulness
Orientation impaired
Concentration impaired
Rambling speech
Past memories fairly intact
Moodiness
Less awareness
More problems with learning new material
Flattening of affect
Takes less part in activities
Activity level will do nothing to defend against the deterioration

STAGE III. DEMENTIAL STAGE
Severely disoriented
Severely confused
Hallucinations
Paranoid ideation
Agitation
Wandering
Needs total supervision
Judgment is severely impaired
Incontinence
Swallowing difficulties
Motor problems
Visual spatial problems severe in nature
Infectious diseases

[1] Reisberg, B., Ferris, S.H., de Leon, M.J., & Crook, T. The global deterioration scale for assessment of primary degenerative dementia. Am. J. Psychiatry. 1982; 139:1136-1139.

THE BOOKS I FOUND MOST HELPFUL

This list of books may seem a little heavy laden with publications dealing with death. Facing Alzheimer's Disease with a loved one is about facing a death sentence from the moment the diagnosis is made, and it is about continuing to face the countless *little deaths* that occur as each and every skill is lost until whatever existed in your relationship with that person lives only in the memory of the caregiver. The stages of mourning happen over and over until the loved one dies. There can't be enough material and support to help caregivers come to terms with the toll this illness takes on everyone involved in this drama.

Carter, Rosalynn with Golant, Susan K., *Helping Yourself Help Others, A Book For Caregivers.* New York. Times Books, 1994.

Mrs. Carter begins her book with the following statement: "There are only four kinds of people in this world: Those who have been caregivers * Those who currently are caregivers * Those who will be caregivers * Those who will need caregivers". The definition of who a caregiver is, that follows that statement, is one of the most succinct descriptions I have read. This is a book everyone facing the prospect of long term care with a loved one must read and possess. She talks about caregiving as a time honored tradition, that although inherent with great stress and isolation, nevertheless holds the possibility of satisfaction if positive attitudes are nurtured and support services and help are attained. No one can do it alone. She provides a list of places to start for information and planning when long term care becomes a challenge in your life. I highly recommend this reading.

Cohen, Donna, Ph.D. & Eisdorfer, Carl, Ph.D., M.D., *The Loss of Self*. New York. W.W. Norton & Company, 1986.

This is a book caregivers can hand to relatives and friends to read in order to enrich their understanding of how the disease affects both the victim and their caregiver. It is not only informative in a very practical and easy to read manner but it is sensitive and to the point about the stages of Alzheimer's Disease and the human needs of the people who face this illness. The personal stories highlighted are described in ways that aren't merely words on paper written by someone safely detached from the impact this illness has on living people. This book stands out in my mind for that reason. It also speaks to the loss of relationships as the illness progresses. I refer to over and over and its one of the first I read after I realized Tom and I were facing Alzheimer's Disease.

Cousins, Norman, *Anatomy of an Illness.* New York. Bantam Books, 1979.
   Norman Cousins examines such topics as creativity and humor as being essential to treatment. Important to anyone touched by chronic illness. This was one of the first books Tom and I read and one I found particularly helpful in meeting the demands and changes Tom's illness imposed on me. It is a book that talks about outlook and attitudes and taking charge of one's life.

Lewis, C.S., *A Grief Observed.* New York. Harper Collins Publisher, 1961.
   Most of us know the story of C.S. Lewis and Helen Joy Gresham through the movies *"Shadowlands"*. This little volume with a forward written by Douglas H. Gresham, is the most poignant expressive, deeply personal accounts of what it means to grieve over someone you love, that I have ever encountered. He gave form to feelings I was unable to express and provided the words that will remain in my heart as the expression of loss I feel, as I face the final chapter with my husband Tom. It is rare that a volume such as this one enters one's life.

Mace, Nancy L., & Rabins, Peter B., *The 36 Hour Day.* New York. Warner Books, 1991.
   A friend whose mother died of Alzheimer's Disease and who obviously recognized Tom's behaviors as being similar to her mother's, put this in my hand amidst my protestations that

Alzheimer's is not what Tom had. This book sat in the back of my closet for over a year before I picked it up and dared read it. It was and still is one of the best basic sources of information about dementia available. This is not a book you need to read from cover to cover the moment you buy it. Speaking from experience, doing so can be a little overwhelming. It is a book you buy and refer to in much the same way we referred to Dr. Spock years ago. It is a starting point on almost every topic relating to Dementia and one of the few books that actually talks about incontinence in the Alzheimer's person in terms of how to deal with it instead of how to make it go away.

Naughtin, Gerry and Laidler, Terry, *When I Grow Too Old To Dream.* Australia. Collins Dove publishers, 1991.
This book is written thorough the eyes and emotions of individual caregivers and patients. The stories are sensitive, uplifting, informative and reflect the uniqueness that is so much a part of the ever changing tapestry of the individuals who have Alzheimer's Disease. What captured my attention was the creativity these caregivers used to cope, the development of strengths that were unexpected, and the sense of life and love and laughter that occurred in spite of extreme conditions. The caregivers who contributed to this book seemed to develop a sense of peace about themselves and their loved ones as the illness progressed. It is important for caregivers to know, especially caregivers entering the early stages of this illness with a loved one, that peace and love can be a continuing part of the relationship even into the last stages. There aren't many publications which tell you this and it's almost impossible to imagine it yourself as life begins to deteriorate. I highly recommend this reading.

Nuland, Sherwin B., *How We Die, Reflections on Life's Final Chapter.* New York. Alfred A. Knopf, 1994.
The author is a surgeon and teacher of medicine and writes that we have sterilized death by removing it from homes and family. He takes the reader through the process of how illness and trauma kills. And so his stories are not just about why someone dies, but how they die and what they physically go through during the last

moments. The portraits of death he offers range from heart disease
to murder. His chapter on Alzheimer's Disease was particularly
helpful to me and the way in which he de-mystifies death through
the telling of the stories in this book really did help dissipate some
of the innate fear I have about facing Tom's death and my own.

Sacks, Oliver, *The Man Who Mistook His Wife For A Hat, and
Other Clinical Tales.* New York. Harper & Row Publishers,
1970.

Tom's neurologist recommended this book to me shortly after
our move to Boulder. It did more to help me understand what was
happening to Tom than everything else I read because it got me into
Tom's brain instead of just viewing it from the outside. Dr. Sacks
relates a number of case studies that involve extreme neurological
afflictions in a way that is both informative and easy to read. This
book is not about Alzheimer's Disease but it has everything to do
with Alzheimer's Disease. I reasoned after reading this volume,
that if the brain can manifest the extremes in behaviors and
misinterpretations exhibited in the case studies Dr. Sacks highlights
then perhaps a brain deteriorating randomly as it does in
Alzheimer's Disease can also manifest similar behaviors and
misinterpretations. It started me thinking about the possibilities of
the world Tom was seeing as opposed to what I saw and helped me
immensely in figuring out what was behind his behaviors and his
losses. Most of all, I stopped trying to make Tom fit into my world,
which relieved a great deal of stress and guilt I was imposing on
myself.

This book gave me a whole new appreciation for the complexity
of the brain. A brain that is capable of dreaming is a wondrous
thing to consider and perhaps the uniqueness of Alzheimer's
Disease is that the dream becomes more real than we know and
perhaps the dream is to be regarded instead of reviled. Living as
closely as I have to this illness I still can't say what Tom
experienced or continues to experience as his illness progresses. I
feel it is time to take Alzheimer's disease out of the realm of senility
and place it where it belongs and that is in the realm of progressive
brain damage. It is the word *senility* that allows too many of us to
convince ourselves that our elderly frail have less worth than the

rest of us because they can no longer relate to our world, our standards, and our needs. It is time to see these people in terms of their humanity as well as their illness. I believe Dr. Sacks is one who lives that ideal in his approach to treatment and this book is one worth reading more than once.

Siegel, Bernie S. M.D., *Love, Medicine & Miracles.* New York. Harper & Row, Publishers, 1986.

Dr. Siegel is well known for his work with cancer patients. His approach to dealing with chronic illness is a mind, body, spirit approach that ultimately strengthens the individuals who choose to face their illness head on. I found the attitudes he proffered applied to Tom's illness as it applies to cancer and other chronic conditions. His message was meaningful to both of us and helped us build a base of hope otherwise denied us by the traditional medical people we encountered in the early stages of Tom's illness.

His meditation tapes and lectures were extremely helpful in my being able to survive Tom's illness after Tom lost the ability to participate in his life.

OTHER SUGGESTED READING

The following are books that deal with positive thinking, and ways of confronting the challenges of caregiving which I found particularly helpful.

Caliandro, Arthur, *Make Your Life Count*. San Francisco. Harper & Row, Publishers, 1980.

Carroll, David L., *When Your Loved One Has Alzheimer's, A Caregiver's Guide.* Based on Methods Developed by the Brookdale Center on Aging. New York. Harper & Row, 1990.

Cousins, Norman, *Head First, The Biology of Hope and the Healing Power of the Human Spirit.* New York. Penguin Books, 1989.

Cousins, Norman, *The Healing Heart, Antidotes to Panic and Helplessness.* New York. W.W. Norton & Co., 1983.

Doernberg, Myrna., *Stolen Mind, The Slow Disappearance of Ray Doernberg.* Chapel Hill. Algonquin Books of Chapel Hill, 1986.

Gardner, Howard., *The Shattered Mind, The Person After Brain Damage.* New York. 1976.

Groverland, Jack, *Miracles Made Easy.* Boulder, Bigtree Press, 16 Canyon View SL, Boulder, Co. 80302, 1985.

Gwyther, Lisa P., *Care of Alzheimer's Patients*. Published by ADRDA and the American Health Care Association. Available from Alzheimer's Association chapters in paperback.

Kubler-Ross, Elisabeth, *On Death And Dying.* New York. MacMillan Publishing Co., Inc. 1969.

Sacks, Oliver, *An Anthropologist On Mars, Seven Paradoxical Tales.* New York. Alfred A. Knopf. 1995.

Sacks, Oliver, *Awakenings.* New York. Harper Perennial, 1973.

Seuss, Dr., *You're Only Old Once.* New York. Random House, 1986.

Simonton, O. Carl, and Stephanie Simonton, *Getting Well Again.* Los Angeles. J.P. Tarcher, Inc. 1978.

Viorst, Judith, *Necessary Losses.* New York. Simon & Schuster, 1987.

For a complete up-to-date list of books that deal specifically with Alzheimer's Disease, call your local chapter of the Alzheimer's Association. They also have many free publications, information about support groups, counseling, and up-to-date information on treatment available. For information on the chapter located nearest you phone: 1-800 272-3900. Or write: The Alzheimer's Association and Related Disorders, 919 N. Michigan Ave., Suite 1000, Chicago, IL, 60611-1676.

OTHER WRITING BY THE AUTHOR

Alzheimer's Invisible Army, The Congressional Record - Senate July 2, 1992 S-9891 and 9892.

T.V. drama had it all wrong on Alzheimer's, The Sunday Daily Camera, Boulder, CO., GUEST OPINION, October 9, 1994.

What All Alzheimer's Disease Families Share, The Sunday New York Times EDITORIAL/LETTERS, November 20, 1994.

CARE CONNECTIONS, Inspiration and Information for Caregivers About Caregiving.

A newsletter edited by Beverly Bigtree Murphy and published under the auspices of the Community Eldercare Coalition of Boulder County, and the Boulder County Aging Division. This publication was developed as the first call for help for caregivers facing the long-term care of a loved one with Alzheimer's Disease, Parkinson's Disease, M.S., Stroke and other long term care issues in Boulder County, CO. *CARE CONNECTIONS* provides information on how to access services in Boulder County, however, the information is transferable to other communities as a guideline for caregivers elsewhere to benefit from. Personal accounts of caregiving experiences are offered and written by caregivers. These accounts are uplifting in manner, sometimes poignant, and sometimes hilarious. The entire newsletter is devoted to enriching the existence of caregivers and letting them know they are not alone in their fears, their grief, and their love.

For information write: *Care Connections,* P.O. Box 471, Boulder, Co. 80306, or make checks payable to Care Connections.

PUBLICATIONS SOON TO BE AVAILABLE

CARING AT HOME FOR AN ALZHEIMER'S LOVED ONE.

A series of bound booklets, soon to be available. For information about this series written by Beverly Bigtree Murphy, and covering long-term home care issues facing the Alzheimer's caregiver write: Gibbs Associates, P.O. Box 706, Boulder, Colorado 80306-0706. Phone & Fax: 303-444-6032. The first two booklets are entitled:

Everything You Ever Needed to Know About Incontinence and Hoped You'd Never Have to Ask!

Altering Your Home, For Their Safety While Keeping it a Home, for Your Sanity.

Other volumes to follow ...

LYRIC CREDITS

AS TIME GOES BY, words and music by Herman Hupfeld
© 1931 Warner Bros. Inc. (Renewed)

DANCING IN THE DARK, by Arthur Schwartz, Howard Dietz
© 1931 (Renewed) Warner Bros. Inc. & Arthur Schwartz Pub. Des/

I CONCENTRATE ON YOU, by Cole Porter
© 1929 Chappell & Co. (ASCAP) (Renewed)

IT HAD TO BE YOU, words by Gus Kahn, music by Isham Jones
© 1924 Renewed and Assigned to Gilbert Keyes Music and Bantam Music Publishing Co. for the U.S.A. only.

LOVE IS HERE TO STAY, by George Gershwin, Ira Gershwin
© 1938 (Renewed 1965) George Gershwin Music and Ira Gershwin Music. All Rights administered by WB Music Corp.

MORE THAN YOU KNOW, by E. Eliscu, B. Rose and V. Youmans
© 1929 (Renewed) WB Music Corp. (ASCAP), Chappell & Co. (ASCAP) and LSQ Music Co. (ASCAP) for the U.S.A. only.

We extend special thanks to Judith Jordan for her contribution toward obtaining copyrights to the songs.